Belief's Own Ethics

Belief's Own Ethics

Jonathan E. Adler

A Bradford Book
The MIT Press
Cambridge, Massachusetts
London, England

First MIT Press paperback edition, 2006

MIT Press books may be purchased at special quantity discounts for business or sales promotional use. For information, please e-mail special_sales@mitpress.mit. edu or write to Special Sales Department, The MIT Press, 55 Hayward Street, Cambridge, MA 02142.

This book was set in Sabon by Achorn Graphic Services Inc., and was printed and bound in the United States of America.

Library of Congress Cataloging-in-Publication Data

Adler, Jonathan Eric.
  Belief's own ethics/Jonathan E. Adler.
    p.   cm.
  "A Bradford book."
  Includes bibliographic references and index.
  ISBN 0-262-01192-1 (alk. paper), 0-262-51194-0 (pb)
  1. Belief and doubt. 2. Evidence. I. Title.
  BD215 .A35   2002
  121′.6—dc21

2001054666

10 9 8 7 6 5 4 3 2

Dedicated to Sheila, Emily, and Jeff

You cannot be believed, Meletus, even, I think, by yourself.
—Plato, *Apology* 26e

Contents

Preface

Traditionally, the primary question of the ethics of belief is "What ought one to believe?" Early on, I advance a view of how to answer this question. The question is to be answered conceptually, in accord with the concept of belief. If the question is to be answered conceptually, belief must be based only on that which can establish a belief as true, which, in the empirical realm, is largely evidence.

On this defense of *evidentialism,* the primary question should be not "what ought one to believe?" but "what *must* one believe?" or "what *cannot* one believe?" So, for example, you cannot now believe that Socrates laughed at noon on his thirteenth birthday because it is obvious that you do not have evidence for it.

In advancing this conceptual defense of evidentialism and drawing out consequences from it, I engaged my main research in epistemology. As the project developed, however, I was surprised to discover that I had to draw on related interests in pragmatics, the study of argument, the psychology of reasoning, and ethics.

The discovery was slow in coming as was the completion of this book. I want to especially thank five dear old friends not only for their comments, but also for their encouragement: L. Jonathan Cohen, Catherine Z. Elgin, Georges Rey, Michael Stocker, and Peter Unger.

L. Jonathan Cohen has been a major inspiration and influence on this book, especially in his account of inductive logic.

To my immense benefit, Catherine Elgin and I have been discussing epistemological issues for over twenty-five years. She has provided me with insightful comments on a hefty chunk of this work. Remarkably, even as our views have come to radically diverge, Kate is still able to tell me what is wrong with my arguments not only from her point of view, but from my own.

I expect that I speak for his many and widely dispersed philosophical pals and colleagues in saying that discussion with Georges Rey is one of our great pleasures. Georges sent me fifty pages of merciless and on-target comments, which we proceeded to argue through for hours upon hours. I am indebted to him for numerous improvements in the text.

Aside from many helpful conversations with Michael Stocker over the ethics of belief, two chapters were read and discussed with him, Jeffrey Blustein, and Christopher Gowans. The four of us have constituted a moral philosophy discussion group that has been meeting fairly regularly for over ten years. I benefited from their criticisms and suggestions, as I have from their good company.

Early on, Peter Unger made me appreciate that the position I defend depends on distinguishing a notion of belief as paradigmatic from various neighbors, which are only approximations to it.

The CUNY Graduate Center introduced me to three outstanding students: Bradley Armour-Garb, Jennifer Fisher, and Peter Ross. Ross gave me exacting comments on early versions of chapters 1 and 6. Fisher provided me with helpful, detailed criticisms on style and substance throughout the manuscript. I had the good fortune to have Armour-Garb, not only as a student, but as a colleague for around two years. In extensive discussion and written remarks he provided me with penetrating and subtle comments on virtually the entire manuscript.

At Brooklyn College and the Graduate Center, I learned much on a number of the topics covered in this work from Arnold Koslow, Michael Levin, and especially, Julia Driver (now at Dartmouth).

Over the last four years I have engaged in regular phone-philosophy with Sidney Morgenbesser. As a philosopher's philosopher, it is expected that he would probe assumptions that we are inclined to take for granted. However, until you talk with Sidney frequently and at length, you could hardly imagine just how many assumptions those are.

Leigh Cauman edited the manuscript with her flair for language, clarity, and good sense.

I also extend thanks for the comments I received on various aspects of this work from: Horatio Alto-Costa, Kent Bach, Tyler Burge, Buzzy Chanowitz, John Deigh, Eugene Garver, Trudy Govier, Richard M. Hare, Christoph Jaeger, Jerrold Katz, Jim Landesman, Isaac Levi, Maureen Linker, Alasdair MacIntyre, Richard Moran, David Owens, David Pitt,

Graham Priest, Paul Saka, Stephen Schiffer, Harvey Siegel, Michael Slote, Roy Sorensen, Ernest Sosa, and Jonathan Vogel. In two talks derived from this work, I received very thoughtful criticism by my respective commentators on those occasions, Gilbert Harman and Timothy Williamson. During the final stages of revision, I received trenchant criticisms from Mark Greenberg, demanding substantial changes. Chapter 1, section 7 attempts to answer a set of his objections.

My thanks to three editors at MIT for their good advice and suggestions: Margy Avery, Judy Feldmann, and Tom Stone.

My thanks to the Wolfe Institute and its director Robert Viscusi for a fellowship that gave me a year to work on the manuscript. Additional thanks to the National Endowment for the Humanities and the Research Foundation of PSC-CUNY for fellowships and grants. A number of chapters draw on earlier articles, and I am grateful to the editors for allowing me do so: *The Journal of Philosophy, Midwest Studies in Philosophy, Mind, Philosophy and Phenomenological Research,* and *The Skeptical Inquirer.*

Aside from L. Jonathan Cohen's *The Probable and the Provable,* a number of contemporary works have influenced me in ways not well captured by endnotes. These include: Robert Brandom, *Making it Explicit;* Donald Davidson, *Inquiries into Truth and Interpretation;* Robert Fogelin, *Pyrrhonian Reflections on Knowledge and Justification;* Paul Grice, *Studies in the Way of Words;* Gilbert Harman, *Change in View;* Isaac Levi, *The Enterprise of Knowledge;* Wilfrid Sellars, "Empiricism and the Philosophy of Mind"; Peter Unger, *Ignorance;* Bernard Williams, "Deciding to Believe"; and Timothy Williamson, "Knowing and Asserting." (References to these works are found in the bibliography.)

Finally, I want to thank my family, to whom this work is dedicated, for making its completion impossible and necessary.

Introduction

1 Intrinsic vs. Extrinsic Approaches

Traditionally, the fundamental question of the ethics of belief is: What ought one to believe? Although this question used to be a central epistemological concern, since the eighteenth century it has been of interest mainly in connection with religious belief. The Enlightenment's answer to the fundamental question is that belief ought to be guided by reason. This answer pressed the question that shifted the ethics of belief from epistemology to the philosophy of religion: Can belief in God be justified or rational, if evidence cannot establish that there is a God?

In contemporary epistemology, the shift to the philosophy of religion is aided by the widespread view that what we actually believe is one thing, what we ought to believe another, and that this latter issue—the properly philosophical one—can be addressed only with explicitly normative notions: rational belief, warranted belief, justified belief, belief when one's only interest is truth. This view concedes at the outset the assumption that has led discussions of the ethics of belief onto the wrong track. (For brevity, I will often use the phrase "the ethics of belief" as a label for a branch of study or inquiry, and not, strictly, as referring to norms governing belief.) The assumption is that the concept of belief alone does not fix the ethics of belief. If this assumption is rejected, one step is taken toward returning the ethics of belief to its place as a central epistemological topic.

In trying to secure this place, I focus on everyday beliefs and ordinary believers, rather than those, like scientists, with a specialized or professional interest in correct judgment. The primary reason for this emphasis is that a number of my arguments, particularly in the early chapters, depend on securing the reader's agreement. The ethics of belief that I defend is already yours too, once certain influential ideas are set aside. They are set aside by examples that are so familiar and dull that they are easily overlooked as worthless to talk about—can you believe that chickens study Shakespeare? can you cease to believe that $2+5=7$? Our evident negative answers to both of these questions cleanly reveal our own commitments.

Specifically, I attempt to elicit admission of your own commitment to *evidentialism,* which is traditionally presented as affirming that the strength of belief ought to be proportional to the strength of evidence. Evidentialism's answer to the fundamental question is that belief ought to be determined by the evidence. It is this answer that is the core of most of the debate. Although in chapter 1 specific arguments for evidentialism are offered, its defense is really the project of the whole book.

Commonly, basic questions in the ethics of belief are posed as questions about what it is *rational* to believe. But once that way of posing the questions is accepted, the issue is biased, if not settled, against evidentialism. For, since rationality attends to the agent or to his acts, it will be easy to envisage circumstances where it is rational for the agent to hold a belief in defiance of the evidence: "Believe that pigs fly in the next four hours, or I'll kill you!" As soon as evidentialists accept the dominant *extrinsic* terms of discussion, their position is compromised. (My usage of "intrinsic" and "extrinsic" is clarified in context. "Internal" and "external" may be preferable, but they already have established usages within epistemology.)

Chapter 1 begins with an ancient challenge to try to believe that:

The number of stars is even. (Burnyeat 1983: 132)

We must fail this challenge, and in the necessity of that failure lies a clue to how to answer the fundamental questions of the ethics of belief. What *cannot* be believed reveals the *conceptual structure of belief,* and the ethics of belief is then derived from this structure. Evidentialism is the *intrinsic* ethics of belief—it is the ethics of belief imposed by the concept of belief itself. Our degree of belief must match our degree of evidential support, since only the evidence can secure the claim to truth of belief.

Because the match is conceptually based, my version of evidentialism diverges from the tradition. As explained further in chapters 1 and 3, under proper conditions, one must believe in accord with evidentialism, and it is a serious error to maintain, as the tradition does, that adherence to evidentialism is an option that one can decide to take rightly or wrongly, wisely or foolishly.

2   The Instability of Moderate Evidentialism

My fundamental thesis is that evidentialism is the basic ethics of belief and that the right way to defend that thesis is conceptually. One form that defense takes is to observe that instances of such thoughts as the following are incoherent:

p, but I lack adequate evidence that *p* (e.g., "It's raining, but I lack adequate evidence that it's raining").

When this observation is combined with related ones, the result is a version of evidentialism stronger than that endorsed by the tradition.

When I began to work on this book, I favored the moderate evidentialism that is pleasingly ecumenical: Evidence should generally determine the strength of belief, but not always. For evident empirical claims—such as that my neighbor's mutt is on my stoop—strength of belief and strength of evidence should match. But for some other prominent beliefs—personal, religious, ethical, aesthetic, controversial—the requirement for adequate evidence should be relaxed.

My position started to shift to the extreme stance defended here in reaction to discrepancies I observed between sophisticated, contemporary anti-evidentialist pronouncements and their actual detailed claims and arguments. The discrepancy was particularly notable in the landmark collection *Faith and Rationality*. The main target of these essays is evidentialism and Enlightenment ideals of guidance by reason, which are rejected in favor of a "Reformist" epistemology:

this tradition has characteristically viewed in a dim light the project of offering evidence for theism. . . . such arguments are unnecessary for putting a person in the position where he is within his rights in being a Christian. Thus well before the evidentialist challenge was issued . . . , it was characteristic of those in the Reformed tradition to have taken up a position in opposition to the challenge. (Plantinga and Wolterstorff 1983: 8)

Here was a volume offering a bold, trumpet call against evidentialism and the Enlightenments demands of reason, and it has been widely so cited ever since its publication. Yet when one actually reads the volume, the boldness withers. I am not alone in being struck by the incongruous combination of bravado and heavy qualification. Richard Swinburne, a distinguished and sympathetic reviewer comments:

Faith and Rationality consists of a number of essays . . . developing a "Reformed epistemology" which . . . is the view that religious belief does not in general require to be justified by arguments, but may be held with perfect rationality without such backing. Or rather . . . the most they purport to show by argument is that the arguments of others to show Reformed epistemology mistaken do not work. When the theses for which they argue are spelled out, they contain many negatives. The opening 77-page paper by Alvin Plantinga sets the tone for the rest of the volume. His paper contains the most developed version of the thesis . . . that *no*body known to Plantinga has shown that there are *no* circumstances in which some person or other may rationally treat "There is a God" as a basic belief. . . . (Swinburne 1985: 48)

My conjecture is that the incongruous combination of boldness of pronouncement and heavily qualified theses is because the Reformists cannot simply dismiss evidentialism. Almost all ordinary beliefs such as that Bill is home or that dogs chase cats need to be grounded on evidence. Instead, the anti-evidentialist selects beliefs that he takes to be manifestly not so grounded—not only supernatural religious beliefs, but also beliefs in the goodness or trustworthiness of others; beliefs in fundamental axioms or principles such as induction; beliefs too basic to be supported by anything more certain or fundamental such as that there are external objects; and others. The suggestion then is that the evidential standard is fine for most beliefs, but not others, particularly the exciting ones.

Even if evidentialism has a hard time with these cases, this line of reasoning is worrisome. It recommends that we sacrifice a doctrine—evidentialism—that works well for a huge range of undisputed data. The sacrifice is alleged to be justified because evidentialism is held to have difficulty in these cases. But these are cases that come to us wrapped in independent controversy and thorny issues. Why not adopt the attitude that the issues raised by these hard cases are beyond the borders of our current, and, perhaps, ultimate, understanding? They do not constitute firm data to reject well-founded doctrines or views.

I have, however, a less abstract reason to abandon the comforting reconciliation of a moderate evidentialism. The reconciliation sat well with me until I asked the obvious question: What is the source of the demand for evidence in the unproblematic cases that is alleged to be inapplicable in the difficult ones? Here is where both anti-evidentialism and my own former moderate evidentialism become unstable. If the evidential standards for these different beliefs vary, the variation must be determined by factors external to belief—the most prominent, as already mentioned, is rationality.

But when one reflects on examples of ordinary, unproblematic beliefs, it is not anything external to belief that is the source of the demand for adequate reasons or evidence. Since one's beliefs are what one regards as true, when we attend to any of our beliefs, a claim is made on us for holding that the belief is true. So it is belief that requires proportional reasons or evidence, not any external source. If so, the ground is removed for variation in the demands of belief according to different kinds of content.

3   Methodological Preliminaries: Abstraction, Assertion, Modesty, and First-Person Methodology

The label "evidentialism" for our basic position is misleadingly narrow, although this is an observation that need not separate us from the tradition. The correct label is the ungainly "epistemic reasonism," where "epistemic" is understood as "pertaining to knowledge." The crucial premise of any argument for evidentialism is that evidence is the link between belief's claim of truth and the condition of the truth of the belief. But the essence of this argument applies to any belief, including nonempirical ones. The evidentialist's claim is that to (fully) believe that p one needs adequate reasons that p. In the schema "S believes that p," "p" could be a sentence of any content (empirical, mathematical, moral, emotional, intuitive), and essentially the same argument would hold. Evidence is just the most familiar kind of *epistemic reason,* and so for convenience it is the notion that dominates discussion.

We have a grasp, even if rough, on the distinction between epistemic and nonepistemic reasons.[1] If Billy tells Mary "My dad is rich," and Mary asks petulantly "Why should I believe you?" Billy can answer by pointing to his father's Rolls Royce. But Mary will not be moved if instead, Billy tells her, "I'll be your best friend." The latter could induce (cause) the belief in Mary, but it could not be a reason for it. Only if backed by epistemic reasons—ones that indicate the truth of the proposition believed—can a belief be justified or knowledge.

Indeed, we may express one facet of our methodological strategy this way: When asked the question "Do you believe that p?"—for example, "Do you believe that Oswald alone killed Kennedy?"—your answer should take the form of answering the question "Is it the case that p?" ("Is it the case that Oswald alone killed Kennedy?").[2] It is immediately apparent that a practical or prudential reason, like "I could not sleep at night if I thought that there was a conspiracy behind the assassination," will not do. Such a practical reason is no indicator that it is true that Oswald killed

Kennedy. Someone else could offer it as a reason to explain why you hold the belief; but you would be unable to acknowledge a disparity between what explains your believing and what justifies your belief.

Even though pivotal notions like "truth," "evidence," "justified (warranted) belief," or "(epistemic) reasons" are problematic, I offer no substantial analysis or extended discussion of them, gladly deferring to the work of others and, more usually, ordinary understanding.[3] Anti-evidentialists affirm that belief can be justified regardless of the evidence, and this is what evidentialists deny. The wide gulf between evidentialism, particularly in the strong form defended here, and its opponents, will not turn on any fine-grained differences over these notions.

Another excuse for presuming upon analyses of central epistemic notions is the *modesty* of the ethics of belief—it does not aspire to fundamental epistemology or "first philosophy." Leaving aside the opening questions, the ethics of belief is wrapped up in projects like distinguishing gullible, prejudiced, or distorted beliefs (or belief processes) from acceptable or admirable ones. (On this project, my main and limited contributions are found in chapters 3, 4, and 11.)

We should expand on this modesty because I invoke it a number of times in order to sidestep some philosophical conundrums and to grant myself data and assumptions. Although I talk a lot about our concern for the truth of our beliefs, I take no stance on the nature of truth. Specifically, you can generally replace remarks like "we care that for any belief p, we have that belief only if p is true" with more innocent ones like "we care that for any belief p, we have that belief only if p." Issues in the philosophy of language and mind in regard to the analysis of propositional attitudes are not addressed, since I presume that findings there will not favor some views in the ethics of belief over others. I take the object of belief ("belief that") to be propositions, as a manner of speaking, not commitment.[4] When I talk of the "concept of belief" I am speaking essentially of what it is to "hold a proposition true," and so the proper analysis of belief sentences and reports, or even the reality of the mental state of belief, is not likely to bear on questions in the ethics of belief.[5]

Although we would be excused for begging off confrontation with such outlandish views as that there are no beliefs ("eliminativism"), we will not be so readily excused from steering clear of providing criteria for what it is that someone—oneself—really believes. Do I believe that $E = mc^2$? In ordinary circumstances, I seem to. But were I among physicists, not only would I be hesitant to express that belief, I would be unsure whether I really believe it or whether I am only inclined to believe it. Surrounded by the physicists, the shallowness of my understanding becomes manifest. In some ways this difficulty is mitigated through our regular appeal to *assertion:* Would I be willing to assert (or state), to some ordinary, nonexpert audience, that $E=mc^2$? (For brevity, I shall assume that assertion is sincere, unless explicitly denied.) If yes, then I believe it. Although the problem of variability to audiences or to circumstances is still only mitigated, I effectively set it aside by leaning heavily on either very simple contents, such as that of "John believes that the cat is on the mat," or the use of schematic or dummy letters as in "John believes that p." Modesty is again at work: The problems posed by specifying one's exact attitude or the content of that attitude do not differentially affect the intrinsic view that I defend.

The most substantial way that the modesty of the ethics of belief enters my arguments is by ruling out radical skeptical alternatives and their surrogates, where radical skepticism denies the possibility of knowledge or reasons altogether. Treating skeptical conclusions as refuting the premises that entail them suggests a dismissive attitude toward skepticism. Of course, it is one facet of my view—and yours—that radical skeptical conclusions such as that I do not know that $2+3=5$ are preposterous. But another, and opposed, facet of my view is that if certain intuitions are compelling—specifically, that to know is to rule out all possible ways of being wrong—then skeptical results follow.[6] Because this is a work in the ethics of belief, it is the former line that dominates. (The skeptic can still find interest in our project; just as a pacifist can find it worthwhile to distinguish aggressive wars from wars of self-defense, even if ultimately he judges them both immoral.)

Since, in epistemological contexts, skeptical reasoning acquires a natural air, I offer recommendations for dispelling that air. The recommendations are especially germane in light of my position that since the claim of full belief is to the truth of its content, a belief satisfies that claim only if it amounts to *knowledge*. Moreover, that position is put forth not with the intent of securing conviction that much that we believe, we believe wrongfully, since knowledge is so hard to obtain. Rather, much that we believe, we believe rightfully, since knowledge is so easy to obtain.

The first recommendation is derived from an attempt to corroborate the claim that belief aims at knowledge by showing that it fits with our common *attributions* of knowledge. Although we all assume that these attributions are by and large correct, if they are not, the corroboration remains: I am not imposing excessive demands, as these remain our ordinary attributions. So whenever I speak of a proposition as known by a person, you can substitute the more cautious phrasing to the effect that we would attribute knowledge to that person.

The second recommendation is a way to parry an innocent-seeming form of skeptical challenge. Consider examples of alleged knowledge of the future, where the skeptic has a field day. Kate told me that her train would arrive at 5 P.M. tomorrow, so I go to the station to meet her at the appointed time. Question: Do I know that Kate will be there at 5? The skeptic accepts my evidence as to Kate's reliability, but he is not deterred: Isn't it possible that there is breakdown or accident on her train or the one before it, greatly delaying service? Isn't it possible that there is an emergency in Kate's family or in her health that causes her to miss the train or cancel the trip? The presuppositions of these and similar questions are ones I seem unable to deny. It seems as well that if I cannot rule out these possibilities, then I cannot know that Kate will be there at 5.

Aside from forceful contemporary responses to skeptical questioning, I would maintain that it is unfair to press these questions here, since the problems raised are not specific to the ethics of belief.[7] Moreover, we would normally attribute knowledge in many of these cases. To appreciate what our practice really is, you should substitute the following: If all the conditions presumed to be working were—the train line is reliable, normal conditions prevail, and accordingly, Kate arrives on schedule—would you attribute knowledge? I think you would: I knew that she would be there at 5, despite my not having checked that there is no emergency in Kate's family or any other of the skeptic's possibilities. If someone saw me greeting Kate at the station and remarked that it was an amazing coincidence that I should be there just when she arrived, I would respond, as would anyone, "It was no coincidence. I knew she would be here at 5." Substitution of the "Wouldn't he know if . . ." or the "Wouldn't we attribute knowledge if . . ." question for the "But isn't it still possible that . . ." question is the recommendation I offer as a way to stave off skeptical interpretations and so avoid distraction.

Given the modesty of projects in the ethics of belief, a wide range of obvious beliefs can be treated as well founded without argument. These are shared beliefs—the earth has existed for a long time; torturing children for fun is wrong—marking out an area of competence for each of us. Given this enormous area of competence, we can secure data as to the rights and wrongs of belief by asking whether in *full awareness* we could hold a given belief. These questions and the responses to them form the core of the *first-person* methodology that is adopted here.

There is an ethical grounding to the condition of full awareness that supports this first-person methodology. If one is acting (believing) rightly, one can acknowledge it without guilt or shame. Though there are exceptions both to the grounding and to the methodology, they do not undermine our use. We use them to support an extreme claim, and the test we impose on that claim is stringent. The claim is that in no case illustrative of the anti-evidentialist position can belief be formed or maintained in full awareness; and the test is the coherence of the resulting thought.

In focusing on what one could believe in full awareness or consciousness, I *abstract* from conditions that obscure the concept of belief, even if these conditions are natural to the process of believing. Beliefs are treated as articulate thoughts, even though they often exist somewhat inchoate in our minds, until pressed into service as assertions (Dennett 1987: 20–21). The most important abstraction is to bracket the normal unconscious workings of belief and the myriad influences on it. In so doing, we create a controlled environment to study belief, as is the standard purpose of *idealization*—to prevent interferences and to effectuate focus on the crucial variables.

However, full awareness of one's belief as what one believes and one's reasons to believe it, although an abstraction from ordinary believing, is not an idealization; it is not a condition, like perfect rationality or frictionless surfaces, that cannot be met. We often and in everyday circumstances have such a full awareness. I openly believe both that I believe that it is raining outside and that I do so because I see the rain through the window.

These methodological starting points are not, however, common ground. Although my largely first-person methodology is unopposed by direct argument, it is disparaged because the dominant methodology is so commonplace as to be almost invisible. The dominant methodology asks what it is rational to believe, and that is a question well answered from the third-person point of view. If Jim's not believing that he is handsome will depress him, without compensating benefit, then it is rational for him to believe it. Yet, from a first-person point of view, Jim cannot take himself to believe that he is handsome as a way to avoid depression. This "*cannot*" is *conceptual*. It would be contradictory for Jim to think that he believes that he is handsome; that his only reason to believe it is that it will lessen his depression; and that the lessened depression does not bear on the truth of whether he is handsome.

Admittedly, many find positions that openly defy evidentialism unproblematic:

I have heard many people say quite sincerely, "I believe that God exists, but by my own lights, I am not justified in believing that God exists." . . . such a person believes that God exists, regards this belief as unjustified, and finds that so regarding the belief does not make it go out of existence. (Kornblith 1986: 119)

One way to explain away such declarations is that ordinary usage of the term "belief" and its cognates, which is central to expressions of devotion, faith, and commitment as well as to mundane attitudes, will be very loose. An intrinsic ethics of belief must explain away such declarations since it leads to the conclusion that it is impossible to maintain a belief in open defiance of the evidence. Although it is mainly in chapters 1 and 3 that I address various candid denials of evidentialism, I here sketch a preliminary procedure for testing whether these declarations really conflict with evidentialism.

To assess whether the above quote reports a viable position, four steps should be taken (the fourth comes later). Step one: Do not think of yourself as in the position of questioning the person here quoted. An obvious problem is that beliefs about God are highly personal. Since it is central to the social fabric to avoid affront, we should not normally criticize such beliefs in everyday settings. Instead, imagine that the questioning of the report is to take place in the privacy of thought, not in public. Step two: substitute other, unexciting contents in place of "God exists," for example, "Tony is in the ice cream parlor," "The cat is on the mat," "It's raining," or "The moon revolves around the earth." The intrinsic ethics of belief prides itself on fit with a vast range of dull, hardly disputable cases, and on refusal to make exceptions for the more difficult ones. Step three: Make sure that what is meant is straightforward belief—in believing one takes the content of the belief to be true (without qualification). There are close neighbors of belief (e.g., belief in, faith, opinion) that are liable to be confused with it. Reports of the exotic beliefs of members of other cultures are, arguably, not beliefs. Often what is referred to in these cases is not treated as fully representational, but as figurative or symbolic (Sperber 1985). More troublesome, full belief and high degrees of partial belief are often confounded, particularly through such assertions as "I believe that Mary is in Scotland." To avoid this trap, replace the assertion of the qualifying "I believe that" by the assertion of the propositional content alone ("Mary is in Scotland"). The latter actually expresses belief. The former is heard as weaker—a hedge, something like "I'm pretty sure that Mary is in Scotland, but don't swear me to it."

These steps filter away many examples that appear as sharp counter-examples to evidentialism and to our intrinsic approach. They help focus us on the demands of belief.

By contrast, the dominant third-person methodology—which takes the ethics of belief to be fixed primarily by answers to the question "What is it rational to believe?"—orients our focus outside of belief. It invites misguided talk of a person's beliefs as constituting his system or conceptual scheme. Beliefs are treated as one's story about the world. The author of the story tries to optimize a variety of goals. It is his choice whether to simplify his story by admitting some helpful falsehoods or to tolerate inconsistencies in order to render his account more comprehensive. Different individuals may respond to "recalcitrant experience" in different ways so as to restore order. There are trade-offs and a plurality of good stories, as each one constructs or shapes his own belief system.

The first-person point of view will have none of the conceptual-scheme view—beliefs as our constructions, constrained loosely like a narrative by coherence and interest, not constrained, like the acceptance of a scientific hypothesis, by what the belief is about. What is remarkable is that the first-person point of view is our point of view, and yet the "conceptual scheme" view is influential.[8] From the first-person point of view, what I believe is just how things are, not how I conceptualize, interpret, or theorize my experience. Belief aspires to be *transparent* to the world. When I believe that p (e.g., the Yankees beat the Mets), then, briefly, things are for me this way: p (the Yankees did beat the Mets). In belief's everyday roles, prominently as guides to action, one sees through one's attitude to the world without seeing that attitude.

Initially, it seems strange that the first-person point of view could break sharply from the belief-as-his-story view that naturally flows from the third-person perspective. But the incongruity only arises if reporting on the first-person view of another is confused with taking the first-person point of view. When I report that Jones believes that Marcia is in Alaska, I make no commitment to the truth of Jones's belief. But, for Jones herself, what it is to maintain her belief is to be committed to its truth. When Jones attends to her belief, what appears to her is simply this: Marcia is in Alaska. The first-person view brings out the *objective* claim inherent in belief.

We come now to step four of our four-step process. This step is not a filtering device, but a test. After sifting through these various filters, ask of what remains: Is it really coherent to believe it? For example, is it something like:

Tony is in the ice cream parlor, but I lack sufficient evidence that it is true?

It seems not.

I take this test to be but an instance of *Moore's Paradox,* which is a chief—first-person—weapon in our defense of evidentialism, especially in chapter 1 (with extended discussion in chapter 7). The statement that forms the core of Moore's Paradox is actually of the form

p, but I do not believe that p.

Moore's Paradox is that assertions of statements of this form are heard as contradictory, yet it is consistent with p that I not believe it. Because of the similarity in our response, as well as to the overt similarity of form, I assimilate the previous statement and test to a strict Moore's Paradox. If I am successful in the assimilation, then I can draw support from the common understanding of Moore's Paradox: Regardless of the content of substitutions for p, any alleged belief of the form "p, but I do not believe that p" will be rejected as yielding a contradiction.

This appeal to your judgment, particularly in regard to questions of incoherence, recurs throughout the book. Presuming that your responses would be similar to my own, I take these responses to support evidentialism and to display your endorsement of it. But since I rely so heavily on your judgment, I need your cooperation. I ask you to respond directly and un-self-consciously to the examples offered. Do not anticipate the conclusions that I seek to reach and, as a result, substitute your own hard cases. If the data derived from these examples do support my case, I am entitled to them. There will be occasion enough to object to the conclusions I reach from the data.

A major aid to judgment as to what can coherently be believed, as already indicated, is to substitute the question "Would it be coherent to *assert* such-and-such?" For example, would it be coherent to assert "Tony is in the ice cream parlor, but I lack sufficient evidence that it is true"? We answer "No," an answer that corroborates our first-person judgments of belief. Moore's Paradox is, in fact, actually presented as a paradox about what it is coherent to assert, not what it is coherent to believe.

Nevertheless, I need to argue that Moore's Paradox is not merely a pragmatic paradox, but a paradox in thought or belief. My argument will go much further, however, since it aims to advance a far-reaching parallel between belief and assertion. A major benefit of the parallel is to secure unclouded judgments about belief by drawing on our judgments about what is assertible.

The first-person methodology is at one with a methodology that asks what the believer can or would (sincerely) assert—where asserting is, roughly, the unqualified saying or uttering (or writing) of a declarative sentence.[9] The underlying parallel is that the requirement of the speech act of assertion is to state what is true, as it is the constitutive claim of belief that its content is true. Since in assertion one is fully aware of what one asserts, one's willingness or resistance to assertion captures one's first-person view of whether one's believing is proper. John cannot assert that "Marcia is in Alaska, but my evidence does not establish that Marcia is in Alaska." The impossibility of such an assertion captures the first-person incoherence of holding the correlative belief.

An irritating problem, however, with the belief-assertion parallel is that "assertion" and "belief" share an ambiguity. Each can sometimes refer to the act or state (asserting, believing) and at other times to the content (what is asserted, what is believed). The ambiguity is often a helpful device of brevity to refer to both features, and I am glad to avail myself of its benefits. But when the ambiguity is likely to cause trouble, "asserting" ("believing") refers to the act or state.

I will constantly revert to the belief-assertion parallel to corroborate my claims. Our own competence as speakers and hearers provides an extensive fund of data for studying the ethics of belief. First-person methodology applied to belief reflects the very ordinary methodology we regularly endorse and apply to the ethics of assertion.

Although both the first-person methodology and the belief-assertion parallel are crucial to my defense of evidentialism, I maintain that they are not tendentious as methodology. They are simply devices for focusing us on the concept of belief. Of course, to effect this focus we observed that it is necessary to engage in some abstraction from the natural workings of belief. A similar abstraction is required for the parallel with assertion. We must abstract the practice of assertion from such important conversational roles as to socialize and to entertain, which relax the requirement of truthfulness and introduce other aims, such as tactfulness.

However, although we need these abstractions to maintain the assertion-belief parallel, on a number of occasions I appeal to conversational expectations to explain-away intuitions and judgments that go against evidentialism and my defense of it.[10] This dual-role of the appeal to assertion—to treat it in abstraction from some conversational expectations and to understand it in its natural home of conversation—are complementary. Both assume that conversational expectations are beholden to many factors that are not epistemic. The dual-role is acknowledged here only to avoid misunderstanding later of those occasions in which I do not look to assertion purified of its conversational functions. But, unless stated otherwise, my regular references to our practice of assertion should be understood as governed by the abstractions just noted. Their purpose is to focus us on the heart of assertion as the presentation of a proposition as true, which exactly parallels the import of belief.

4   Chapter Summaries

The role of assertion in arguments for evidentialism is prominent in chapter 1 (and developed elsewhere, with the belief-assertion parallel outlined in the appendix to chap. 10). The appeal to assertion converges on more direct arguments to the effect that recognized violations of evidentialism give rise to incoherences.

The evidentialism defended in chapter 1 has been deemed offensive for the prominence it gives to evidence in determining belief. It diminishes our own role in choosing our beliefs. The implied view is that belief is voluntary.

In chapter 2, I argue against *voluntarism,* but I deny that opposition to voluntarism implies that we are not responsible for our beliefs. Belief is not up to me, but that does not exclude my responsibility for it. It is not up to the student, but up to the teacher, what grade the student receives. Nevertheless, if the teacher grades fairly, the student is responsible for her grade.

The main premise of the argument against the possibility of voluntarism is derived from its role in an argument by Bernard Williams (1973: 136–151, "Deciding to Believe"), and that premise figures, as well, in arguments for evidentialism. The premise is that you cannot regard yourself as holding a belief because you choose to. The reason is simple enough: Choice cannot make the belief true. I also take this premise to rule out the possibility of weakness of belief on the model of *weakness of will.*

The conclusions of chapters 1 and 2 depend mainly on the premise that you cannot take yourself to believe without adequate reasons. But do I literally mean that it is impossible to hold a belief in overt defiance of evidentialism? In chapter 3, I defend an affirmative answer. Previously, I sketched a four-step process to help explain away blunt dissent from evidentialism. In chapter 3, however, a complementary tack is taken. The condition under which believing in defiance of evidentialism is incoherent is the condition that there is simultaneous recognition of one's believing and of one's impoverished epistemic position. But in many cases of defiance of evidentialism this condition goes unsatisfied.

The main claim of chapter 3 is that the incoherence test—the test of asking whether one can maintain a belief in full awareness of one's epistemic position—uncovers the error in many cases of distorted belief (beliefs formed out of distorting processes such as prejudice or wishful thinking). The argument depends on the assumption that distorted beliefs violate principles so simple and useful that we repeatedly commit ourselves to them through everyday actions and assertion. If under full awareness we are *explicit* about these commitments, distorted beliefs are exposed, thereby unmasking the incoherence.

Chapter 3 is called "Normative Epistemology," in analogy with "normative ethics," as contrasted with "metaethics." Normative ethics offers moral advice and sets out moral duties, leaving to metaethics the task of the analysis of central ethical concepts. In normative epistemology, we offer advice and set out duties toward improvement of one's beliefs. We are interested in what one ought to do to be a better believer.

Chapter 4 contributes to normative epistemology by exposing fallacies that are committed both by believers and by theorists of belief. The main fallacy is to argue from the lack of a proposition's disproof to the real possibility that it is true, and then either to the wrongness of rejecting it, or, more strongly, to the permissibility of believing it. Broadly, the fallacy is a version of the popular *argument from ignorance*. Obviously, if any such reasoning worked, evidentialism as conceptually defended would fail. You should not be able to take any belief of yours as justified where the only ground is that it is possible that it is correct.

A handy, though contrived, illustration of arguments from ignorance is this: It hasn't been shown that the universe wasn't created. So it's possible that it was. If it's possible that the universe was created, then it cannot be wrong to believe it. So it is permissible to believe that the universe was created. Such arguments I claim are persuasive because they exploit ambiguities in ordinary usage of "possible" and conversational expectations of cooperation.

In chapter 4 I discuss William James's "The Will to Believe" (1951), probably the most famous article in the ethics of belief. The title of the article suggests that discussion of it belongs in chapter 2. But, in fact, the article is not concerned to defend the possibility that we can choose our beliefs. It presupposes that possibility and proceeds to argue that under certain conditions, we are entitled to choose to hold certain beliefs. James is not then merely using an argument from ignorance; he is defending it with the avowed intent of refuting evidentialism.

In recent years, a new topic has been deservedly placed on the agenda of epistemology—*testimony* and trust. Sadly, the reason it has been placed on that agenda is misplaced urgency. The argument goes: If we must rely on trust (the word of an informant) for much of what we believe or know, then when we accept what an informant tells us, our grounds for what we thereby come to believe will be trust in him, rather than evidence.

The reasoning assumes that the only place where evidence can affect the acceptance of testimony is as specific evidence of the trustworthiness of the speaker, and such evidence is not usually available to the hearer. In chapter 5 I argue that this assumption is false and unnecessary. We should reject the implied contrast between trusting someone and having evidence to take his word. We have vast, easily obtained *background* beliefs that serve as reasons or evidence to support our acceptance of the word of the speaker. This appeal to background beliefs is promoted throughout, as an answer to various charges that evidentialism's requirement of adequate evidence or reasons is too demanding.[11]

The appeal to background evidence to defend the empirical support we have to accept testimony is a prelude to the attempt in chapter 6 to show that our background beliefs (or evidence) are themselves well founded. Specifically, they are *tacitly confirmed* in their role in the formation of expectations, which are, effectively, predictions subject to verification.

The claim that our background beliefs are well confirmed would not be controversial except that I offer it as an answer to the *infinite regress problem,* which is one of the two fundamental problems of epistemology (the other is its kin, radical skepticism). The infinite-regress problem is that if beliefs require reasons to be justified and if reasons are beliefs, then some beliefs must be held without reasons, on pain of a debilitating regress. (Alternatively, if some beliefs are inferred from others, not all can be.) If some beliefs lack reasons, or are not inferred from others, then how can they be well founded or justified? But if they are not well founded, how can they transmit that property to what is inferred from them? The most well-known views in epistemology—foundationalism, coherentism, reliabilism, skepticism, Wittgenstein's "groundless" beliefs—can all be presented as responses to the infinite regress problem.

In addressing the infinite regress problem, I might be thought to be ignoring my earlier insistence on the modest ambitions of the ethics of belief. But discussion of the regress problem is forced on us because the most influential objection to evidentialism is that it implies or requires an unacceptable doctrine, namely, foundationalism. Foundationalism tries to stop the regress by affirming that there are basic beliefs that are self-justifying or that are justified but not by (other) beliefs. If the connection holds, then as goes foundationalism, so goes evidentialism. While endorsing the alleged connection, Nicholas Wolterstorff hastens to remind us of the "growing consensus that [foundationalism] is not a plausible criterion of rational belief."[12] In chapter 6, I attempt to dissolve the regress problem in order to liberate evidentialism from foundationalism.

In chapter 7, I apply some of our major theses to three important paradoxes of belief: Moore's, which I will have already relied on, the Lottery, and the Preface. Specifically, I argue that the transparency of full, as contrasted with partial, belief provides a unifying thread among these paradoxes. The crucial factor common to the latter two paradoxes is that the contradiction that both lead to depends on a *conjunction principle*. Roughly, if someone believes each of a set of propositions, then that person believes their conjunction. The solution to both paradoxes that is immediately suggested is to reject the conjunction principle. Invoking transparency, I argue that these solutions are impotent, since the contradiction is derivable without use of the conjunction principle. I proceed to defend an alternative solution. The argument draws explicitly on the first-person methodology, and in the final section I expand on this methodology's value.

The primary purpose of chapter 8 is to develop a forceful challenge that could be raised to evidentialism—that our acquisition and maintenance of beliefs are normally responsive to circumstances or conditions that are not evidential. What if the circumstances in which many of our beliefs are formed do not permit extensive inquiry or investigation, and yet we still need to form beliefs? Think of our responses to how others act toward us. If, at a dinner party, a guest cuts you off while you are speaking, you come to resent it. You judge (come to believe) that he was rude to you. The resentment takes the form of an unqualified or full belief. Although the judgment is quickly formed, it is not abnormally formed. The emotions engaged require a spontaneous judgment, leaving little opportunity to investigate whether, for example, the acquaintance was either not brusk at all (you were being overly sensitive) or that he had an excuse of especially pressing business.

If this kind of case is representative of the *constraints* on us to form full beliefs, then serious challenges to evidentialism follow. In unremarkable circumstances, our belief-forming processes are not responsive to evidence alone, and we have no difficulty in admitting that we do hold these beliefs while recognizing that we acquired them casually with little search for evidence. In chapter 8 I develop different ways of posing these and related challenges, especially of the need for faith where evidence is lacking. At the end I hint at some ways of responding to these challenges, which are pursued in later chapters.

Chapter 9 begins to set up my response to the various challenges to evidentialism. It is a chapter that initially looks backward to clarify previous claims and to support evidentialism. The focus of sections 1 and 2 are on the distinction between *full* and *partial* (or degrees of) belief, which will have already been called on. It is tempting to think that anything one can do with full belief, one can do with degrees of belief, even if less securely or confidently. But this, I argue, is not so. There are central roles that can be sustained only by full belief, not by any lesser degree of belief. Assertion offers one example, but a more obvious one is that only full beliefs are candidates for knowledge, not any degree of partial belief.

Next, I begin the forward-looking task of answering the challenges posed by constraints, and of confronting the broader challenges that coalesce in the charge that evidentialism is too demanding: We would lose too many warranted beliefs if we tried to live up to its demands for adequate reasons. Part of my answer draws on recent work in epistemology, which holds that standards for the adequacy of reasons vary according to circumstantial (contextual) differences. It is obvious that a presidential advisor should invest more time and resources in determining whether foreign aid ought to be given to assist in a civil war in Asia than do you or I as ordinary citizens. But contextual variation does not answer all these related challenges. In the last two chapters I attempt to meet the remaining ones.

Chapter 10 confronts a problem that has hovered over our discussion since the beginning. Each of us can think of many cases in which we openly express beliefs and doubts about them. Yet, according to the strong claims I have attributed to full belief, one ought to have reasons adequate for knowing what one fully believes. How can one satisfy—and regard oneself as satisfying—these strong claims and still have doubts? I firmly believe that public funds should not be used to pay for private education, through "vouchers," yet I have doubts about it. Such an unremarkable position has to be carefully unpacked before it raises a problem for evidentialism. As noted earlier, we have to be sure that we are speaking of full, not partial, belief, among other purifying tests. But after these tests are applied, cases of full belief with (avowed) doubt remain. In chapter 10 I attempt to show their compatibility with evidentialism, arguing that some reasons to doubt do not amount to straightforward objections or undermining evidence. These doubts are directed to *confidence,* and only derivatively, if at all, to belief itself. If you discover that a political belief of yours is unexpectedly not held by someone whose views you respect and who broadly shares your political outlook, you have reason to lessen your confidence in that belief. But you have no reason yet that undermines your belief.

If full belief is compatible with certain doubts, we can learn from them. Specifically, we can learn from those doubts about which beliefs to hold with more suspicion, though without renouncing them. These doubts also provide motivation to *self-correction* or self-control, a central topic of my final chapter (11). Important motivation is provided as well by extensive studies in cognitive psychology, which I will have alluded to a number of times prior to this chapter.

Nevertheless, there is a conceptual roadblock to self-control or self-criticism or self-correction as applied to particular beliefs: How is it possible to have reason to criticize any of one's beliefs without thereby abandoning it? Even after we have navigated our way around this conceptual roadblock via arguments in chapter 10, an important tension remains. Viewed from the natural perspective in which we hold a belief, each one appears justified. But standing back—from a detached perspective—we expect that some of these beliefs, or some of a particular kind, are erroneous or poorly formed, and we care to discern which.

5   Your Questions and a Guide to Locating My Answers

This book aims to defend a radical view, and to defend it in part by securing your endorsement of it. The first two sections above briefly indicated how I intend to defend that radical view and tried to explain why a more moderate position ultimately appears unsatisfactory. The methodology section that came next offered various strategies for separating your real, everyday ethics of belief from your professed view. But I do recognize that your professed view, or at least that of many of you, does diverge from evidentialism or my conceptual defense. In this closing section I want to give voice to that professed view, even if doing so covers some of the same ground as the above chapter summaries. I will set out questions that I hope articulate your various discomforts with the central doctrines defended here, as well as some of your straightforward objections or challenges to it. Aside from some clarificatory remarks, I shall respond only by indicating the locations in the book that address those questions.

1. The basic test is whether one can in full awareness hold beliefs in defiance of evidentialism. The claim is that one cannot. The "cannot" is held to be conceptual because the thought itself would be contradictory. OK,

but where is the contradiction? If someone alleges to believe that there are unicorns and admits to lacking good reasons for it, where is the out-and-out contradiction—the relevant "*p* and not-*p*"? (See chap. 1.)

2. I admit that many hold beliefs in defiance of evidentialism. Is it plausible that in all or even most of these cases one is hiding or obscuring one's reasons or in some way avoiding full awareness? Do I mean literally that one cannot hold such beliefs under the stated conditions? (See chap. 3.)

3. We hold beliefs with avowed doubts. But if evidentialism requires support for beliefs roughly adequate for knowledge, how could the avowed doubts be possible? A person could believe that Abraham Lincoln was among the greatest U.S. presidents, while admitting doubts about it (e.g., he knows that his study of American history is very limited). Sometimes one of the above four steps will dissolve the worry. It is, however, not credible that this cleansing process will always work. The person could hold the belief fully, and admit the doubts. In fact, we often applaud persons who can take so self-critical a perspective on their own beliefs. So the question remains. (See chaps. 10 and 11.)

4. There is another form of doubt that we carry with us and apply to most any belief. The doubt may stem from viewing ourselves as fallible or from reading psychological studies that show pitfalls and foibles in much of the reasoning that issues in belief. There are domains in which I form beliefs knowing that I tend to be gullible (as when I deal face-to-face with salespersons). These doubts do not point to specific beliefs as mistaken, but they do tell us that *some* of our beliefs are mistaken. So don't we regularly have beliefs of which we openly avow doubts? (See chaps. 7, 10, and 11.)

5. We openly hold beliefs for reasons or evidence in some situations that we would not in others. In ordinary conversation I accept a neighbor's word that the Ford Taurus is safer than the Toyota Camry. But if I become set to purchase one of these, I will not rely just on the neighbor's word, but I will check other sources like *Consumer Reports*. How can I allow for such variation in the sufficiency of reasons for the very same belief? (See chap. 9.)

6. We often say things like "I *refuse* to believe that Emily lost my favorite jacket." We change and make up our minds—I can go from ambivalence as to whether a crew cut would look good on me to just deciding (all-out believing) that it would look good on me. Does not the previous very ordinary refusal, as well as the latter type mental activity, signal a voluntariness to belief? (A bit of qualification on this evidence is provided in section 3 above. Some observations in chap. 9 on latitude in belief are pertinent. The main discussion is in chap. 2.)

7. Although evidence is held to be only one kind of epistemic reason, evidence does not seem to capture all that overtly and properly moves belief,

even when we stick to empirical beliefs. What of matters like simplicity? The challenge embedded in this question I take to be complex. The part that most defies evidentialism is of a pragmatic sort touched on above: When evidence appears to oppose entrenched beliefs, the believer has a number of choices as to how to respond, and these choices are determined by the weighing of a variety of factors like simplicity, not logic alone. (This part of the challenge is addressed in chap. 1 with further discussion in chaps. 9 and 10.) The other part of the challenge is not addressed here, though it is addressed by others: to explain exactly how matters like simplicity are linked to judgments of truth or approximations to it.

8. How does evidence alone sustain belief, even under the special conditions set out earlier? For evidence itself consists in beliefs, and so to justify any one belief would require evidence, which itself would require still further evidence, since it amounts to other beliefs. Isn't evidentialism committed at its roots then to an infinite regress? (See chap. 6.)

9. Even if evidence was all that moved belief under the condition of full awareness, how are we to understand ordinary believing, which is regularly gained and lost not under that condition? (See chaps. 1, 8, and 9.)

10. More exactly, how do I account for the automatic ways we constantly acquire beliefs as through memory, perception, or testimony? There is hardly awareness of the process, let alone the time and resources for gathering and evaluating evidential reports. (See chaps. 5 and 6.)

11. The absence of awareness and yet the possibility of justification for the resulting beliefs seems to fit well with an *externalist* account of epistemic relations. On these accounts, epistemic relations like justification or knowledge hold or not according to whether certain relations in the world actually obtain (prominently, whether the processes under which a belief was formed are reliable). But evidentialism appears to be a thoroughly *internalist* view, which demands, counterintuitively, that the agent must be aware of the sources of his beliefs if he is to justify them. Is evidentialism thoroughly internalist, and if so, how does it meet externalist criticisms? (Briefly, I think that the contrast is overdrawn—internal justification is successful only if external relations hold; and external processes that regularly yield full beliefs cannot be wholly beyond the grasp of the agent. See chap. 6.)

12. The transparency of belief to its content holds of many simple beliefs, especially those that are guiding action—we see (believe) that there is a bear coming out from behind the tree in front of us, and we instantly respond. We look though our attitude to its content, rather than looking to the attitude itself. But this is not true of other beliefs—we often attend to our beliefs as what we believe and comment on it accordingly. I may affirm "I believe that in some circumstances capital punishment is justified" (or,

"From my point of view . . .") not to imply a less than full commitment, but to acknowledge that those I am addressing hold a contrary view. What then of this reflective aspect of belief? (Some of the answer to this question is a matter of emphasis—I concentrate on transparency for purposes of opposing the chief lines of dissent from evidentialism, without denying the reflective aspect. See above section 3 and chap. 1. Issues and puzzles raised by our capability to hold a reflective or detached view of our beliefs are taken up in chaps. 7 and 11.)

13. I pick out as central a notion of belief that is distinguished from degrees of belief and from neighboring notions (faith, belief in, commitment). Why should this notion be accorded centrality? The concept of full belief as I analyze it has extremely strong implications that do not seem to fit with our considered opinions of belief. Even if the concept of full belief does have these implications, why should we not introduce a new concept "schmelief" that lacks these implications and is more in line with our ordinary, considered opinions? (As already indicated above, it is crucial to the arguments throughout, especially those in chaps. 1, 9, and 10, that full belief is our ordinary concept of belief. Chap. 9, specifically, draws out contrasts between full and partial belief that are contrasts in role or function, especially that only full belief can be what is expressed in assertion.)

1

Getting Off the Wrong Track

Any account of the ethics of belief should fit tightly with the crucial fact that it is not possible to regard oneself as both holding a belief and holding that one's reasons for it are inadequate. This is illustrated by the ancient challenge to believe that:

The number of stars is even. (Burnyeat 1983: 132)

We cannot meet this challenge.

Evidentialism, an ethics of belief advocated by David Hume, John Locke, W. K. Clifford, and many others, coheres well with the impossibility of our meeting the ancient challenge. Stated in its traditional version, evidentialism is the thesis that *the strength of one's belief ought to be proportional to the strength of one's reasons.* Locke writes:

For he governs his Assent right, and places it as he should, who in any Case or Matter whatsoever, believes or disbelieves, according as Reason directs him. He that does otherwise, transgresses against his own Light, and misuses those Faculties, which were given him to no other end, but to search and follow the clearer Evidence, and greater Probability. (Locke 1975: 688)[1]

Thus evidentialism explains the crucial fact that we cannot meet the ancient challenge. The explanation assumes that we grasp evidentialism's requirement of adequate reasons (or evidence) as a conceptual condition for believing properly. Since we know that we do not have adequate reasons for believing that the number of stars is even, then we cannot, in continuing awareness of that knowledge, believe that the number of stars is even. However, this version of evidentialism is stronger than the traditional version stated above. The traditional version is unable to explain why one *cannot* believe that the number of stars is even; it explains only why one ought not believe it.

In part I of this chapter I defend the stronger version of evidentialism by arguing that it follows from the concept of belief. This *intrinsic* approach is contrasted in part II with the dominant *extrinsic* approaches. Early in his influential essay attacking evidentialism, Alvin Plantinga writes, "Why should we think a theist must have evidence, or reason to think there is evidence, if he is not to be irrational? Why not suppose, instead, that he is entirely within his epistemic rights in believing in God's existence even if he supposes he has no argument or evidence at all?" (Plantinga 1983: 30). In this brief passage, Plantinga implies both a blunt rejection of what I've been calling the crucial fact and his affirmation of rationality as the proper criterion for evaluating norms for belief.

In contrast to the intrinsic approach that I defend, Plantinga advances— or assumes—an extrinsic approach to the ethics of belief. Extrinsic approaches lead discussions of the ethics of belief onto the wrong track in their claim that answers to the question of what one ought to believe are determined by criteria external to belief, most prominently, rationality. In part II of this chapter, I examine four doctrines deriving from extrinsic approaches.

The right track, taken by intrinsic approaches, is to ask what the concept of belief itself demands. On an intrinsic approach the answer to Plantinga's second question is that the theist simply cannot hold such a belief if he attends to it when affirming that "he has no argument or evidence at all." The impossibility of holding such a belief, which is implied by the crucial fact cited above, is of primary importance because it is a *conceptual* impossibility. Only secondarily, if at all, is the belief irrational.

I   The Intrinsic Ethics of Belief

1   From the Subjective Principle to Evidentialism

The crucial fact can be formulated as the *subjective principle of sufficient reason:*

When one attends to any of one's beliefs, one must regard it as believed for sufficient or adequate reasons.

The "must," which governs the whole statement, is essential. Without it, perhaps, our taking ourselves to have adequate reasons is merely a gratuitous, even if widespread, expectation.

The main reason to believe that the subjective principle of sufficient reason is a fact is that we find ourselves compelled to follow it. The compulsion is due to our recognition, when attending to any particular belief, that we are entitled to the belief only if it is well founded. That we do follow it is then a reflection of our grasping the demands of belief, not merely a curious psychological truth about us.

We also attribute acceptance of the subjective principle to others, at least for what they *assert,* and in setting out the grounds for that attribution we capture in brief the intuitive argument for evidentialism. If Sally (the speaker) asserts that p (e.g., "Hamlet is playing at Lincoln Center") to Harry (the hearer), then, normally, Harry takes Sally to have good reasons to believe that p. For otherwise Harry will not accept that p as a result of Sally's asserting it. Since Sally should not assert that p unless she has good reasons to believe it, Harry takes Sally to recognize that she has good reasons to believe p. The requirement that assertions be backed by good reasons, since they claim the truth of what is asserted, is just the analogue of the requirement that beliefs be backed by good reasons, since upon awareness they claim the truth of what is believed.

We would not impose the subjective principle on ourselves by inclination. We would surely prefer to avoid the burden of sufficient reasons or evidence—this is true especially of those who hold wild or paranoid beliefs, such as that the fluoridation of water is a Communist plot. But even they accept the burden, as is shown by their own (tortured) defenses of these beliefs.[2] They will gladly adduce evidence for their belief if questioned. Similarly, as already suggested, even those who reject either evidentialism or the subjective principle typically restrict their rejection to certain contents of belief (e.g., "There is life after death," "Picasso is a greater artist than Duchamp"). For unproblematic contents, such as that the cat is on the mat or that there are tigers, either they do not reject, or they outright endorse, evidentialism or the subjective principle, correspondingly restricted.

Well-known experiments in social psychology reveal the workings of the subjective principle of sufficient reasons, despite their studying judgments whose underlying processes are inaccessible. For example, in one of a large number of studies, an array of identical stockings was set before subjects, and they were asked to select their favored pair.[3] Subjects preferred 4 to 1 the pair that was right-most in the array. Typically, in these studies, subjects explained their actions and presumed judgments (that this [right-most] stocking is preferable to that stocking) with what we regard as rationalizations, such as that the stockings selected "looked better." Since their confabulated reason (that this pair looked best) claims adequacy, it explains their judgment. From their point of view, no further reasons are operative.

In general, across a wide spectrum of related psychological studies, subjects are influenced to form beliefs whose causes they deny or cannot know. Yet, they offer reasons for their relevant beliefs, and, though from our point of view these are rationalizations, subjects feel compelled to offer them. The felt need to rationalize is plausibly explained as reflecting the demands of the subjective principle.

As these studies also show, the reasons demanded by the subjective principle are *epistemic* reasons, rather than, say, reasons of advantage. In subsequent interviews, following the stocking-choice experiment, subjects dismissed as preposterous the suggestion that their reason could be that the preferred stocking was right-most. The suggestion was dismissed, presumably, not because it proposed a merely weak or bad reason, but because what it proposed could not be a reason at all—that is, an epistemic reason, one that can imply the truth of a person's belief. We regularly employ a distinction between epistemic and nonepistemic reasons. One's wanting to be a Hollywood star may induce the belief that one is a Hollywood star. But it is not a reason that can justify believing it true.

The subjective principle asks us to attend to our believing a proposition. The condition that we attend to our believing, or become fully aware of it, is for theoretical purposes, not a practical proposal that believing should be self-conscious. Most belief is, of course, acquired nonconsciously— think of the multitude of beliefs or updatings of old beliefs that are continuously formed as one navigates the world. A central way for a particular belief-state to become active is for its content to play a role in guiding action, and then, as observed earlier, it is not our believing that we attend to, but the proposition believed (the belief). In themselves our beliefs do not strictly enter claims of truth (or knowledge). A claim requires an active presentation, which believing, particularly if nonconscious, cannot accomplish. However, when we merely attend to our having a belief, such a claim is made, and that is the claim whose conditions of satisfaction are fundamental to the ethics of belief.

To attend to the belief as the subjective condition requires demands more than awareness of the content, which is the usual way in which belief guides action. It is to be aware of the belief as believed, and to ask oneself "why" in regard to one's believing.[4] We respond by looking for reasons for the truth of what is believed. (Or, to speak more naturally, we look for reasons for believing that it is true.)

When we do attend to a particular belief, there is no guarantee of success. Sometimes, as when we become aware of a distant memory—for example, that in a local baseball game fifteen years ago I hit a game winning double—we do not take ourselves to have adequate reasons. It seems plausible that the memory could be the product of later suggestion or wishful thinking. What is crucial is that, once we are suspicious of the veracity of the memory, we cease to hold the belief (suspend judgment), even if we still regard it as probably correct.

The point of introducing the subjective principle is not to attempt any argument from our believing ourselves to have sufficient reasons to our actually having them. Obviously, one can wrongly take oneself to have adequate reasons. The purpose is to argue that we impose the demands of the subjective principle on ourselves because these correspond to the demands of belief. That the content of the belief is true is not settled by our believing it. There is a gap between our attitude that the world is a certain way and our position to secure the correctness of this attitude. This gap can be bridged only by evidence or reasons, which link the believer to what is believed.

2   The Incoherence Test

We take both the arguments from the subjective principle and the direct argument for evidentialism to stem from the conceptual nature of belief because overt denials of their conclusions are *incoherent* (a stark contradiction). The *incoherence test* says that p is incoherently believed by anyone X just in case p is believed by X, but, if X became fully aware of his epistemic position in regard to p (his believing that p is true, and his assessment of his evidence or reasons to believe it), X could not continue to believe that p (since the corresponding thought would be an overt contradiction).

The test draws on parallels with incoherences underlying *Moore's Paradox*.[5] One cannot assert statements of the form

p, but I do not believe that p.

For example,

It is raining, but I do not believe that it is raining.

The assertion is heard as contradictory, even though both conjuncts may be true. A rough account of the contradiction (to be improved on in chap. 7) is this: Assertion expresses belief, and belief is the holding true of a proposition. So the assertion would present the speaker as simultaneously holding both that p and that she does not believe it. But then she is believing p and also believing that she does not believe it. But if she is believing p and attending to it, then she must believe that she believes it.[6] The whole thought in this single consciousness would now be that I both believe that p and that I do not believe that p. But no such belief is possible, since its content is an overt contradiction.

The unassertibility revealed in Moore's Paradox is explained by an underlying incoherence in thought (Shoemaker 1996). It is not explained pragmatically, by, say, conversational expectations, such as the conventional implication of "but" that a contrast is to follow. The incoherence derives from assertion as the conveyer of truth, as belief is the attitude that its content is true.

The necessarily failed attempt at belief in the opening example corresponds to the following Moore's Paradox–like thought or assertion:

The number of stars is even, but I lack sufficient evidence that the number of stars is even.

In detail, the incoherence is:

I believe that the number of stars is even. All that can secure for me the belief's claim of truth is adequate evidence (reason) of its truth. I lack adequate evidence. So I am not in a position to judge that the number of stars is even. So I do not judge it true. So I do not believe that the number of stars is even.

The incoherence takes the form of an explicit contradiction (between the opening and closing propositions).

The contradiction is not a further belief.[7] The initial statement is implicitly rejected by the end of the reasoning. That there is no further belief is the lesson of ordinary cases of uncovering evidence that undermines a belief. The contrary evidence thereby erases the belief. There are not separate stages—recognition (of undermining evidence), decision (to surrender the belief), and execution (by ceasing to believe).

My analysis depends only on the recognized lack of adequate evidence, not on the extreme lack that the opening example actually illustrates. In that example, we do not merely take ourselves to have less than adequate evidence to believe that the number of stars is even; we take ourselves to have no evidence at all. However, despite the egregious nature of this particular example, it still serves to make the general point. The same incoherence arises from recognition of less than adequate evidence as it does from cases where the evidence is recognized as starkly inadequate. Instances of the following are heard as Moore's Paradoxes as well:

p, but I lack (sufficient) evidence (reason) that p.

For example, Jeffrey's at camp, but I lack sufficient evidence that Jeffrey is at camp. The correlative explanation, in line with the subjective principle, is that one cannot believe both that one believes that p and that one believes that one lacks sufficient (or any) reasons that p. For consider an (enlarged) instance of this form of Moore's Paradox in a student's assertion:

I'll receive a grade of A in logic, but I lack adequate reasons that I will. Although I have received grades of A on all my tests and papers, I have not received a grade on the final exam.

We hear this assertion as a contradiction. If the student had just asserted that he will get an A, then if the hearer were to learn of his reasons, the hearer would no doubt have been critical: "You shouldn't have said that you will get an A, but only that you are very sure."

The incoherence test exposes not only what cannot be believed, but also what must be believed. We discern this necessity from the attempt *not* to believe that, for example, there are stars, and the failure is again conceptual:

I do not believe that there are stars. But the evidence that there are stars is overwhelming. No further inquiry is needed. So I judge that there are stars. There are stars. So then I believe that there are stars.

Assuming that full awareness is the right condition for grasping the demands of belief, we can roughly sum up: When that condition holds, what one "can" believe when attending to a proposition one "must" believe; and what one "cannot" believe is what is "impossible" to believe. Less cryptically, combining what we learn from each of these incoherences in thought:

Necessarily, if in full awareness one regards one's evidence or reasons as adequate to the truth of p then one believes that p, and if in full awareness one attends to one's believing that p then one regards one's evidence or reasons as adequate to the truth of p.

The first conditional moves from one's judgment of the strength of one's evidence to belief; the second moves in the reverse direction, from awareness of one's belief to one's judgment of the strength of one's evidence.[8] The consequent of the first conditional does not affirm merely that " … one *regards* oneself as believing … ," but that one does believe. Once one judges that the evidence or reasons are adequate, one thereby does hold the belief, and that one does so is apparent. On this understanding, the antecedent of the second conditional is just a stylistic variant of that consequent (of the first conditional). The combined conditional is effectively an equivalence.

So we cannot recognize ourselves as believing p while believing that our reasons or evidence are not adequate to its truth and conversely. The "cannot" is a conceptual, not merely psychological, inability. The notions of higher orders of infinity or electrons shifting levels, with no intermediate position, boggle many minds. But the "cannot" or "unbelievability" that concerns us here is not rooted in (contingent) empirical or psychological barriers. By contrast, we hear familiar tales of, for example, those who have abandoned their fundamentalist religious upbringing, but who claim that they cannot believe, say, evolution by natural selection, despite now being persuaded by the evidence for it.[9] Even if these cases do describe psychological impossibilities (inabilities), they remain conceptual possibilities, ones that can be (and are) overcome by others.

3   Who Am I to Say What You Can Believe?

As I interpret the results of the incoherence test, just as you cannot assert, you cannot think that you have the belief corresponding to any of the following:

It's 3:25, though it's obvious that it is not 3:25.
Or, … , though I'm just guessing.

Or, . . . , though I have evidence that it is not 3:25.

Or, . . . , though I vaguely recall setting my watch ahead ten minutes.

But who am I to say what you can believe? If the implication of this question is that I exercise neither control of your beliefs nor know them intimately, then the implication is irrelevant. If my reasoning is right, then the corresponding thoughts would be contradictions. But no thought corresponds to a contradiction, any more than there can be a contradictory fact.

But the pointed question may be read another way: If the incoherence test is a genuine test, how can I (JA) know (a priori) that it will turn out that all instances that express avowed deviations from evidentialism generate a contradiction? The answer is that the incoherence test is a vivid way to present the conceptual argument for evidentialism. However, the argument must stand on its own. The test simply builds confidence in that argument through applications whose findings rule out explicit violations of evidentialism. On a large range of ordinary cases like those above, there is agreement that the assertions are heard as contradictory. The heard contradiction is most naturally explained as due to what would be a contradiction in the implied thought. Since the contradiction is expressible by appeal to variable "p," the contradiction is not restricted to certain contents of belief.

Actually, though, the cases usually raised against evidentialism are not the dull ones like "It's 3:25," but the interesting ones like "The spoon was bent by psychokinetic powers," "People are basically good," and "The comet-impact account of the extinction of the dinosaurs is correct." These are the cases in which something important is at stake, yet, let us suppose, evidential indeterminacy is unavoidable, at least for the foreseeable future. It is in these cases that persons want to insist that avowed deviation from evidentialism is possible.

To respond to the implied objection, I need to clarify the role of the incoherence test in the argument for evidentialism. The large range of cases in which there is intuitive agreement on the outcome of the incoherence test neutralizes the incredulity that attaches to our strong form of evidentialism. Beyond this, the test cannot advance the argument for evidentialism The argument for evidentialism is a conceptual one, to which empirical evidence is inappropriate.

If the conceptual argument is secured, then we can return to the recalcitrant cases, many of which we can explain away without resorting either to dismissal as borderline cases or to blunt denial of sincerity. Rather, we can question whether the exact conditions for the incoherence test are met, especially the condition of full awareness, as contrasted with the merely informal conditions governing the various cases that I presented.

Even though the full awareness condition requires an abstraction from psychological reality, it does not prevent us from addressing the concept of belief. The ongoing parallel with assertion is crucial here, for asserting presupposes full awareness of one's act and epistemic position.

The failure to impose the full awareness condition explains why the claim as to the incoherence, and so unbelievability, of many beliefs is so hard to take literally. Here is reasoning that suggests the stark implausibility of our incoherence claim: "If the idea that all bees die in the winter is incredible, this means not that such an idea cannot be believed, but that it ought not to be. It cannot mean the first, because some people do believe it. They believe it, but they ought not to" (Helm 1994: 16–17). But this is a fateful misstep, however well motivated. It is the misstep of Locke, Hume, Clifford, and other traditional evidentialists, as well. Given how much divergence and conflicts there are among beliefs of different persons under conditions of shared information, it is reasonable to infer that there is a large element of choice in believing. So traditional evidentialists resign themselves only to offering advice as to how to render those choices more rational or moral or intellectually honest.

But taking the observations of believing in defiance of evidentialism at face value is the analogue of taking as a basic datum for testing theories of motion that heavier objects do fall faster (in free fall) than light ones when dropped from equal heights. The normal condition is not the right—ideal—condition. The normal condition of believing is that of nonconscious influences and distraction. But when we want to discern what belief demands we should look at it without these interferences, which is accomplished by imposing the full awareness condition.

Am I stacking the deck? In a class I taught on writing, a young woman wrote that she had suffered from anorexia nervosa. She would practically starve herself to lose weight for the purposes of appearing more attractive. Yet, she was then, as now, visibly thin, as was evident to her as to anyone who knew her. We can reconstruct one central thought of hers so as to pose a challenge—a putative counterexample—to our coherence test for evidentialism: "I believe I'm overweight, but I can see that I am not."

Waive the difficulty that qualification by the "I believe . . ." rather than the flat-out assertion "I'm overweight" signals, as already noted, not full belief, but only a weak, partial degree of belief. The pertinent observation here is that the condition reported is of a person who is suffering a mental disturbance. Despite the single assertion reporting on her own attitude, it is credible that the disparate thoughts are not held in a single consciousness—that, in short, the assertion does not represent the recognition in full awareness of a belief and her having opposed evidence to it.

But the attempt to block such counterexamples by emphasizing this difficulty may still be held to stack the deck. Have I not granted to myself a maneuver to evade any alleged counterexample by simply denying requisite awareness, and thereby rendering claims of incoherence untestable? But this pointed question is unfair. My basic claim could hardly be more testable as philosophical claims go: There are no cases in which a person in full awareness (as in assertion) both acknowledges that they hold a belief and that their evidence is insufficient for its justification. Given the boldness of this claim, if it is false, it should be easy to bluntly refute.

Consequently, I want to repel the previous pointed question by one of my own: If the basic claim is false, why is it so hard to show its falsity through simple cases like "Our car is in the driveway, but I do not have evidence that it is in the driveway"? The question gestures at my suspicions that the very need to search for esoteric cases, like those afforded by thoughts of the mentally disturbed, tacitly concedes the main claims. If there is no compelling connection between the concepts of belief, truth, and evidence, then counterexamples to the basic claim should be plentiful. The need to search beyond the simple, blunt cases concedes the connection even as it tries to refute it.

What occurs with mental disturbance is an obscuring of the concept of belief. We abstract away from these interferences by imposing the full awareness condition. The rationale for the first-person methodology follows: Once we clear away interferences, what is apparent is the concept of belief and our belief-practices, and then one's believing in recognized deviation from evidentialism vanishes as data and even possibility.

4   Adequate Reasons

In the various formulations of evidentialism and the arguments for it, there has been an unfortunate vagueness in the phrase "adequate reasons" and its kin. A number of times I have hinted at an interpretation in which the adequacy is adequacy to justify or warrant the belief, so that if other conditions are satisfied, the belief amounts to *knowledge*. However, that interpretation goes out much further on a limb than is necessary for the basic issues of the ethics of belief, and so I argue for it only briefly.

The interpretation is supported if instances of the following count as versions of Moore's Paradox, as our response to them indicates:

p, but I do not know that *p*.[10]

For example, the cat is in the yard, but I do not know that the cat is in the yard. Since Moore's Paradox is taken as implying that one should assert *p* only if one believes *p*, then, by parity of reasoning, one should assert *p* only if one knows *p*. Earlier we offered corroborative evidence: The standard form of challenge (or query) to a speaker's assertion that *p* (e.g., the cat is in the yard) is for the hearer to ask "How do you know that *p*?" There is a tight connection between the requirement of knowledge and the mutual expectation (of speaker and hearer) that what is asserted is backed by adequate reasons.[11] (The expectation will be suspended when, for example, the assertion is mutually recognized as controversial.) The tight connection that I conjecture is that satisfaction of the expectation of adequate reasons is taken as satisfaction of the condition of knowledge. In recognizing myself as believing that *p*, the sufficient reasons I take myself to have for believing it are sufficient for knowing it. It is only from such a position that one can look through one's believing to the proposition believed, that is, *transparently*. Any weaker set of reasons warrant only a weaker attitude than full belief, and thus one can look only to the partially believed proposition via one's attitude, that is, not transparently.

Another consideration favoring this construal of adequacy, though also going further, is that it accords with our first-person view. That is, we take ourselves to have adequate reasons or evidence to believe that *p*, rather than merely believing it strongly or to a high degree, just when we treat it as what we know. The first-person view leads us to the more tendentious claim that the relation of reasons or evidence and the truth of the belief in question is one of necessity. Given our reasons or evidence, it must be the case that *p* is true. The reasons are conclusive.[12]

Consider the following ordinary exchange:

Joey (6 years old):   Dad's home.
Mary (his 8-year-old sister):   No, he's not. Why do you say that?
Joey: The Olds just pulled into the driveway, Dad must be going through the basement.
Mary: No. Mom just came home. Dad took the train to his office. He brought his car into the mechanic earlier, and then after work, Mom picked it up.

Joey is taken aback at Mary's denial. Had he allowed for the serious possibility that his reasons held, but that his dad had not returned home, he would neither have drawn his conclusion ("Dad's home"), as contrasted with "Dad is almost certainly home," nor would he have been taken aback. Since Mary turns out to be right, Joey learns that his judgment of the adequacy of his reasons is mistaken. But there would be no cause for correction if his mother's being home, rather than his dad, was only highly unexpected or a serious possibility. So the original thought I ascribe to Joey is that it *must* be the case, given his evidence, that his father is home.

Although Joey's "must" is genuine, it is not only relative to his evidence but expresses a restricted necessity (Lycan 1994: chap. 8). Joey takes his evidence to exclude such possibilities as that his father took a walk around the block after pulling his car into the driveway, not such unlikely possibilities as that his father sold his car to a stranger, who just happened to pull the car into the family's driveway.

The ordinary first-person judgments in this and previous cases will be appreciated as support for my position if we bracket our theoretical musings on knowledge (or conclusive reasons). For one thing, we are coached to understand knowledge as a difficult achievement. In bracketing these understandings, to borrow from our methodological discussion in the introduction, we assume that the requirements of knowledge are those requirements that accord with the roles that the concept of knowledge plays in our practices. These roles, especially in backing assertions, are easily missed in abstract reflections. The same bracketing is required for getting to the nature of belief. Our reflective grasp of the concept of belief is subject to conflation with related concepts (belief in, inclined to believe, faith, opinion, assent), as well as to overintellectualization, by salient, but problematic, content (e.g., "The universe did not exist before the Big Bang," "Pederasty is unnatural," "Psychic healing helps cure persons of disease").

But it is within our ongoing epistemic practices or activities that our actual view of knowledge, conclusive reasons, or belief is revealed. In abstract reflection, our basic claims are defeated from the start—the standards for knowledge are too high to be commonly satisfied, and belief is too common a phenomenon to be subject to high standards. By contrast, our ordinary understanding and practices treat knowledge as easy to achieve, and so it can realistically serve as the aim of the ordinary phenomena of belief.[13]

It turns out, as a final reason favoring this construal, that if knowledge is analyzed via justification, then the simplest account is one in which those reasons or evidence are conclusive. The account yields a neat resolution of the much discussed *Gettier problem* (Gettier 1970). This problem is that, however strong a person's justification that a proposition holds, it leaves open, on the usual analyses, the possibility that the proposition is false. But from a false proposition, a further one can be deduced, which is only accidentally true for that person. It is then alleged that there is justified true belief but not knowledge of the proposition deduced. However, if justification is conclusive, then it is impossible for a belief to be justified but false. (Recall, however, from our discussion of the case of Joey, that this impossibility is restricted and relative.)

Analyses of knowledge or justification that require conclusive reasons are usually dismissed because, with inductive reasons especially, the evidence cannot entail the conclusion. No amount or variety of finite evidence for the proposition that "all swans are white" entails that proposition. But the fallacy is to assume that the only necessity is logical or analytical necessity (and so, correspondingly, that the only possibility is the broadest kind of possibility—logical possibility or self-consistency).

What I find particularly attractive about the conclusive reasons account is that it conceives knowledge as an ordinary and common achievement and yet acknowledges that what is achieved meets high standards. As previously indicated, this is the basic claim for full belief that I will defend throughout—that it is ordinary and common, yet the standards to be met are high.

It should be evident why, in adopting this position, I go much further out on a limb than is required. Anti-evidentialists of various stripes do not just deny evidentialism. They affirm that belief is proper without any reasons or evidence, or in the absence of undermining reasons or evidence, or with reasons or evidence adequate only for a probability greater than half. The denial of any of these theses does not require that evidence or reasons be adequate for knowledge, let alone that reasons be conclusive. To deny any of these positions, it would be enough to require that one properly believes that *p* only if one's evidence or reasons very strongly support the truth of *p*.

In defending evidentialism on the strongest construal, I obviously present it with the greatest challenge. If it goes through on this construal, it certainly works on the weaker, more popular, construals. Those with doubts about the centrality of knowledge can still adopt my arguments against anti-evidentialist theses by substituting their own weaker readings of the demand for reasons or evidence. (I will, in fact, use the crucial term "justification" in the standard way as requiring reasons adequate for knowledge, though without commitment to the claim that such adequacy amounts to conclusiveness.)

However, I do not want to end this section on the suggestion that the adequacy of reasons for full belief as adequacy for knowledge or conclusive reasons is merely a position adopted for the sake of argument—to set the highest challenge to evidentialism. The position dovetails nicely with crucial claims, particularly the connection to assertion cited above and that when one attends to one's full belief that *p* one looks through one's attitude to the proposition believed. This transparency feature mirrors the central *factiveness* of knowledge: If *X* knows that *p*, *p* is true. Correspondingly, in attending to one's belief that *p*, one treats it as the case that *p*.

In this section, I have largely, but not fully, allayed the complaint that my use of "adequate reasons (or evidence)" is a kind of persuasive definition, forcing dissenters to the unenviable position of defending belief on *in*adequate reasons. But in understanding "adequate reasons" as "adequate for knowledge or something close to it," I have offered a substitute that answers the complaint, though not fully.

The phrase will still rankle those who argue that we have good reasons to hold some beliefs without evidence, even when the beliefs are empirical. These theorists hold that we each believe, for example, that perception or induction is reliable, but that we have no evidence for these beliefs.

This position I have argued against via assertion, intellectual responsibility, the connection with knowledge, and its lack of intuitive acceptability. These theorists will claim that the fact that a person cannot believe that *p* while recognizing that her evidence is inadequate does not imply that a person cannot believe that *p* while recognizing that she has no evidence.

But this claim is not first-personally endorsed: we take ourselves to have, and to need to have, good evidence or reasons for taking perception or induction to be reliable. The no-evidence theorists feel compelled to take their position as the only way to respond to the *regress problem* for justification. In chapter 6 I attempt to liberate them from the regress problem and so the felt compulsion to exempt certain beliefs from the demand for reasons or evidence.

5   Full and Partial Belief

In arguing for evidentialism I have partly acquiesced to a widespread indifference to the distinction between full belief, the all-out acceptance of a proposition, and only partial or qualified belief (e.g., "almost sure"). But doing so forecloses some natural lines of reasoning favoring evidentialism. In the case of partial (or degrees of) belief, evidentialism is virtually self-evident. If one's degree of belief that p is greater than half, one's (subjective) probability of p on one's evidence is greater than half, and conversely.[14] Traditional evidentialism, at its most general, claims:

One ought to have a degree of belief n that p if and only if one's reasons or evidence support the truth of p to degree n.

We almost imperceptibly conflate the two sides of this equivalence (the left side concerned with the strength of our attitude and the right side with the extent of evidential support). We read smoothly the following declaration by Hume, just preceding his pithy expression of evidentialism ("a wise man, therefore, proportions his belief to the evidence"): "in our reasonings concerning matter of fact, there are all imaginable degrees of assurance, from the highest *certainty* to the lowest species of moral *evidence*" (Hume 1977: 73; my emphasis).[15]

By ignoring partial belief in arguments for evidentialism, we put aside how the strong demands of full belief are an extension of demands hardly contestable for partial belief. We also put aside challenges both to evidentialism and to anti-evidentialism. The evidentialist has the challenge to explain how an argument rooted in proportionality can allow for a threshold to the all-or-nothing concept of belief beyond which further (positive) evidence or reasons cease to have an impact on the strength of belief. (The discussion below partly answers this challenge, although the distinction between full and partial belief is addressed mainly in chap. 9.)

But the anti-evidentialist faces a much more serious challenge. What account of full belief will allow for the sharp discontinuity he posits, if he accepts evidentialism for partial belief and full belief as the end-point of degrees of belief? The anti-evidentialist assumes that, when we get to the highest strength, we do not require correspondingly greater evidential strength, if we need evidence at all. Yet, in that case, the claim of truth is greater (than for any degrees of belief), and it is that claim which is the source of evidentialism's proportionality demand.

This final observation deserves explicit formulation:

(I)   If the belief-like attitude A toward p is (epistemically) stronger than A' in the same situation, then, if the available reasons are insufficient to justify A', then they are insufficient to justify A.[16]

Principle (I) formulates the common-sense idea that as one's claim of the truth of p is more forceful, then, correspondingly, one is committed to stronger reasons or evidence in its favor. By reference to (I), I indicate the free ride that anti-evidentialists extend to themselves when they fail to specify whether their theses are meant to hold for full or degrees of belief.

For illustrative purposes consider two related extrinsic doctrines, the first of which is treated below:

(1)   We are permitted to *believe* that p (e.g., John is in Alaska) unless we have adequate reason for supposing it false. (Alston 1983: 116, 119)

(2)   If a *belief* (e.g., The red button flashed on the camera) arises immediately (non-inferentially) from perception (memory, testimony) under normal conditions then we are entitled to hold it (i.e., the belief is justified or warranted or is knowledge).

Both of these are so-called Reidian views, which treat belief acquisition or maintenance as a *default*—we are entitled to it unless there is special reason to object. Each has as the implied contrast, "We do not need reasons for believing it."

Principle (I) suggests a test of these doctrines. Substitute within them explicit reference both to degrees of belief and to the contrast clause:

(1′)   We are permitted to have a *high degree of belief* that p (John is in Alaska) unless we have adequate reason for supposing it (probably) false. We do not need reasons that support p to that high degree.

(2′)   If a *high degree of belief* (e.g., that the red button flashed on the camera) arose immediately (non-inferentially) from perception (memory, testimony) under normal conditions then we are entitled to that high degree of belief. We do not need reasons that support it to that high degree.

In each case, the degree of belief selected is the purposely vague "a high degree of belief" (e.g., "almost certain"). My objection turns neither on difficulties of specifying a precise degree of belief nor on demands for commensurate evidence that follow were one to form a precise degree of belief. Theses (1′) and (2′) are just on their surface less natural and less plausible than (1) and (2). (1′) and (2′) violate the thesis that strength of conviction of a claim can be satisfied only by a matching strength of evidence, which underlies (I). But, following (I), if the lack of reasons proportionate to a high degree of belief implies that the actual degree of belief is unjustified, this lack will likewise imply that the corresponding full belief is unjustified.

Still, this objection to (1) and (2) will not be persuasive without some account of why instances of (1) and (2) do strike us as plausible, whereas (1′) and (2′) do not. The explanation, or a good part of it, is a *pragmatic asymmetry*. Expressions for full belief are unqualified assertions, but expressions for partial belief are explicitly introduced by *epistemic qualifiers* like "I am almost sure that . . ."[17] or "On the evidence, it is probable that . . . ." Because of their *marked* or burdensome nature, qualified assertions call for the articulation of reasons. Those for unqualified—normal, unmarked—assertion do not.

The pragmatic asymmetry proposed is that expressions for full belief may be (default) asserted without asserting one's reasons, whereas expressions for partial belief cannot. The pragmatic asymmetry does not violate (I), since the pragmatic asymmetry is over the demand to *present* one's reasons, not over their strength. In fact, in accord with (I), the assertion of *p* presumes backing by reasons adequate for knowledge that *p*. These reasons will then be stronger than the reasons demanded to explain one's qualified attitude.

The conclusion I reach is that the intuitive plausibility of (1) and (2) in contrast to their analogues for partial belief gain from this asymmetry and that it is an unearned gain. For, in accord with (I), the demand to justify a full belief is greater than the demand to justify any degree of belief in the same content. Since we cannot hold any of the parallel default theses—no reasons required—for partial belief, then by (I) we shouldn't hold them for full belief. Those who have promoted the above default theses, under the sway of this pragmatic asymmetry, have confused, I think, not gathering or not showing reasons with not having them. I follow up on this theme in chapter 6.

Extrinsic approaches, which are taken for granted by anti-evidentialists (and many evidentialists), have an uneasy relation to the full/partial (belief) distinction. The unease explains why they rarely treat it directly. Anti-evidentialists are in a bind. On one hand, if they construe belief as a matter of degree, then it is extremely difficult to deny evidentialism for degrees of belief.[18] On the other hand, if they construe belief as full belief, they will need to borrow from the arguments that enforce a distinction between full and partial belief. That distinction is compatible with principle (I); but, as we just observed, anti-evidentialist default theses, like (1) and (2), violate (I).

II Extrinsic Ethics of Belief

6 Critique of Four Extrinsic Doctrines

I shall set out for critical examination four widely accepted doctrines characteristic of extrinsic ethics of belief:

1. The ethics of belief, and evidentialism, specifically, are committed to substantive views of rationality and enter substantive claims on issues in epistemology and moral theory.

2. The ethics of belief is lax. The requirement of adequate reasons or evidence is diminished or abandoned. Characteristically, those who find evidentialism too demanding advocate Reidian views, in which beliefs are "innocent until proven guilty" (Wolterstorff 1983: 164). William Alston advances the view (cited above) that "we are permitted to believe that p unless we have adequate reason for supposing it false" (1983: 116).[19] Variations on this theme allow that it is right or permissible to believe that p if p is not demonstrably false or if p is not shown to be false or in the absence of any specific reason to oppose p. The burden of proof is on those who would deny entitlement to believe, not on the believer. If my belief cannot be refuted in any of these ways, I am entitled to it.[20]

3. The "ought" of what it is right to believe is the "ought" of what it is right or best for a believer to do. The ethics of belief is a branch of practical or prudential ethics.

4. Methodology for the ethics of belief is either normative, and hence can be indifferent to the facts of actual believing, or else descriptive, its prescriptions bounded by the facts about us as believers, particularly our finitude or limits.

In addition to these four doctrines, two further ones are closely associated with extrinsic approaches. Under the first doctrine, it is claimed that evidentialism implies or requires *foundationalism*.[21] ("Almost always when you lift an evidentialist you find a foundationalist," Wolterstorff 1983: 142.) Foundationalism holds that any corpus of beliefs is essentially structured into basic (foundational) and nonbasic (inferred, derived) beliefs. Basic beliefs provide grounds for the nonbasic ones but do not themselves require evidence. Although this fifth doctrine is an instance of the first, it requires separate treatment, which it receives in chapter 6.

A sixth doctrine is *voluntarism*—belief is subject to choice or to the will. This doctrine goes along with the third and fourth. If the ethics of belief allows for "permission" to believe, and its "ought" is that of moral action, then we require the ability to exercise that permission and to comply with the prescriptions. Contrary to this ascription to evidentialism,[22] the basic argument for it is incompatible with voluntarism, though discussion is deferred until chapter 2.

The first doctrine—that the ethics of belief presupposes substantive views of rationality and views on issues in epistemology and moral theory, e.g., foundationalism—ignores the innocent reflections that issue in evidentialism.[23] Evidentialism is arrived at by generalizing on so unremarkable a practice as asking "Why?" when someone affirms belief in a proposition. The expectation is that, in response to the why-question, reasons or evidence will be provided.

Nevertheless, there are many routes to this first extrinsic doctrine. The most obvious is that discussions in the ethics of belief are dominated by the familiar terms of ethics: "ought," "should," "permissible," "wrong," "justified." These terms are incorporated into talk of epistemic duties, obligations, and responsibilities. Criticism of belief is expressed in the terms of immorality ("blameworthy") or irrationality.[24]

However, as just observed, this first doctrine is suspect on its surface. The common formulation of evidentialism, as the view that the strength of belief should be proportioned to the evidence, stands on its own. From the mere presentation of the position, we immediately grasp its rationale. The presentation does not dangle, waiting on an elaborate defense. In section 1, I argued for evidentialism on conceptual grounds, explicitly assuming no substantive views of rationality, epistemology, or ethics. The dominance of the above ethical terms in discussions within the ethics of belief is partly a product of the wrong methodology and starting point I criticized in part I. But it is also a product of the limited normative vocabulary available. We are hard pressed to select simple terms to enter normative claims other than the standard ones of ethics. In contrast, the intrinsic approach takes the basic evaluative terms for the ethics of belief to be "cannot" and "must," as in the incoherence test. The place for terms like "right" or "proper" is derivative, and, more so, terms like "ought" or "irrational."

The second doctrine (the ethics of belief is lax) as well as the third (the "ought" of the ethics of belief is the practical "ought" of action) follow from taking the ethics of belief to be determined by what it is rational to believe. Thus the "ought" of the ethics of belief is taken as based on practical, ethical, or prudential considerations.[25]

The second doctrine reflects weak demands for reasons or evidence. Recall the view that

we are permitted to believe that *p* unless we have adequate reason for supposing it false. (Alston 1983: 116)

According to this view, if you find yourself, for whatever reason, with the belief that the number of stars is even, you are entitled to continue to believe it. For you will surely not find adequate reason for "supposing it false." (That the evidence is roughly 50/50 or, effectively, null is adequate reason not to believe it. But it is not adequate at all for believing that it is false, i.e., believing that the number of stars is not even.)

But counterexamples are to be found in more moderate examples, such as the earlier one of the student who, let us assume, is convinced that he will receive a grade of A. Given his strong performance in the class, he has no reason to suppose that he will not receive an A. Nevertheless, once he comes to appreciate that he might not do extremely well on the final, he ceases to hold the belief. His response is mandated: It is not just wrong or impermissible for him to hold the belief; in full awareness, it is not possible.

Another form taken by a lax ethics of belief is to propose weak conceptions of belief. Richard Swinburne holds that:

normally to believe that *p* is to believe that *p* is probable. (Swinburne 1981: 4)

If this is a proposal about the meaning or analysis of "belief," then, for reasons already canvassed, it amounts merely to stipulation. If you judge it only probable (more likely true than false) that the bus leaves at 7:40, then that is your degree of belief, and you would deceive or lie if you asserted "The bus leaves at 7:40" rather than "Probably, the bus leaves at 7:40." You cannot think "p, but there is a strong probability that not-p."

Admittedly, ordinary expressions sometimes do support this path toward a lax ethics of belief. An amateur investigator might claim to believe the comet-impact hypothesis of the extinction of the dinosaurs based on very forceful evidence. Yet, he still regards the evidence as inconclusive, and he freely admits that there remain some troubling data for his hypothesis. Without disputing that the use here of "belief" is natural, I propose that the investigator really only believes the hypothesis to a very high degree. His attitude here is not akin to the unqualified way he fully believes that, say, the dinosaurs are extinct. The assertion that

The comet-impact hypothesis is true, but the evidence so far is inconclusive.

seems to use the second conjunct to actually withdraw the unqualified assertion of the antecedent. The more accurate assertion is the qualified

The comet-impact hypothesis is almost certainly true because the evidence so far is strongly supportive, but not conclusive.

This investigator's own practices favor the latter reading. The investigator pursues further studies of the hypothesis with the question of its truth left open.

The appeal of a lax ethics of belief depends on a stubborn conflation of the extent to which the evidence supports a belief with the strength of that belief on the evidence. It is a conflation of an epistemic relation with a psychological state or attitude. One instance of this is to confuse the evidence's being "inconclusive" for the proposition believed with its failing to be determinative in regard to one's attitude. But if it is inconclusive in the former way, it remains decisive that one must withhold belief.

However, the conflation shows how readily we slide between the two, and that their affinity is at one with the subjective principle of sufficient reasons. The natural phrase "reasons (evidence) for belief" embeds the conflation. One's reasons or evidence are of the content of one's belief, and it is only by virtue of the evidentialist proportionality claim, which is taken for granted, that these are thereby reasons for belief. The subjective principle is sufficiently second nature that our strength of belief, which follows only on the judged strength of evidential support, comes to be identified with it. Evidentialism claims that these are conceptually connected, not one and the same.

The third doctrine holds that what one ought to believe is determined by the full range of practical considerations bearing on how one will act guided by that belief. A recent article sounds this standard theme:

> there are occasions in which it is permissible, morally and rationally, to form beliefs not on the basis of evidence, but on the basis of pragmatic reasons. (Jordan 1996: 409)

One reaches the third doctrine by mistakenly reasoning from the fact that belief is always the belief of some agent (some doer) to the conclusion that what one ought to believe is derivative from what is right (best, optimal, rational) for one to do, all things considered.[26]

If what is meant is that the "oughts" of the ethics of belief can be overridden or outweighed by the demands of morality or prudence, then it is just a truism. You ought to speak civilly, though not if someone threatens to kill you if you do.[27] But it becomes nontruistic when the "ought" and related ethical terms ("permissible") are taken as directed at belief, not primarily at the individual who holds the belief. On certain occasions, morality or rationality require or allow pragmatic reasons to take precedence over evidence.

The oft-repeated example that is supposed to favor this doctrine is of a wife who overlooks weak evidence of her husband's infidelity. She expects that if such evidence were to undermine her belief in his faithfulness, it would destroy their marriage. She judges that the expected value of keeping her marriage together, if the evidence is misleading, well outweighs that for ending the marriage, if the evidence is correct. The verdict is that it can be rational for the wife to continue to believe that her husband is faithful in defiance of the evidence. From these and related examples, it is concluded that if there is behavior

> which one ought to prevent oneself from engaging in, and if one can ... prevent this behavior by adopting a certain belief, then one ought to adopt that belief, apart from the epistemic warrant or lack thereof for that belief. (Meiland 1993: 520)

Thus the relation of evidence to what one ought to believe "needs to be justified by a practical argument" (524).

A telling concession of those who advocate the third doctrine is that the justifiably suspicious wife might have to deceive herself in order to maintain the belief in her husband's fidelity. But advocates respond: "this only shifts the question—from whether it is wrong to believe on the basis of insufficient evidence to the question of whether self-deception is always wrong" (516). But why should self-deception be required at all unless the agent recognizes her prospective beliefs as violating their own claims? The answer is that it should not. When we imagine self-deception lifted, the person can no longer maintain the belief, since she has now exposed an incoherence, of the kind set out above. (Briefly, for the wife, the incoherence is "My husband is faithful, but I have evidence that he has been unfaithful.")

The rationality that I have focused on is rationality of action. Some, however, would introduce as more pertinent the notion of *epistemic rationality*, taking the best means to the end of gaining truth. This notion is much less natural and much less studied than rationality of action (taking the best means for reaching a given end).[28] Still, I expect that some understandings of epistemic rationality would favor evidentialism as well. But this is true neither of dominant views of epistemic rationality nor of those that give comfort to extrinsic approaches.

The thesis that draws the sharpest break with evidentialism claims that *consistency,* although an important advantage of a set of beliefs, is only one virtue among others. Here is a recent expression of this broadly pragmatist theme: "there are criteria for rationality other than consistency, and that some of these are even more powerful than consistency. . . . These criteria are all independent . . . pulling in opposite directions. Now, what should one do if, for a certain belief, all of the criteria pull toward acceptance, except consistency—which pulls the other way? . . . it seems natural to suppose that the combined force of the other criteria may trump inconsistency. In such a case, then it is rational to have an inconsistent belief" (Priest 1998: 420). If this is correct, then, here, as elsewhere, I insist that it should be possible to engage in the reasoning advocated openly. But it isn't. From the first-person point of view there is no coherent thought of the form: "p, q, r . . . are each true. However they are inconsistent. That is, at least one of them is not true. But that's OK because the collection has compensating cognitive benefits, and it would be foolish to sacrifice all the rest of these, merely for consistency. So 'Yes,' each of these is true and yet one of them is not true."[29] Overlooking this incoherence is a product of abstracting consistency from its centrality as a constraint on belief. Consistency is not just a "virtue" of a set of beliefs. Each of a set of beliefs makes a claim to truth, not to simplicity, fruitfulness, or other cognitive virtues.

That claim can be satisfied only if the joint truth of those beliefs is possible; that is, only if the set of beliefs is consistent.[30]

The fourth doctrine assumes that the methodology of the ethics of belief is either descriptive or else normative. Either you infer the norms of belief from what human agents are capable of following, or else norms for belief dictate what it is right or wrong to believe, regardless of what believers actually do. The intrinsic ethics of belief rejects this dichotomy.[31]

Appeal to the "is/ought" distinction, or to the "naturalistic fallacy," in order to argue for purely normative approaches ignores relevant modal facts. It erroneously assumes that the facts ("is") to which normative claims can be indifferent are mere contingencies. But when the "cannot" is conceptual, this reasoning fails. Similarly, contrary arguments for naturalistic approaches assume that the "cannot" in the contrapositive form ("'cannot' implies not 'ought'") is that of inability. The result is an approach to the ethics of belief that is hopelessly dependent on peculiarities of human psychology, rather than applicable to any (potential) believers.

The "cannot" of the intrinsic ethics of belief is conceptual; it derives from the incoherence of recognizing both that one holds a belief and that one's reasons for that belief are inadequate. The incoherence is a contradiction, so the point is that there is no such thought, not merely that such thoughts are irrational. The "cannot" is strongly normative, generating not simply "not ought"s, as entailed by the "'ought' implies 'can'" thesis. Not only is it not the case that one ought to believe that the number of stars is even, but one *ought not* to believe it. The restriction governs any believing creatures, not merely humans, for underlying the incoherence is a conflict between the conceptual nature of belief and one's epistemic position.

7   Assertion and an Everyday Bridge between First- and Second-Order Judgments

You cannot believe that there is an even number of stars, when you recognize that it is belief that you are aiming at, as required by the full awareness condition. One lingering worry over the full awareness condition is that it is arduous to realize idealization; a deeper worry is that the incoherence test and the argument that inspires it confuse *second-order* with *first-order* incoherence. If it is incoherent to believe that *p*, recognizing *p* as what I believe, that is a second-order incoherence. How is it supposed to follow that the belief that p itself—the first-order belief—is incoherent? I hope to relieve both worries by recalling our ongoing parallel with assertion.

Assertion presupposes full awareness of one's act and epistemic position. Assertion is that speech act in which the speaker presents the hearer with the content p, not the speaker's attitude toward it. However, the hearer recognizes not just the content of the assertion, but that of the speech act as that of an assertion. Analogously, the background condition satisfied when one attends to one's belief is that the content is held as true, not merely that the content is thought or entertained.[32]

The parallel supports the deaf ear we seem to be turning to those who insist that they do hold full beliefs in avowed defiance of evidentialism. A hearer, Harry, will accept a speaker Sally's assertion that p (e.g., The #2 express stops at Franklin Ave.) because Harry takes Sally to believe p. The backing of the assertion by the speaker's belief is a backing of p, not the speaker's attitude. If Harry challenges Sally with the question "how do you know?" Sally successfully meets the challenge by offering her reasons that p, not reasons about the nature of asserting (or believing).

What happens if the speaker's reasons and attitude pull apart? Harry believes that if Sally lacks the attitude but satisfies the epistemic condition then he will still accept Sally's assertion. But not conversely. For it is only the reasons that provide the guarantee that Harry seeks.

Assertion provides us with a model of a pervasive epistemic practice where the full awareness condition is presumed to be met. The hearer accepts the speaker's assertion because the hearer takes it as what the speaker believes. So in the common and ordinary speaker-hearer relation, a necessary bridge for the hearer to accept the speaker's word is a second-order one. That bridge is generated virtually automatically, requiring no notice or cogitation.

Our model for the ethics or epistemics of belief is that of the ethics or epistemics of assertion. When one attends to a belief, one regards it as asserted by (and to) oneself. (We thereby abstract away from social obstacles to assertion such as those due to matters of privacy, as our parallel requires that we abstract away from conversational expectations like politeness.) In asserting to oneself, one simultaneously occupies the role of speaker and of hearer. In these dual roles, the anti-evidentialist cannot assert to himself that his alleged requirements or conditions for belief are satisfied. The evidentialist can. But I have argued that, under the idealization of full awareness, if (and only if) one's ethics of belief is correct, one can state explicitly—assert—that its requirements are fulfilled. So I infer from the incoherence of the second-order position in overt defiance of evidentialism that the first-order beliefs, which yield that incoherence, are wrong or improper.

8   Summary: The Traditional and the Conceptual Approaches to Evidentialism

Traditional evidentialism implies that when one's belief is not in accord with the evidence then one is engaged in believing unwisely or irrationally. More simply, one is not believing as one ought. But, of course, one can deliberately act unwisely, irrationally, or against what one ought. Indeed, it seems senseless to recommend wise or rational behavior, unless there is an option of not complying with the recommendation. Yet, as we have observed, anti-evidentialists thrive on this approach, even if they dissent from what the tradition regards as wise or rational or one's duty.

The evidentialism I am defending rejects not only or not primarily the implication, pursued in chapter 2, that belief is a matter of choice or the will. Rather, I am concerned to reject the implication—more detrimental in large part because it is taken for granted—that the relation between belief and evidence is a contingent one, which requires shoring up from tendentious doctrines of ethics, epistemology, or rationality. In particular, we do not specify the basic doctrines of the ethics of belief in "deontological" terms of "ought"s and duties. The objective version of evidentialism for full belief is not one about how one ought to believe (rationally, wisely, or ethically). Rather,

One's believing that p is proper (i.e., in accord with the concept of belief) if and only if one's evidence establishes that p is true.

On the conceptual or intrinsic approach, normative judgments ("ought"s) are not directed to belief as they are on extrinsic approaches including that of traditional evidentialism. If, under ideal conditions, I cannot help but believe (not believe) when I recognize that the evidence establishes (fails to establish) that p, it makes no strict sense to say that I ought (or that it is not the case that I ought) to believe p.

Because judgments of what one cannot believe are conceptually grounded, they are simultaneously normative and descriptive. The main doctrines in the ethics of belief are testable. We test them against the data of what we do (and so can) actually believe when we focus on the claims inherent in our believing a proposition and whether our epistemic position fulfills those claims. As previously noted, what we cannot possibly believe, we cannot actually believe. So evidentialism corresponds to the facts. When we attend to any belief in clear light, it describes how we judge.

The argument from the subjective principle to evidentialism is both normative and descriptive because it is conceptual. In reconstruction that argument is this:

1. Necessarily, if in full awareness one attends to one's believing that *p*, one regards it as believed for adequate reasons.

So, 2. One cannot recognize oneself as fully believing that *p* (rather than believing *p* to a high degree) and that one's reasons for belief are inadequate (yielding less than full support).

3. The reason that one cannot so recognize oneself is that the thought would be a stark contradiction.

So, 4. The "cannot" is conceptual, not merely an inability, and the concept that generates the contradiction is belief.

5. The impossibility of believing implies that in first-person awareness we recognize the demands of belief, and that those demands are for adequate reasons of the truth of what is believed.

So, 6. One believes that *p* in accord with the concept of belief only if one has adequate reasons that *p*.

So, 7. One ought to believe that *p* only if one has adequate reasons that *p*.

The reconstruction makes it plain that our argument does not move from an "is" (of the subjective principle) to an "ought" (of evidentialism). First, it simply could not move from an "is" to an "ought" (licit or illicit) because the premises are avowedly not purely factual and the main conclusion (6) is not a prescription or "ought" judgment. Premises (1) and (2) are not mere descriptive truths. They do not claim merely that we do, in fact, think of ourselves as having adequate reasons. Rather, they claim that we cannot (in full awareness) believe otherwise. The main conclusion of our argument (6) is a version of the primary form of evidentialism. It does not contain "ought" and it is not a directive to action. The prescription for action (7) is derivative, and even then, as observed earlier, it must be understood as subject to qualification and overriding by further "ought"s. Second, the subjective principle leads us to evidentialism only by way of exposing demands of the concept of belief. The concept of belief explains the modal character of the subjective principle. The subjective principle does not directly ground evidentialism; the concept of belief does that.

The epigram of this book provides an illustration of these interconnected claims. It comes from the *Apology,* when, during crossexamination, Socrates in exasperation censures his chief accuser: "You cannot be believed, Meletus, even, I think, by yourself" (Plato 1981: 26e). Meletus has charged Socrates with "corrupting the young and of not believing in the gods in whom the city believes, but in other new divinities" (Plato 1981: 24b). Socrates prods Meletus, in front of the jury, into admitting that one of the accusations is that of atheism: "you do not believe in the gods at all."

The unbelievability that Socrates ascribes to Meletus is on conceptual grounds. Attribution of incoherence to Meletus's beliefs follows on the beliefs he attributes to Socrates. Meletus ascribes to Socrates beliefs that contradict each other—that there are gods and that there are no gods. The impossibility of holding those beliefs reflects back on Meletus, denying believability in his own attribution to Socrates. The ascription is normative: Meletus is "guilty of dealing frivolously with serious matters" (Plato 1981: 24c). But the accusation is also descriptive. Once Meletus's commitments are brought to his attention, he cannot, and now does not, maintain them.[33]

2

Can One Will to Believe?

Traditionally, denials of evidentialism were a step toward assigning to the individual responsibility for his beliefs. It is not up to the evidence to decide what a person ought to believe; it is up to the person. The assignment was understood as implying *voluntarism*—the view that we can choose our beliefs. On extrinsic approaches, what is rational or desirable to believe can be believed as the outcome of a decision.

Recently, some who take an extrinsic approach have denied that belief is voluntary. They are moved by the way beliefs just arise in us automatically or habitually, without choice or act of will or intention. You turn your head and notice a collie emerging from an alley. You are compelled to believe that there is a collie emerging from that alley, without pause or room for deliberation or choice. The resulting extrinsic position seems, however, committed to the unhappy triad that the ethics of belief is governed by considerations of rationality; that, where terms of appraisal like "rationality" apply, voluntarism holds; and, yet, that voluntarism is false.

But my concern here is not whether recent views can extricate themselves from this bind, nor even with whether extrinsic approaches require voluntarism. Rather, my concern is whether voluntarism is true and whether it is implied by intrinsic approaches. The recent theorists who deny voluntarism are glad to ascribe it to evidentialism. For, as just indicated, their reasoning is that since evidentialism claims that one's beliefs ought to be based on evidence, it implies that epistemic or ethical appraisal of believing is possible and so presupposes voluntarism.

In chapter 1, we disarmed this argument by rejecting its major premise. The rudiments of the ethics of belief are conceptual. Its pivotal modal terms are "must," "cannot," or "can," not those of deontology: "ought," "obligatory," or "permissible." So even if ethical appraisal issues in "ought"s, which govern voluntary acts, evidentialism is not committed at its rudiments to treating belief as subject to our will.

Nevertheless, the issue of voluntarism is too central to the ethics of belief for our curiosity to be satisfied merely because no connection between evidentialism and voluntarism (let alone a connection of entailment) has been established. In examining whether there is a connection much depends on how voluntarism is understood. I will understand it as affirming that one can choose or control one's belief as one can choose or control one's raising of one's hand. Thus I deny voluntarism so understood. My main reason for this denial is the kind of incoherence that follows from overt violations of evidentialism. If evidentialism is consistent, far from implying voluntarism, it is incompatible with it (section 1). The denial of voluntarism does not, however, exclude *responsibility* for one's beliefs (section 2).

In section 3 of this chapter, I consider the related question of whether there can be weakness in belief on the model of weakness of will (in action), or *akrasia*. Although my negative response is again fated by prior commitments to evidentialism, I take the opportunity to observe some contrasts between the relation of reasons to belief and the relation of reasons to action, which bear on later discussions. The brevity of this chapter reflects that the positions taken—particularly, the denial of voluntarism and the denial of weakness of belief—follow largely from premises already introduced in chapter 1.

1   Voluntarism and Williams's Argument

Voluntarism is the view that we can control our beliefs, as we can raise our hands. The issue is not whether we can voluntarily influence or indirectly control our beliefs. It is undeniable that we can induce a belief by attending to one-sided sources, biasing ourselves toward a sought-for opinion. On the positive side, we can develop dispositions or habits to be open to contrary evidence or criticism, and to evaluate that evidence fairly.[1] The arguments of chapter 1 (and 3 below) imply that, in full awareness, we represent our belief-forming dispositions and habits as responsive to reasons for and against our beliefs. So there is a corresponding duty to develop these dispositions and habits. There is no dispute that this development is under our control and that we are responsible for it.

Discussions of whether we can decide to believe focus on the acquisition (or surrender) of particular beliefs, and I shall fall in line with those discussions. But the focus skews the data. For, in general, control over belief, as we control our imagination, is not something we would want or that would serve us well. By contrast, we would often want control over various biological functions for purposes of improved or more pleasurable functioning (e.g., hunger, sex). Of course, there are any number of individual cases in which we would want control of belief. We could lose unpleasant beliefs (that I am too short to be a good basketball player) and ones that just clutter our brain (that the phone number for a mattress company is 1-800-mattres), as well as gain desirable ones (that Mozart is alive and composing). Nevertheless, standing back from these particular cases, we recognize that with such control our beliefs would be a poorer guide to the world. Belief in this regard is more like love. In particular cases, we do want the control—we don't want to love someone who will be bad for us. Still, overall we recognize that the control would distort the point of our capacity for love. We want opportunity for spontaneous feelings and discoveries about ourselves. Our love should depend on who we are—warts and all—not on who we would like to be. So we wouldn't generally want the control, even if we could have it and even if we knew that with it, we could avoid serious mistakes. Given the enormous role of belief in guiding our actions, the parallel conclusion holds for belief and more forcefully: If belief is responsive to us it is responsive to the wrong object.[2] Although I do not offer these ruminations as independent argument for our opposition to belief at will, it speaks favorably of that opposition that it harmonizes with these negative conclusions about the desirability of the control overall.[3]

When we speak of the control of will over belief, we are speaking of *direct* control.[4] There are three (overlapping) features of this direct control, whose paradigm cases would be raising one's hand or imagining the Eiffel Tower (or imagining that the Eiffel Tower is in Central Park). First, and most obvious, we control what we do. We raise or lower our arm as a simple exercise of will. The belief follows, without mediation, as a result of the willing. Again, no indirect method is employed as it is in executing a plan to swallow a "pill" that yields the belief and induces forgetfulness that one took the pill. Second, the belief arises immediately, through *basic actions* (Danto 1968). To perform the act of typing the letter "c" I need to perform the prior act of moving my arm. But the latter act, the act of moving my arm, I perform as a basic act. I perform it without performing any prior act. If belief were subject to decision, then, on this construal of voluntarism, the connection between decision and belief would be like-wise, as unmediated as the connection between a decision to imagine (e.g., the Eiffel Tower) and the imagining. Third, the action we perform is a (causal) result of an intention to perform that action, as holds for raising one's hand or imagining that the Eiffel Tower is in Central Park. Although I would express my intention in these cases as simply that I intended to, e.g., raise my hand, the expression would be short-hand for "raising my hand as a result of this very intention" (Searle 1983: chap. 3).

This third condition is in keeping with the conceptual arguments of chapter 1. Indeed, the incoherence of the following covers a good part of the argument against believing at will:

Mork and Mindy are good friends, but I believe that because I choose to.

This thought is incoherent, as would be any instance of:

p, but I believe *p* because I choose to.

The incoherence that we take to block voluntarism is a version of Bernard Williams's crisp demonstration of the conceptual impossibility of believing at will. Williams's main argument is this:

> If I could acquire a belief at will, I could acquire it whether it was true or not; more-over I would know that I could acquire it whether it was true or not. If in full consciousness I could will to acquire a "belief" irrespective of its truth, it is unclear that before the event I could seriously think of it as a belief, i.e. as something purporting to represent reality. At the very least, there must be a restriction on what is the case after the event; since I could not then, in full consciousness, regard this as a belief of mine, i.e. something I take to be true, and also know that I acquired it at will. With regard to no belief could I know—or, if all this is to be done in full consciousness, even suspect—that I had acquired it at will. But if I can acquire beliefs at will, I must know that I am able to do this; and could I know that I was capable of this feat, if with regard to every feat of this kind which I had performed I necessarily had to believe that it had not taken place? (Williams 1973: 148)[5]

Williams's argument supposes that we can believe at will, for the purpose of showing that the assumption leads to a contradiction. Consequently, he rejects the supposition.

The heart of Williams's argument is that the exercise of will does not satisfy the claim to truth of belief. So the crucial premise is that it is not possible to regard oneself as holding a belief, while recognizing it as due to the exercise of the will.[6] Variants of this premise are obvious influences on the arguments in chapter 1. If, or to the extent that, believing at will involves a recognition of one's exercise of the will as the source of the belief, the conclusion is that it is not possible to believe at will.

The obvious reason to endorse Williams's conclusion, as well as the premise that implies it, is the most impressive. When we try to believe at will, we fail, and not from any mere inability. Our failure seems to mark a genuine inconceivability. Pick haphazardly an ordinary proposition such as "Plato would not like peanut butter," and attempt to believe it directly, just as a result of a decision. Also, randomly select among propositions that you do believe, and simply try to cease believing them. You cannot do either, and it would not help to imagine, in the former case, that you desire the belief, or in the latter case, that you are averse to it.

Reasonable voluntarists accept the failure. They allow that we cannot just believe that the Eiffel Tower is in Central Park or cease to believe that $2+3=5$. As I discuss in chapter 4, William James, that great enemy of evidentialism, allowed that choice is not possible in similar cases: "Can we, by just willing it, believe that Abraham Lincoln's existence is a myth . . . ?" (James 1951: 90). His implied answer is "no."

In considering these and similar cases, voluntarists are apt to *restrict* the scope of what is subject to a decision to believe. Not all contents are open for voluntary believing. Voluntarists can allow that it is not possible to knowingly believe, for example, a contradiction, let alone will it, and there are further restrictions of possibilities they can endorse (Raz 2000). More important, as with our discussion of the alleged rationally self-deceived wife in chapter 1, coming to believe or ceasing to believe in clear defiance of one's evidence needs to be accomplished nonconsciously. Indeed, this restriction is tacitly made in prominent criticisms of Williams's argument. The criticisms involve various ways that a belief at will could be surreptitiously induced.[7] So, for example, critics successfully deny Williams's inference from our not being able to know in each case that we acquired a belief at will to our not knowing that we had the ability at all. We could have that knowledge in other, more circuitous, ways, they object.

In sum, reasonable voluntarists admit that their view does not extend to much belief-formation. In particular, when beliefs arise or cease as the direct outcome of processes like perception or memory, our decisions can play no role (James 1951; Ginet 2001).

On my view, these restrictions are tied together and amount to wholesale concessions. I introduced the restrictions via the blunt cases where the will is powerless to form a belief (Homer is alive in Soho), surrender a belief (kangaroos can hop), or resist coming to a belief (there is a book in front of me). The lack of power seems to make sense only as a conceptual impossibility. It is not at all "up to me" that Mork and Mindy are good friends, so it is not up to me to believe that the statement that they are is true. Belief is not up to me the way raising my hand or imagining the Eiffel Tower is up to me, since the truth of what is believed is not up to me.[8]

Voluntarists must assume, by contrast, that these decisive cases are explanatorily *basic.* The indisputability of what the evidence indicates satisfactorily explains why belief is compelled. They then advance the conclusion that where the evidence is not decisive, voluntary belief is possible. This is clearly James's view, and it seems to be that of Carl Ginet as well: "it is psychologically possible . . . for a subject to come to believe something just by deciding to believe it, where the subject has it open to her also to not come to believe it" (2001: 74). I, of course, reject the view that the commanding nature of the evidence in these cases is explanatorily basic. A deeper explanation is needed and available in terms of the concept of belief.

In chapter 1 I observed that cases that appear to support a lax ethics of belief are those in which the evidence for a proposition is inconclusive. A gap is thought to open for the will to generate a judgment (a belief).[9] But the claim of a gap where the evidence is inconclusive seems plausible only when we attend to the derivation, not the epistemic position in regard to the belief. Where the epistemic position is one in which the evidence only partially supports the conclusion, then, correspondingly, we cannot fully, but only partially, believe. Nevertheless, for the sake of argument let us revisit the cases where the evidence is not decisive.

Consider the phenomena of "making up one's mind."[10] There is strong evidence, let's posit, that my friend Irene lost a book that I lent her, but I hesitate to judge that she did. The ambivalence weighs on my mind, and finally, with no further evidence, I judge that she did—my mind is made up and I made it up. We may imagine, as furthering the voluntarist challenge, that I am recognizably drawn to so making up my mind because I am angry about the missing book, and if I do not blame Irene, it is likely that my anger will not find a suitable outlet. Can we not correctly describe this as a case of deciding to believe?

The example does capture a familiar phenomenon. We sometimes need to make up our minds, and that can be a voluntary act (judgment). Were believing at will possible, it should be a familiar phenomenon, since it is not credible that we do or could really have this ability, but that so far we have not discovered or implemented it.

With qualifications to come, I admit that to judge all-out that Irene lost my book is to satisfy the conditions for believing that she did, a claim in line with the conclusions given in chapter 1. So there is an act under my control—namely, judging true—that issues in full belief. (This conclusion preserves the symmetry with ceasing to believe. Recall that if I judge that there is undermining evidence—such as a conflicting observation—of something I believe, I thereby cease to hold that belief.)

But we should remain suspicious as to whether making up one's mind and related phenomena amount to deciding to believe, though that may be how we describe them. The data is equivocal. First, since to judge that inquiry should successfully end issues in belief, ending inquiry and believing are very closely associated. The judgment that inquiry should close, at least for complex inquiries, is voluntary and often highly indeterminate, not susceptible to rule or algorithm. Correspondingly, different investigators will, unsurprisingly, end the same complex inquiry at different times. Second, when the evidence is positive, but indecisive, and there is a lack of clean and accessible conditions of falsification, the seeming decision to believe may actually be only a decision to induce belief. Imagine in the lost book case that there is a new system that can remotely track "zebra" codings (a "lojack" system for books). Knowing that the system will kick in within twelve hours, I now find it much more difficult to just make up my mind that Irene lost my book. In the original case, where I will probably never know definitively whether Irene lost it or not, my seeming decision to believe may simply exploit my personal knowledge of how easy it is to influence my beliefs surreptitiously. I am not deciding to believe; rather, I am deciding to place myself in a position where I will come to believe.

Voluntarists may be puzzled by the form that my criticism has taken—ruling out cases here and there hardly makes sense when all that they take themselves to need is a single case of voluntary belief. However, this response fails to appreciate the real purpose in my challenges to the data that voluntarists offer. The purpose is to clear away cases that foster an illusion that obscures the conceptual argument earlier invoked, and that does claim to cover all the cases.

However, along these lines lurks a difficulty for the conceptual argument. What is the status of Williams's assumed premise that "I would know that I could acquire it [the belief I decided to believe] whether it was true or not"? What if a believer just holds the false view that where the evidence is fairly supportive, but still indecisive, it is in our discretion as to whether to believe or not? Couldn't that person simply will to believe in overt recognition of the inadequacy of his evidence? If I answer "yes," then I seem to have backed into the bizarre position that one cannot will to believe, unless one holds the false view that one can. The better answer is that the ignorance or error posited is not really possible, although one can readily be distracted from recognizing one's knowledge. The key support for this answer follows from the conceptual argument: The resulting belief would be *unstable.*

Previously, I claimed that full belief requires competence with certain rudimentary epistemic discriminations. A believer must have at least a rough grasp of the distinction between epistemic and nonepistemic reasons. In particular, he must see his own desires and decisions as generally fitting in the latter category. For they are always with him. He believes that he is under 6′ tall, but he desires to be taller. He does not believe that there is life on Mars, but he desires it. The value of one's system of belief as a guide to action would dissipate unless one is generally unresponsive to one's own desires and interests as a basis for belief. Any healthy believer knows that the belief that p depends on what p is about, not on himself (or his desires).

Still, the grasp can be obscured in particular cases. But then belief will be unstable—the underlying incoherence is only temporarily held off. The nature of the instability is illuminated in Daniel Dennett's reflections on "brain writing": "Let us suppose we are going to insert in Tom the false belief: 'I have an older brother living in Cleveland'" (Dennett 1978: 44). Dennett goes on to observe that when Tom is asked simple questions like what is his brother's name, he will find himself having to give the bizarre answer that he does not know. Thus the instability. Notice that even if Tom is not asked by others, if he merely attends to the belief, such simple questions will immediately occur to him. The integration of a belief with neighboring ones normally arises just with awareness of its content. Dennett thinks that the result of this exercise poses a major, but not an insuperable, barrier: "This does not show that wiring in beliefs is impossible, or that brain writing is impossible, but just that one could only wire in one belief by wiring in many (indefinitely many?) other cohering beliefs so that neither biographical nor logical coherence would be lost" (1978: 44). But if we wire in many other cohering beliefs, we generate more possibilities for conflict with other beliefs and related actions. If we brain-write in a name, address, and phone number for Tom's brother, what is going to happen when Tom engages in the ordinary act of trying to contact his brother? "Brain-writing" seems viable only for isolated, inconsequential beliefs, like the memory of an unimportant historical date or beliefs that will guide action without being forced to consciousness. These restrictions are severe, and, once again, attest to the conceptual connection of belief, truth, and evidence.

With this clarification on the nature of the instability as a natural extension of Williams's argument, let us return to the cases where the evidence is indecisive—cases that are the life-blood for the reasonable voluntarist. Once again William James concedes to us, however unintentionally, that these cases are not really so special. Besides conceding that in many cases we cannot just will to believe, James also restricts the candidates available for willing to believe to those that "*cannot* by . . . [their] nature be decided on intellectual grounds" (1951: 95, my emphasis). Thus James mentions only two classes of cases to which he extends his blessing for voluntary belief, morals and religion.

However, our reasonable voluntarist wanted the blessing to extend much further. He wanted it to apply not only to the cases where evidence cannot decide a matter, but to many of those cases, like that of Irene, where current evidence does not decide it, though further evidence might. In viewing these cases as open for us to believe or not, the voluntarist, again, posits a gap where the will must intrude (lest we be deprived of many ordinary beliefs). But in so doing he is ignoring our knowledge that the indecisiveness is a passing limitation. Undoubtedly if theorists can ignore this knowledge, so too can individuals. But here the instability problem lurks. If I know that I will learn decisively within twelve hours whether Irene lost my book, it no longer seems open for me to just make a decision. That is one way of getting at the instability: "Irene lost my book, although in twelve hours I may learn otherwise."

The direct conceptual argument and the argument from instability are convergent because they are both developments of Williams's crucial premise that one could not recognize the result of an exercise of will as a belief. This crucial premise does not, however, carry the whole burden of argument for Williams. Williams's argument is meant to show that believing at will, even in the absence of full consciousness, is impossible. But to the extent that we need to be unaware of or hide from ourselves, or hide from what we are doing, to that extent we weaken the value of control. Though you may still be able to accomplish the same ends—believe the same contents—with these indirect means, your success will be more dependent on resources outside your will. So the real heart of Williams's argument resides in its crucial premise, which implies that the proposal of voluntary belief violates the concept of belief. That is why it cannot be accomplished in full awareness that one is acting on that proposal.

2   Nonvoluntarism Does Not Imply Nonresponsibility

Nonvoluntarism is generally taken to rule out responsibility, since one is not responsible for what one does not control.[11] But the "since" clause is dubious. Happiness is not subject to one's decision—it is not up to you whether or not you are happy. But you are still responsible for your happiness. After all, who else could be? It is not merely that you are responsible for the efforts to make yourself happy or to believe correctly. What determines your happiness or your beliefs, luck aside, is your doing.[12]

The nonresponsibility view is incompatible with our ordinary judgments. We blame people who believe that whales are fish, that some UFOs are alien spaceships paying regular visits to earth, that a neighbor littered the sidewalk when she did not. Although the blame is attached only when these beliefs are visible or acted on, the blame is for the belief itself. We think it blameworthy for people to hold such beliefs, given the available evidence. We excuse beliefs in ways that imply the appropriateness of ascribing responsibility. If, to repeat an earlier example, a young woman believes herself overweight when she is noticeably thin, she is excused because of her mental imbalance (anorexia nervosa). The excusing force is not limited to the way she acts (by practically starving herself). It must extend to the believing itself, since it is the belief that guides her action.

In regard to the example in the previous section, if someone says to me that "You should not believe that Irene took your book," they are ascribing responsibility to me. However, this example may be thought to back-fire, since it is credible, though contentious, to hold that I am responsible for an act only if I could have done otherwise. But if I could do otherwise, then I must have control over my belief, contrary to the conclusions of the previous section.

Aside from the contentious assumption that responsibility requires that one could have done otherwise, these examples are subject to the equivo-cation considered in the previous section. The blame equivocates between applying just to belief and to the hastiness with which inquiry is ended. Thus, if I responded to the accusation by insisting that my evidence did show that Irene took the book, the accuser would likely respond some-thing like "I am not claiming that you should not believe it, given how you construe your evidence. I am saying that you should not have so construed your evidence."

We think of ourselves as responsible for who we are, for our character or personality (Taylor 1982). We are bound to think this way, since these are the sources of the acts that we take ourselves to perform freely and respon-sibly. Yet, it is a deep puzzle how we can be responsible for our characters or personalities, if that requires, as it appears to, that we select our charac-ter or personality in a deliberative act. (How could the selector be me?)

A ground rule for addressing the issue of responsibility for beliefs is that we may avail ourselves of whatever assumptions are necessary for free will and responsibility generally. Consequently, we can presuppose that we are responsible for the selves that we are, even though we cannot truly select the selves that we are. By parity, we should not exclude the possibility of responsibility for our beliefs merely because we do not select them. The comparison is closer than so far suggested, since the kind of person one is is in good part a matter of what one believes.

In a recent article, Robert Adams (1985) argues for our responsibility for nonvoluntary states of mind. Adams excludes from his account of re-sponsibility simple responses (e.g., thirst), but also certain talents (e.g., musical). Adams writes: "among states of mind that have intentional ob-jects, the ones for which we are directly responsible are those in which we are responding, consciously or unconsciously, to data that are rich enough to permit a fairly adequate ethical appreciation of the state's intentional object and of the object's place in the fabric of personal relationships." For Adams, if we feel wrongful anger or resentment toward someone, we are to blame for those feelings.[13] Adams rejects the view that blame implies that one could have done otherwise. To Adams, "it seems strange to say that I do not blame someone though I think poorly of him, believing that his motives are thoroughly selfish. Intuitively I should have said that thinking poorly of a person in this way *is* a form of unspoken blame" (1985: 21). Adams allows that it is not right to punish for such states but notes there are other forms of censure, for example, reproach, in blaming someone.[14]

By restricting his claims to mental states that respond to "rich" data, Adams weakens the driving intuition of those who infer nonresponsibility from nonvoluntariness. The inference treats our voice in belief-formation as analogous to our voice in pancreatic function. The comparison is starkly ill suited, since the autonomic functions are not reachable (or penetrable) by the higher cognitive powers of the mind, strikingly unlike the nature of belief. Moreover, for many of our beliefs we do have the ability to influence and shape the dispositions underlying their acceptance. If you are quick to ascribe ill motives to others, you have probably had many occasions to discern and evaluate this pattern of your attributions and you can undertake to control them accordingly. The modification does not require direct control over your believing.

Even if one cannot choose to believe otherwise, beliefs are capable of *responsivity to reasons,* and that is crucial for responsibility. A person is responsible for an act when, roughly, if there were reasons to act otherwise, he could appreciate and respond to them.[15] Thus, assume that Jones does his laundry because his shirts are dirty. But had he been told that his money was running out on the parking meter, he could appreciate the latter reasons and act appropriately (delay doing his laundry). Jones's belief that he should now do his laundry gives way, and on a reasoned basis, to the belief that he should now put money in the meter.

Responsivity to reasons is presupposed in such ordinary and pervasive activities as conversing and arguing with one another.[16] If the speaker offers the hearer a reason to believe that p, the speaker expects that the hearer can appreciate and be moved by it. The credibility of p will then be raised for the hearer, unless he has grounds to object. If so, he will present them to the speaker, expecting him to respond in turn. Reason responsiveness in belief is a mutual expectation of conversation and argument, and so, too, is responsibility for our beliefs.

More fundamentally, in conversation our assertions are presentations of what we endorse. So we are responsible to others for their being true. But, as well, our assertions express our beliefs, and in asserting them we are essentially aware of them as our endorsements. In chapter 1, I noted that a similar awareness is the entry point for understanding the concept of belief. Admittedly, the awareness of the belief as what we believe is not under our control as is our asserting (or what we assert); and there is no possibility in belief that parallels the wide difference between an awareness of what one thinks to assert and the actual asserting of it.[17] Still, much of our awareness of our beliefs is not simply what just "pops" up to us, but a result of our directing our mind and activities. If we maintain a belief on becoming aware of it, we enter a claim to truth on ourselves. Effectively, we assert the belief to ourselves, and so incur responsibilities that parallel those we incur when we assert our beliefs to others.

3   The Possibility of Weakness of Will for Belief

Up to a point, the comparison of responsiveness to reasons for belief with responsiveness to reasons for action works. But it stops working at the endpoint of belief and action. Responsiveness to reasons is all we want for freedom and responsibility in belief, but not so for action. We have free will not to act on our preferred option. But the failure to act on one's judged best reasons (weakness of will or *akrasia*) has no parallel in belief, since we cannot in full awareness believe against our best judgment on the evidence. So there is no parallel possibility for belief as there is for action.

Actually, "weakness of will" is used to pick out several phenomena. Throughout most of this section, I shall be concerned only with strict weakness of will, acting against one's best judgment. One judges that it is worse to eat a brownie ice cream sundae than to refrain; yet one deliberately eats it anyhow.

Another phenomenon that is also referred to as "weakness of will" is a failure to follow through on one's intentions or plans (Holton 1999). I intend to mow the lawn, but instead just stretch out my breakfast and read the newspaper on the porch. We carry out an intention when the content of that intention plays a causally efficacious role in bringing about the action.[18] There is no analogue for believing, and this sharp disanalogy foreshadows a negative conclusion for weakness of believing construed strictly. We hardly use the phrase "intend to believe." Believing is not the outcome of carrying out an intention, since I cannot take the content of that intention to cause the belief, and so I cannot act to fulfill that intention.

Strict weakness of will is more puzzling than the other phenomena, and it dominates philosophical discussion. The puzzle is this: If one acts for a reason, then one acts for one's best reason, if one can choose freely. But in weakness of will one acts—deliberately—for an inferior reason. But how can this be? Why would one act deliberately for an inferior reason?

If this does not sound puzzling, notice how tempting it is to redescribe the earlier example of the ice cream sundae as follows: Although the person had judged that eating the sundae is worse, at the moment of action, he was overcome by anticipation of the sweet taste. He altered his judgment with hardly any notice, so that the eating came to be preferred to the refraining. So he deliberately ate it. This redescription fits in with a common way in which we are tempted away from rational action—immediate goods or benefits are disproportionately favored over those that require a delay before receipt (Ainslie 1985). But once we offer this redescription we are no longer dealing with weakness of will, strictly construed.[19] What makes something a case of weakness of will is that the agent acts against his best judgment.

Cases of strict weakness of will are tempting to redescribe in this way because they are not rational according to the agent's own judgment, yet he acts deliberately. But if weakness of will is possible, its lack of rationality is not a lack of *motivational intelligibility*. We can all make sense of the anticipation of the pleasure of eating the sundae overwhelming, without reversing, good judgment. The nearer reward is overvalued, even given equal certainty of outcomes.

In his ingenious "How Is Weakness of Will Possible?" Donald Davidson (1982) attempts to answer his title question without whitewashing any of the puzzling elements of weakness of will—deliberate action that is clearly against one's better judgment, yet which is motivationally intelligible. His account has been explicitly invoked as a model for weakness of belief (Heil 1984). Without addressing this application directly, I will explain why I doubt that the model can carry over to belief.

Davidson's presentation draws heavily on an analogy between practical reasoning (to action) and theoretical reasoning (to belief). However, in a crucial respect, I find the analogy misleading, and, when the matter is cleared up, putative cases of weakness of belief seem unable to preserve motivational intelligibility.

For Davidson, one determines, in deliberation, the best course of action "all things considered." The rational agent will form an all-out or detached judgment to act, corresponding to his all-things-considered assessment. However, in cases of weakness of will, Davidson argues, the all-out judgment does not correspond to the all-things-considered judgment of what it is best to do. To judge, all things considered, that doing *A* is better than doing *B* is consistent with an out-and-out judgment that *B* is better than *A* (a judgment "detached" from its all-things-considered evaluative grounding). The weak-willed person then does *B*.

Theoretical reasoning is likened to practical reasoning because the former seeks to determine which hypothesis is best supported by the available evidence.[20] The analogy implies that, just as the objective of practical reasoning is to discover which option is best all things considered, the objective of theoretical reasoning is to discover which hypothesis is best supported on the total available evidence. It is this implication that is misleading. For the objective of theoretical or empirical reasoning is determining whether a hypothesis is true, not whether it is best supported. Knowing that one's evidence is the total available and favorable is insufficient for accepting the hypothesis as true. The unconditional or detached assignment of a degree of belief is not truly the endpoint of cognitive inquiry. If we do not judge this evidence adequate, doubt is not yet resolved. What it is best to do is what is better than all the alternatives on the available reasons. But what it is best to believe is only what is genuinely worthy of belief, not what is currently better than the alternatives. There is no warrant for moving from any comparative judgment alone to the corresponding full belief. But it is full belief that is the goal of our epistemic reasoning, even if we often have to settle for less. (More on this theme in chap. 9.) Once we realize this break in the analogy, the motivational problem surfaces rapidly. Since the final judgments Davidson draws are comparative ones, conflicting reasons, like conflicting desires, can retain their force. Thus it is coherent to think of a dispreferred reason (a desire) as still exercising a pull away from doing what one judges best. But when the judgment is of the truth of a proposition, as with full belief, all reasons are thereby comprehended. No opposing pull remains.

It is helpful for clarifying this conclusion to follow Williams (1973, "Ethical Consistency") in contrasting conflicts between beliefs with conflicts between desires. When beliefs conflict, they weaken one another, since both cannot be correct. When one belief is favored by the evidence, the disfavored belief evaporates, since it has been determined not to be true. But when desires conflict, as with desires to pursue careers both in medicine and ballet, the conflict does not itself weaken either. When one is acted on, the other retains a hold, experienced as regret.

Extend the contrast to reasons. Informally, desires are standard reasons to act. A desire disfavored or overridden in determining action does not then evaporate, but retains motivational force. But the evidence that initially favors a belief, if subsequently undermined, is just nullified as mistaken or misleading. If the initial evidence at the scene of a crime is a scarf, which resembles one that the butler wore, then that evidence, let's say, favors the butler's guilt. But if we subsequently discover that the butler was out of town at the time of the crime, the scarf exercises no further pull on us, even if we cannot discover what it was doing there.

In the absence of any epistemic pull, contrary to one's best judgment, weakness of belief lacks motivational intelligibility. But the lasting pull of disfavored reasons to act—desires—can secure motivational intelligibility for weakness of will. Thus the Davidsonian model of weakness of will is not transferrable to weakness of belief.

4   More Extreme Cases

The main conclusion of the previous section did not rest on the imposition of a full awareness condition. The disanalogy turns, rather, on a discrepancy between the goals of practical and theoretical reasoning. The imposition of a full awareness condition is problematic here because weakness of will (and belief, were it possible) does seem to involve some lack of connection among, or transparency of, the contents of the mind. To assume full awareness in the case of practical reasoning would be to assume away the phenomena. Without that condition, we can admit cases close to incontinent belief without threat to our main argument.

We can be distracted from our relevant reasons. Finding Cynthia strikingly attractive distracts me from my knowledge that she is very disorganized, and I proceed to judge (believe) that it would be good for her to become treasurer for my company. Still, this distraction is more extreme than in weakness of will. One can act on a disfavored reason, such as a craving for a hot fudge sundae, even while acknowledging that it is disfavored.

More extreme cases of being moved by hidden reasons correspondingly break the analogy with akrasia more sharply. Depth psychology offers cases in which a patient intellectually appreciates her plight, but that appreciation does not penetrate to alter belief, for example, in compulsive handwashing or anorexia.[21] The description of these cases that we are assuming is that the person all-out judges that, for example, his hands are dirty and yet fully believes that they are clean. The alternative description is that as these thoughts come together in awareness, they clash and cannot both be sustained. The person may avow the judgment, but it does not have its normal consequence of issuing in a genuine belief. The anorexic avows that she is not overweight, given the evidence, but she does not fully endorse that assessment.[22] The compulsive may go ahead and wash his hands, but the action is not fully deliberate. What looks like the sustaining of both judgment and belief may only be vacillation between them in and out of the subject's awareness, and we conflate different moments in describing them as a single moment in which both are sustained.

By their extreme nature, these cases differ from garden-variety weakness of will. Weakness of will is merely loss of control by reason, not a breakdown in mental health. It is a common and expected phenomenon, given conflicting pulls in our mental life and our limited understanding and control of it.

Even when confronted with these extreme cases, however, we needn't reconsider the conceptual connection between belief and reasons that we have posited. One cannot think "I have adequate reasons that *p* is true, but I refuse to believe it." (Or worse, "I believe it false.")[23] Even in less extreme cases, if someone affirms something akin to "I know that the evidence against cousin Betty is overwhelming, but I still do not believe that she did not recycle that empty can," the straightforward reading does not correspond to the actual attitude. By affirming the latter conjunct, the speaker hints at suspicions as to the quality of his evidence. The speaker is entertaining the possibility (and hope) that further evidence will be exonerating. He is having second thoughts—drawing back from the first part of his assertion ("I know that . . .").

Earlier, I noted that sometimes "weakness of will" is used in a less problematic way than to pick out actions that are strictly against one's better judgment. Traditionally, an important use is to refer to a failure to judge in accord with principle or reason. The brownie sundae is bad overall for reasons of health, but judgment favors the pleasing taste, and now action gladly follows judgment. There is no disparity here between what one judges all-out best and what one does. For this type of weakness of will, a parallel weakness is possible for belief. It is a close analogue of the (Platonic) failure of reason to exercise due control over the force of pleasure.[24] In chapter 11, the possibility of this kind of weakness of belief is defended. However, the imposition of the analogous self-control is laced with perplexities. The control is supposed to apply to one's beliefs, suggesting a weakness or fault in one of them; yet, for the analogy to work, each of them must be regarded as well founded.

3

Normative Epistemology: The Deceptively Large Scope of the Incoherence Test

1 Objection: Intrinsic Ethics of Belief Is Too Weak

The fundamental claim of this chapter is that a wide range of beliefs formed or maintained by distortive processes fails the incoherence test discussed in chapter 1. This claim might be thought dubious because the operation of that test assumes that the believer recognizes his own problematic position, whereas when people form or maintain beliefs illicitly, they rarely recognize themselves as doing so. Quite the contrary, as suggested by the subjective principle of sufficient reasons itself. The fact that one cannot *regard* oneself as believing *p* without adequate reasons does not entail that one does not do so. Rather, one may regard one's reasons as adequate even though the reasons are in fact inadequate.

My reply is that incoherences may exist, even though the believer does not recognize them, most prominently through *self-deception* and its kin. This reply is crucial to defusing many of the apparent counterexamples to the repeated claims in chapter 1 to the effect that certain purported beliefs cannot be believed because they generate incoherences in first-personal thought. The manifest problem for my claim is that much that cannot be believed is actually believed, which is a contradiction. The way to respond, in accord with arguments in chapter 1, is to ask what would follow if the person became fully aware of his belief and his epistemic position. If the epistemic position is recognized as inadequate for the truth of the belief, there is incoherence. Correlatively, as full awareness is blocked or diminished, it becomes easier for a person to believe what is unbelievable. The incoherent thought behind so egregious a belief as that the number of stars is even we found to be quite complex. It is unsurprising, then, that we readily overlook analogous incoherences in less egregious cases, where no flag goes up signaling a blatant lack of credibility. The result is that the incoherence test has much wider scope than it appears.

As just observed, the most prominent way in which we obscure to ourselves unwanted beliefs is through self-deception. However, I shall argue that self-deception always grates against reason; and that in many of the standard cases that are supposed to show the rationality of self-deception, their purported rationality dissipates on closer inspection. The classification of self-deception as a form of motivated irrationality is exactly right.

In fact, circumvention of the constraints imposed by the truth claim of belief does not require the sophisticated mechanisms of self-deception. Everyday ignorance, confusion, and especially *distraction* are often enough. Distraction is also enough to evade the simple but far-reaching, positive recommendation for believing that I advocate below. That recommendation is just to be *explicit* about one's beliefs and reasons.

The recommendation reduces disappointment with this chapter's strategy for extending the incoherence test. The extension holds only under full awareness. But now the critics, who cast the original doubt as to the force of the incoherence test, may reformulate their objection as follows:

OK, many distorted beliefs are maintained by hiding an underlying incoherence, and that shows that the conceptual defense of evidentialism has further application than it appears to have. But still the test is of little use in actually exposing distortions, since the condition of full awareness is difficult to impose. Even when it seems to be imposed, the person whose belief is distorted, may report that he has applied the test and passed it, when he has not.

This objection asks too much. If believing can be readily distorted, and if the distortion violates the believer's own claims, then, it should be difficult to expose.

Once we separate the question of whether an incoherence is present and the question of whether we have good grounds for attributing it, a limited practical value can still be found in our extension of the incoherence test. If incoherence does underlie a distorted belief, it must be that the distortion violates commitments of typical believers. So, explicitness about those claims and commitments is a device to expose the distortion.

But this practical value is limited. However sure an observer is as to the nature of another's distorted belief, it is difficult for the observer to guide that person to a recognition of it. Even sincerely avowed recognition need not suffice to eliminate the distortion.

2 The Inherent Irrationality of Self-Deception

To deceive oneself is to induce oneself to believe a proposition as a means of hiding or of obscuring an incompatible belief.[1] That is a very rough statement, but good enough for our purposes of refuting claims that no a priori judgment can be made as to the rationality of self-deception—it depends on the circumstances. Since what is hidden or obscured is what the agent regards as the truth, the intrinsic ethics of belief implies an inherent irrationality to self-deception, even if it is readily overridden in light of the agent's whole range of needs and interests.

Realistically, of course, we have numerous interests besides truth. We will not sacrifice all else for a smidgen of more evidence or greater certainty. But we should not be content with the latitude that this truism affords. The strength of the intrinsic ethics of belief as a critical tool is actually exhibited in our resistance to self-deception and in our reluctance to avail ourselves of its manifest benefits, in all but the most innocuous of cases.

As the truism says, however, truth is only one among many of our interests. If a contest offers a prize of $10 for guessing the number of jelly beans in a large transparent jar, you might spend two minutes trying to estimate the number. If the prize is $1,000,000, you will spend much, much longer. Yet, in both cases you are interested in being right. In the second scenario, however, the benefits of being right are significantly greater. Accordingly, you are willing to forgo more of your other interests, such as the social pleasures of a long lunch with friends. In an attempt to win the much greater prize, you are willing to invest more of your time and resources. The additional investment amounts to imposing on yourself higher standards (of sureness or certainty).[2] Similarly, if a drug risks only a stomachache, then the safety tests that it is subjected to are far less extensive than if the risk is death. In general, when the rewards, benefits, or risks diminish, standards diminish in turn. Being right matters less. From these unremarkable observations, a worrisome line of thought concludes that truth is not a dominant motive when potential gains or losses are not severe.

Although truth may be one interest of ours among others, only it constitutes the claim of belief. When these other interests determine or influence belief, one believes wrongfully, as is shown by one's conceptual inability to openly admit their role in belief formation. But the converse is not true. Beliefs based on what fulfills the claim of truth (namely, evidence) can be openly believed, even if the belief is undesired.

The problem that Descartes presents as inspiring his *Meditations* could hardly be posed for any attitude other than belief. He writes, "Some years ago I was struck by the large number of falsehoods that I had accepted as true in my childhood, and by the highly doubtful nature of the whole edifice that I had subsequently based on them" (1996: 12). Among our attitudes, only belief ("accepted as true") could spark the Cartesian inquiry. It is an unremarkable condition on any normal life that many of our hopes, guesses, thoughts, desires, and wants will be frustrated or mistaken. Even for many desires that are achievable and whose value is great, like winning a lottery, loss is accepted with equanimity. If we restrict ourselves to desires that we actively pursue, failure is often hardly a source of concern. We want to go to an entertaining movie, but the movie we go to isn't. That's life. But Descartes's problem does grab us. The failures that concern Descartes are serious, and a source of reproach.

The problem should not be dismissed by casual admissions of our fallibility. Our beliefs are by and large correct only if their sources are reliable. The sources of our vast, routinely formed beliefs are few—perception, testimony, reasoning, memory. Error in some beliefs suggests defects or flaws in their corresponding sources and thus the potential for a dangerous spreading effect. Descartes expresses this danger, while overstating it (as he immediately acknowledged): "Whatever I have up till now accepted as most true I have acquired either from the senses or through the senses. But from time to time I have found that the senses deceive, and it is prudent never to trust completely those who have deceived us even once" (1996: 12). So although many of the beliefs that we passively acquire in droves are matters of complete indifference, for example, that my neighbor's tie is blue, their falsity cannot be regarded with equal indifference. If the belief is based on viewing my neighbor's tie in good lighting conditions and from close by, and nevertheless I discover that it is false, the discovery poses a problem for my reliance on my perceptual faculties.

A rewarding thought experiment shows that Descartes's problem is also not solved if we retreat from believing to thinking that one believes. Robert Nozick asks us to imagine the possibility of a machine—the "experience machine"—allowing anyone hooked up to it to endlessly dream a life that goes as well as desired (Nozick 1974: 42–45; similarly, Blanshard 1974: 421–422). Since the dreamer is not permitted to withdraw from the machine once he is attached, he does not recognize himself as dreaming. So he accepts his dream as real. Despite its design to yield maximally pleasurable experiences, Nozick rightly conjectures that we resist entering the scenario because of its utter lack of reality. The thought experiment implies a similar conclusion about belief. It is not enough that the world appear to us to match our beliefs, which the machine could accomplish. What we want is that there really be a match.

Truth or knowledge as the aim of belief fulfills the function of reason. In an important article (to be discussed further in chap. 5), Tyler Burge writes: "Reason necessarily has a teleological aspect, which can be understood through reflection on rational practice. . . . One of reason's primary functions is that of presenting truth, independently of special personal interests. . . . The Humean reply that reason functions *only* to serve individual passions or interests is unconvincing. Reason has a function in providing guidance to truth, in presenting and promoting truth without regard to individual interest. This is why epistemic reasons are not relativized to a person or to a desire" (1993: 475; see also Velleman 1989: 44–45). If reason seeks truth, then it is not to be identified with an instrumental reason that acts only by calculating from factual input what means are best to realize various purposes or ends that are simply given to it. On this view, reason has no concern with determining ends or purposes.[3] The Humean picture fits badly with how much we are moved by intellectual curiosity and wonder. In ordinary conversation, when we are told of anything unexpected, we ask "why?" As shown by ancient art and religion, our ancestors asked why at a very abstract level, and they asked it about matters far detached from biological drives or practical needs.[4]

We care about the truth of our beliefs intrinsically, but, more obviously, extrinsically.[5] Beliefs guide our actions, and the truth of our beliefs typically explains the success of actions they inspire.[6] F. P. Ramsey puts forward the idea that "A belief . . . is a map of neighboring space by which we steer" (Ramsey 1978b: 134; see also Armstrong 1973: part I, esp. chap. 1. Ramsey's idea is divisible: A belief is informational [a map], and we endorse or project it [as a guide]). You want a Ben and Jerry's hot fudge sundae and believe that there is a Ben and Jerry's shop two blocks east. If the belief is true and you appreciate its connection to your goal, you will form a plan to go there. Acting on the plan, you will fulfill the desire. If the belief were false in the most usual ways (e.g., the shop is located elsewhere), the plan would fail.

Self-deception and its kin appear to argue against a deep concern with truth whether extrinsic or intrinsic. The studies in psychology discussed earlier suggest that these phenomena are very common (Nisbett and Wilson 1977). In these studies, subjects comment confidently on the origins of beliefs formed in experimental settings without real access to these origins. But the studies do not show that we constantly confabulate reasons to back erroneous judgments. The studies do not cast doubt on our accuracy about an enormous number of very obvious judgments (Nisbett and Ross 1980: 211; Dennett 1987: 52). "Why did you buy that new pair of stockings?" "I ripped my last pair." We do not need introspective access to our belief-formation processes to make such judgments with accuracy and confidence.[7]

These studies also do not offer paradigm cases of self-deception, because subjects' erroneous judgments are neither the product of ego-defensive ("hot") motivation nor do they play an active role in action, where learning through feedback is available. (I return to this limitation in section 7 below.) By contrast, consider a garden-variety example of self-deception. A father deceives himself, let us assume, that his daughter's poor grades are due to the teachers' misunderstanding and resentment of her offbeat brilliance. But the tale loses realism unless the father still acts in ways that indicate that the deceit is not wholehearted. He hires tutors for his daughter, checks her homework more carefully, and disciplines her studies more vigorously. (A similar conjecture applies to the example of the wife who seeks to obscure to herself evidence of her husband's infidelity. Does she really not even check more carefully whether, for example, their bank accounts have been drained?) Typically, when a self-deceptive belief guides action, its rationality diminishes for the subject with his extended reliance on it. Perfect self-deception, where one completely loses the uncomfortable belief (as a consequence of the self-deceptive project), is then rarely optimal self-deception (the condition that best realizes the goal that motivates the agent's self-deceptive project).

This diminishing rationality is a consequence of the inherent irrationality in wanting to believe falsely.[8] What one really wants is not just to have the belief in question, but that its content be true. The father wants his daughter to be brilliant, not merely that he have that placebo belief. Even while the father is pulled to hide from himself his daughter's failure, we expect an opposed pull from the belief that he hides from himself.

The nature of the wrongness in self-deception is illuminated, if overstated, in Kantian terms. Self-regarding duties are a crucial test of a Kantian ethics, for in self-regarding behavior, we seem to have no problem with autonomy or consent (as we do with, say, lying). Kant's claim, however, is that as rational beings we have an intrinsic value that ought not be violated even by ourselves. An "inner lie" is for Kant worse than an "external" lie because the man who lies to himself "makes himself contemptible in his own eyes and violates the dignity of humanity in his own person" (Kant 1991: 225 [429]). Effectively, we cannot consent to our own project of self-deception. This moral criticism of self-deception appears to be sanctimonious overkill for behavior so ordinary, often inconsequential, and typically not guided by evil intentions. I try to build up confidence for a tennis match by concentrating on the games I won against an opponent, while diverting attention from my losses, knowing that the outcome will be a biased belief. Surely, this is morally harmless, if a moral matter at all, an analogue of "white lies."

Four considerations mitigate the moral charge against such ordinary cases of benign self-deception. First, there will always be cases in which the wrong in two acts is the same even though the costs and consequences are widely disparate (e.g., taking home stationery from the office for personal use versus pickpocketing). The blame is thought of as arising from our intentions, as the locus of our control. Intentions can be relevantly the same, even when the costs and expected consequences are quite different. Second, to judge an act wrong is not thereby to ascribe a correlative flaw in the agent's moral character. Everyday wrongful acts, like wearing fur coats or cheating on taxes or speeding, are minor marks against character in large part because they are widely practiced and socially tolerated. Third, the extent to which it is worth exposing or admonishing an act of self-deception is not settled by its being inherently wrong. We are tolerant of failings due to normal human frailties, where little harm is done. Otherwise, leading a merely decent ethical life would appear too demanding. Fourth, there is a socially endorsed norm not to treat such confidence-building thoughts as that I will beat Peter in tennis today as claiming literal truth. This is why tact, politeness, and many "white lies" are not considered culpable deceit.

Self-deception distorts one's own grasp of the world, thus denying one's own claim in belief while promoting it. The instability of self-deception shows that the self-deceiver is beholden to belief's claim of truth in his very need to evade it. One must engage in a manipulation of oneself that works only if it is partial and largely isolated from action and neighboring beliefs. The self-deceiver, like the liar, needs to be vigilant to avoid confrontation with evidence that points toward the belief he wants to hide. Thus the project is self-undermining. The self-deceiver must hide from himself the fact that he is trying to avoid sources of undermining evidence. But to avoid them successfully he needs to retain some cognizance of both his project and the belief he is trying to avoid. Again, then, perfect self-deception could not be optimal self-deception.

Self-deception is a refusal to spell out to oneself one's claims tied to a particular belief (Fingarette 1969). Under full awareness the spelled-out thought would be contradictory, and so the self-deception is destabilized.

3   Negligence and Believing the Unbelievable

Self-deceptive projects are subject to blame, since the unawareness of inconsistency is due to some kind of intellectual negligence or irresponsibility.[9] But much of our ignorance of inconsistency is innocent. There is nothing incoherent about presenting a set of axioms that contain a hidden contradiction or inconsistency, as Russell's Paradox showed for Frege's axioms. Inconsistency among beliefs is expected for finite beings with large sets of disparate beliefs.[10] We regularly and unproblematically fail to recognize inconsistency among our beliefs. When I learned that a journal rejects nine out of ten articles, I believed that its standards were very high. When I learned that a journal accepts 10 percent of its submissions, I thought that its standards were not very high.[11] In the noninnocent cases, the inconsistency is a failing within the person's grasp, even if it is not recognized except under full awareness. The condition of full awareness lifts the veil imposed by self-deception, or subtler kinds of intentional inattention, to expose the internal failing already present.

The scope of the incoherence test extends further when persons are under an obligation for heightened scrutiny of a belief owing to having invoked that belief in behalf of, say, political action or to advise others. If one believes in astrology, for example, that belief typically plays a very active role in informing one's actions and in advising friends, acquaintances, and customers. This role standardly increases one's responsibility for correct judgment and, accordingly, for scrutiny of one's belief.

The beliefs most prominent in discussions of the ethics of belief are those we affirm, defend, or act on, and so these are beliefs for which we have a heightened responsibility. Religious beliefs became central to debates over the ethics of belief because of their importance in peoples' lives. Consider, again, the example from the *Apology* discussed at the end of chapter 1. The accusation against Meletus—that he "cannot be believed . . . even . . ." by himself—stems from his own original charge that Socrates believes in new gods (other than the gods of the city). Socrates presses Meletus to interpret his complaint—is the charge that Socrates has heterodox religious beliefs or that he is an atheist? Meletus opts for atheism.[12] The result is beliefs that are contradictory. (On the assumption that to disbelieve that *p* implies not to believe that *p*, we have an out-and-out contradiction.) There is no difficulty in recognizing the inconsistency, nor is it minor. It is a direct denial of the focal belief that expresses the original charge.

Socrates' cross-examination exposes Meletus to a pragmatic self-refutation. One is entitled to assertion provided that one genuinely believes what one asserts. But what Meletus affirms is unbelievable. So he fails to meet the minimum condition for the entitlement. In the case of Meletus, the instability of his relevant beliefs surfaces as soon as Socrates brings attention to them. Yet similar instability on immediate critical attention applies to familiar beliefs that are widespread, persistent, and seemingly stable. A small sampling, mainly from my classes and academic environs, include:

(1) All that happens is a matter of fate. (Alternatively, and equally incredible: We are each responsible for all that befalls us.)

(2) One's values are determined by one's society (or parents).

(3)   Human physical attractiveness ("good looks") is subjective ("Beauty is in the eyes of the beholder").

(4)   The world is a mental (or social) construction.

(5)   Science advances by rhetorical victory, not through prediction, testing, and observation of an independent world.

(6)   One is entitled to use words, or (abstract) words like "truth," only if one can define them.

(7)   We act only on selfish motives.

(8)   Language determines thought.

(9)   Generally, one should express—never hide or disguise—one's feelings.

Despite appearing to be more stable than Meletus's unbelievable beliefs, (1)–(9) readily succumb to a clear awareness of what is claimed and their obvious implications. Take (4). When a colleague of mine heard another express such a view, she asked, "Didn't many people die of infection before we grasped (and so could construct) the world of microbes or viruses?"[13] No straightforward answer was forthcoming. Or consider (6). Reflect on various sentences that you readily understand. You will find that you are unable to define most (or any) of the terms in them.

None of (1)–(9) can be believed with even dim awareness of their immediate implications in specific cases. The internal incoherence requires only a critical scratching of the surface. In fact, I expect that many devotees of these beliefs would now disavow the above formulations as simplistic, though I stand by their accuracy to common expression.

Aside from the obviousness of the implications, how blameworthy an individual actually is for maintaining these beliefs depends on the appropriate level of intellectual scrutiny. In the case of the *Apology*, three factors conspire to set a very high level. First, and most crucial, the costs of error are high: Meletus's beliefs are offered in support of his (legal) accusation against Socrates. Second, he puts these beliefs forward to others. Our responsibilities rise when we assert beliefs to others, placing demands on their time and effort, while recommending that others accept and act on them. Third, the relevant beliefs are salient, especially epistemically salient. They are the kind of beliefs—such as the controversial opinion that Socrates does not believe in gods—that ought to be justified, rather than presupposed or taken for granted. Epistemic salience orderings are along two dimensions: vulnerability and importance. In advance, we expect opinions to be more vulnerable than simple, readily checked, factual claims. The more important or forceful claims of an argument, those that least permit modification or accommodation, are those that are high in order for critical examination and challenge.

If these factors are typical of what affects the proper level of self-scrutiny, agents will grasp their import since it is manifest or obvious from their very action or understanding of the context. So, where a belief has survived as a result of intellectual negligence, then, on full awareness, the agent will recognize that he ought to have subjected the relevant beliefs to further tests or critical reflection, but that he did not. Yet, in his use of those beliefs he represented himself as scrupulous and responsible. The result is a recognized inconsistency or incoherence.

4   Distraction and the Unbelievable

Even under heightened responsibility, it may be questioned whether beliefs like (1)–(9) arise and persist only through self-deception. These beliefs are maintained and affirmed without the tension that is symptomatic of the inherent irrationality of self-deception, and yet their suspect nature is on the surface. Self-deception is too sophisticated a mechanism to cover a large range of cases of believing what I claim to be unbelievable.

My response has to be that there are very simple mechanisms for obscuring awareness of one's epistemic position in regard to a particular belief. Self-deception may be among them, contrary to the suggestions in the previous paragraph. The complexity of the mechanisms of self-deception, as well as the intricacies of a good analysis of it, do not require corresponding sophistication in its use; otherwise the "Emperor's New Clothes" could not be so handy a parable.

However, rather than develop this view of self-deception directly, I shall conceive the question posed as representing a broader position, and one that I will start to challenge here and pursue further in later chapters. The position is that our "on-line" self has control of its contents, especially the beliefs guiding its judgments, and fully understands them. The position blocks the natural response to the original question in regard to the incoherence test: We can persist in incoherence with little effort because the test requires concentration, which is easily avoided. We have limited consciousness of relations between beliefs. We sort beliefs into separate categories for ease of memory and quicker access.[14] (Recall my earlier example—thinking of a journal that rejects nine out of ten articles as tough, yet thinking of a journal that accepts 10 percent of its submissions as not tough.) But the essential cognitive economies that categorization promises would be of no avail unless accompanied by very limited awareness of our beliefs, even when inferentially related. Like categorization, beliefs activated to guide reasoning or action appear to consciousness under a guise or focus or mode of presentation, which restricts our awareness of the interrelations between them and other beliefs.

Even when one intends to so examine one's believing and even while engaging that intention, one can be distracted. Distraction can, of course, be a mechanism of self-deception, yet be instigated by a more overt intention than in paradigm cases of self-deception. If I do not want to threaten my comfortable belief that I played well in a basketball game, I distract myself from the coach's review of the game by concentrating on a crossword puzzle. However, what really recommends distraction as an explanation is that it commonly operates without any intention.

Along with simple credulity in accepting the pronouncements of others, the way I suspect that distraction operates in cases like (1)–(9) above is that those who hold any of these beliefs do so on the basis of a hazily conceived abstract line of thought. Once convinced that there is an argument that implies the proposition believed, it seems pointless to subject it to test or critical reflection. This explanation in regard to denials of evidentialism is that if you take yourself to have an argument that some beliefs must simply be basic or groundless, then you will readily be distracted from your own expectation that each of your beliefs is held for good reason.

A similar account is familiarly applied to a complementary position. Under rarified but forceful skeptical reasoning, we can sincerely, but falsely, claim to have abandoned a belief. In Meditation I, after Descartes reaches the extreme point at which he takes himself to have good reason to cease believing such obvious matters as that $2+3=5$ or that there is a sky, he realizes that he is unable to do so. He calls on resources for obscuring to himself his own beliefs. Descartes overreacts by treating these propositions as not just doubtful, but false. He conjures up his "malicious demon" as an extreme form of self-help in this project. Finally, Descartes reminds us that the project is not beholden to practical demands. The project is a purely theoretical inquiry into knowledge, so that belief's indispensable role in guiding action is bracketed. These efforts belie presentation of Descartes's "method of doubt" as leading to a wholesale suspension of belief. Teachers know this from their classes. When skeptical arguments are found persuasive, a student's response may well be that he has ceased believing, say, that he is in a classroom (since he may only be dreaming it). Yet, this avowal is without conviction.

Less specialized cases are easily envisaged. Consider an instance of (6) above, that to understand a statement one has to be able to define its terms. At the *Louvre,* Jones exclaims, "The *Mona Lisa* is beautiful." His ersatz Socratic friend responds, "What do you mean by 'beauty'?" Jones falls silent and perplexed. He was sure he knew what he asserted, yet now he finds that he does not even know what his words mean. The question is expected to be relevant, and it certainly appears to be. But, if it is relevant, it presupposes that Jones ought to know the meaning of "beauty," and know it well enough to articulate it so as to back his assertion. Since, however, Jones is unable to meet this challenge, he thinks he loses entitlement to his assertion. He ought to cease to hold the belief and he (sincerely) claims to do so, but that never truly occurs. Behind his expressed belief is a stable background of beliefs that rejects the challenge. Jones does not attend to this background, so on the surface he treats the reasoning against his belief as persuasive. But he does not fully endorse it. Thus he maintains his belief, despite his avowals. The abstract question distracts Jones from his belief's continuing hold on him.[15]

If we can be distracted by abstract argument or questioning from recognizing our own beliefs, it is unsurprising that the incoherence test can be flouted. The incoherence test calls on us to attend to our epistemic position in regard to the proposition believed. The attending requires concentration, and so it is ripe for distraction. Indeed, it is a commonplace of cognitive psychology that even when we attend to an object or event or assertion, we regularly do not notice details that we nevertheless register. You are introduced to a new colleague, and almost immediately after separating you cannot recall her name or the color of her hair or whether she was wearing a jacket. You see her jacket, but you do not see that she is wearing a jacket. Nevertheless, given a set of choices as to the color of her jacket, you will score much higher than chance, even while sincerely denying any memory for it.

The workings of distraction are enough to remove the paradoxical ring of the idea of believing what is unbelievable. Although the demands of belief on us can be met through our own practices, they are evident only on examination. Normally, belief plays a pervasive role in guiding action and inference, but we do not attend to it. Application of the incoherence test requires effort and concentration from which we are easily distracted. Further, as I will now discuss, the test also requires explicitness about the details of one's epistemic position that are ordinarily kept implicit.

5   Just Be Explicit

[A]ll the facts harmonize with a true account, whereas the truth soon clashes with a false one.

—Aristotle, *Nicomachean Ethics*

In Reason's fight against thought debased by prejudice and propaganda, the first rule is that . . . commitments that are potentially controversial should be made explicit as claims, exposing them both as vulnerable to reasoned challenge and as in need of reasoned defense.

—Robert B. Brandom, *Making It Explicit*

We have been discussing self-deception, distraction, and like mechanisms as ways to maintain beliefs that mask incoherence. In light of the mechanisms that interfere with well-formed beliefs, what recommendations can we offer to impede their operation and facilitate believing well? In this section, I want to supplement the negative recommendations not to be self-deceived and not to be incoherent with the positive recommendation to be *explicit.* The positive recommendation furthers the two negative ones. It is more difficult to obscure to oneself a belief that one has stated openly to oneself and especially to others; and if one is explicit about a set of related beliefs it is more difficult to overlook them in a test of their coherence.

The recommendation of explicitness is endorsed, however, only when it is applied cautiously and discriminately. Explicitness is burdensome, and among its burdens are ones that detract from inquiry and reasoning. This theme moves to the forefront below in section 8.

After some initial illustrations to suggest what needs to be made explicit, I develop the central argument for the wide scope of explicitness as a way to ferret out incoherence. The argument depends on five assumptions, stated below, which amount to the following: the principles violated in distorted belief are central to our evaluative practices and so are likely to be implicit and overlooked.

For purposes of simplifying discussion, let us assume that explicitness is intended to be used rightly—it is guided by concern for the truth of one's beliefs. Under this restriction, we lighten our load by ignoring the ways in which explicitness can be used to distort belief by overloading, or distracting self-criticism.[16] Additionally, I will talk of implicitness or explicitness (full stop) without specification of what one is implicit or explicit about, on the expectation that appropriate completions are easily supplied.

To be explicit is to articulate or formulate or express what has been implicit. Explicitness highlights and clarifies claims, assumptions, or commitments, while increasing the visible range of beliefs with which any particular belief must cohere. In articulating, formulating, or expressing, we bring beliefs forward as claims, rather than as elements in the background of our understanding. Hazy thoughts are forced into the mold of definite statements. The result of analyzing a loaded or abstract term ("equality," "rational," "justice," "discrimination") or substituting specific theses for the labeling of a position ("liberal," "conservative," "radical") is to generate determinate claims.

The reconstruction of an argument into an ordered set of premises and conclusion, where premises are broken down to simple statements and inferences (or subconclusions), is a paradigm of explicitness. Terms are standardized and logically gratuitous devices of rhetoric or persuasion removed. The bare structure of the reasoning stands forth. Assumptions hidden by the smooth flow of reasoning from premises to conclusion are articulated. Criticism is facilitated both by easing the demands on memory and by providing more precise, narrower targets to direct objections.

Fallacious reasoning typically depends on inexplicitness. The fallacy of "many questions" occurs when the given options to answering a question commit one to a disavowed presupposition. What is presupposed is paradigmatically what is implicit. The stock example is the complex question "When did you stop beating your wife?"

Deductive reasoning is particularly valuable here as a device of explicitness. As Alasdair MacIntyre retells the story: ". . . Charles II once invited the members of the Royal Society to explain to him why a dead fish weighs more than the same fish alive; a number of subtle explanations were offered to him. He then pointed out that it does not" (MacIntyre 1988: 88;

see also Hamblin 1970: 38–39). The hapless investigators are misled by the pragmatic stress on finding an explanation, which presupposes that what is to be explained is fact. The presupposition is accepted, but not noticed. If, instead, "A dead fish weighs more than the same fish alive" is actually deduced from "There is an explanation of why a dead fish weighs more than the same fish alive," then confrontation with this obvious presupposition immediately brings to attention the question of whether it is truly a fact.

Logical fallacies such as the fallacies of affirming the consequent or denying the antecedent are confused with valid patterns of reasoning when they are dressed up with specific content. But the underlying pattern itself, if baldly—explicitly—expressed, would usually be recognized as fallacious. It is tempting to hear the following as formally valid: "If the library is open, the post office is too. The library is closed. So there is no point in going to the post office." But the temptation dissipates if the cloaked formal pattern is stated explicitly: If p, then q. So, if not-p, then not-q. (An additional benefit of the abstract formulation is the use of variables ["p," "q"]. This brings salience to the large scope of claims implied, while begging for substitutions likely to generate counterexamples.)

Recent epistemology provides a pertinent example of rendering explicit important hidden assumptions through the formulation of underlying generalizations. The skeptical argument derivable from Descartes's worry in Meditation I over the possibility that he may be dreaming has been argued to assume a "closure" principle, a version of which is the following:

If I know that p and I know that p entails q, then I know that q.[17]

As applied to Descartes's argument the reasoning is by contraposition: You know that if there is a book in front of you, you are not dreaming it. But you do not know that the book that you think you see in front of you is not really something you are dreaming. So you do not know that there is a book in front of you.

The highlighted conditional is not evident, yet it does not require any new inferences. By virtue of his reasoning, Descartes is committed to a rule licensing the move from antecedent to consequent. It need not be the principle cited above. But that one recommends itself for its simplicity and intuitive plausibility. Though the abstraction requires effort, it is effort directed at understanding Descartes's reasoning.

In general, explicitness bolsters the two other, more basic, recommendations. As we are more explicit, we increase the possibilities for detecting incoherence and diminish the opportunities for self-deception or successful distraction. Rendering explicit underlying generalizations in reasoning, as with the above "closure" principle, heightens vulnerability by generating a greater range of claims to which one's specific belief must cohere. Self-deception depends on hiding or obscuring commitments, which is harder to do if these are clearly stated to oneself or others. The wife in the tale of (allegedly) rational self-deception will have a much harder time denying her evidence if she has notated it or communicated it to others.

I turn now to arguing more systematically for the importance of explicitness in expanding the test of incoherence through endorsing four assumptions—a fifth is introduced later:

1. In many everyday domains we have extensive commitments, through action, and especially assertion, to widely accepted evaluation (and meta-evaluation) criteria, including impartial procedures, deference to experts, and testing claims by drawing implications from them.
2. Since we use these criteria often and in varied circumstances, they generate precedents that are forceful constraints on further uses.
3. These evaluation criteria, as well as the extensive precedents in their use, are in good part implicitly believed (or likely to become implicitly believed).
4. What is implicit is easily overlooked.

By the first assumption, we are committed to a range of ordinary procedures and criteria for the evaluation of putative beliefs. The conjecture is that criticizable distortions of belief are criticizable because these criteria are ours and they are violated. Serious or criticizable distortions of belief I understand as not merely hastily or fallaciously formed beliefs or those due to ignorance of, say, statistical inference, but beliefs that are either blatantly unwarranted or unwarranted but persistent despite opportunities to confront counterevidence or counterargument.

Although commitment to criteria of evaluation alone may not fix their applications, by the second assumption there is not much latitude or indeterminacy except in unanticipated cases. You cannot appeal to the *Consumer Reports* guide for purchasing a stereo but deny its value for the assessment of the hot sports car you want, if your goals are broadly the same (the best product within your price range). The constraint credibly assumes that if you know of its value for the one purchase, its similar value for the other is evident.

The last two assumptions help to diagnose why the distortion of beliefs, despite covering incoherence, readily occurs and persists. By the third assumption, the unavoidable procedures and criteria tend to be hidden as implicit beliefs. The fourth assumption introduces the obvious barrier to criticizing these violations. What is implicit is easily overlooked. The job of explicitness is to bring them forward, and thereby to facilitate the exposure of underlying incoherences.

For an illustration, consider the recent bestseller *The Bible Code* (Drosnin 1997). The author reports on a formula that is supposed to be a key to decoding hidden predictions in the Bible.[18] Specifically, the author emphasizes the prediction of the assassination of Israeli President Yitzhak Rabin. The author places great weight on this prediction for its precision and its (alleged) occurrence in an ancient text. (The focus on the assassination enormously understates how extraordinary this prediction would have to be, coming thousands of years earlier. Think of the stupendously vast improbability of predicting the birth of a single child with a particular DNA-sequence, given all the chance circumstances and complexities of any successful fertilization.) Consequently, the author takes the truth of the prediction to highly confirm the hypothesis that the "code" foretells the future.

The author depends on our appreciation of the strong confirmatory value of surprising predictions that turn out to be true, without stating it. Similarly, the author intends for us to infer his impartiality and empirical approach from his frequent profession of agnosticism. However, at no point in the rest of the book does he offer any other precise prediction of events subsequent to the book's publication. Although the code operates in ways that render it difficult to predict events unanticipated by us, it remains feasible and crucial.

Had the author been explicit about the very criteria he exploits (confirmation increases with precision or surprise value of a prediction; an empirical, impartial approach to evaluation of predictive claims) his glaring failure to abide by them would be manifest. In invoking these criteria to support the code, he commits himself to their relevance and value. But he then, inconsistently, neglects them when it comes to seriously testing the code.

6   Internal Commitments

The argument in the previous section depended on an additional fifth assumption, most evident in the first assumption above: Certain commitments are to be counted as beliefs for purposes of determining incoherence, even when they are not strictly beliefs. The main reason favoring the assumption is that the commitments we are concerned with are commitments to the truth of propositions (or sentences), and that is the core claim of belief or assertion. So far as our incoherence-of-distorted-belief argument goes, the big question with this assumption is what are to count as one's implicit or implied commitments.

The term "commitment" is sometimes brought into service as a replacement for "belief" because theorists want to capture logical and inferential dependencies that need not be matched by any belief. You can believe p and p imply q, without believing q. Although this is the most familiar illustration, it is only a small sampling of the "nonfecundity" of belief: One can believe that p, and almost nothing else follows. You can believe that tomatoes are good in salads without believing or even disbelieving that fruits are good in salads, even though tomatoes are fruits. Commitments are introduced to allow for a belieflike attitude that has the requisite fecundity. If a logical consequence of what you believe is false, then a commitment of yours (to what you believe) fails and it follows that your belief is false.

The purpose of theorists in so introducing the notion of commitment is to mark out a terrain of *external* demands on our beliefs that delineate their logical or conceptual implications. These are external demands because they need not correspond to anything that the person would acknowledge. This notion of commitment is not useful for our purposes. For, even if there is a contradiction among a set of the person's beliefs and these commitments, it will not be an incoherence, for there need be no obscured grasp of this contradiction.

The shift away from belief to the external demands of commitment seems hasty. As I use the term "commitment" here, it applies, first, to consequences or implications of one's belief that the agent *should* or *ought* to appreciate. The demand is internal—grasped—by the agent, since in failing to do as he ought either he would recognize himself as acting wrongly or, if he doesn't, then there is negligence. Second, it applies to assumptions necessary for the intelligibility of one's actions. For assertion, it would include presuppositions requisite for understanding what is asserted.

Descartes is internally committed to the above closure principle (or something like it), if it is necessary to his argument. He is committed to it, even if his argument can be understood well enough without it.

Genuine internal commitments are within the agent's grasp or responsibility, and so are to be counted effectively as beliefs. When a person uses an impartial procedure or appeals to an expert to inform his judgment, I ascribe to his action a commitment to an extensive range of further applications of these procedures and appeals—effectively, to beliefs that these procedures and appeals are proper for a wide range of applications. The person might not have thought so—he may have no real corresponding belief—and, surely, his behavior will leave a great deal of indeterminacy regarding his intentions. Nevertheless, his actions are purposeful, and he is internally committed to those propositions necessary to make sense of his actions, which includes consonance with his own related beliefs. The author of *The Bible Code* can not appeal to the precise prediction he both ascribes to the code and recommends to his readers, as confirmation of its validity, without commitment to precise prediction as a general test. That internal commitment together with his related beliefs is incoherent, and the author dodges the corresponding impossibility of belief only through self-deception or distraction.

7   Further Defense and Applications

The Bible Code provides, of course, an extreme example of irrational belief. Rather than rely heavily on an extreme illustration, we need to develop the argument that the five assumptions cited above do indeed connect distorted belief and incoherence. Widespread use of the relevant simple criteria follows on their practical unavoidability. Appeal to the judgments of experts, respect for the opinion of peers, trial-and-error experimentation, assessment of prospective new beliefs by conformity to well-established facts, consistency with one's prior judgments and their rationale, impartiality and fairness in evaluations, and so on, are procedures and criteria on which we all regularly depend. You can easily verify or falsify this claim for yourself.

But if you do verify it, you will verify the second assumption as well. We build up a large set of precedents in the criteria and procedures to which we are committed, which fix much of their further uses insofar as the weak assumption that like cases are to be judged applies. So latitude to treat new cases differently, as not subject to prior criteria or procedures, decreases. Of course, the actual uses will not be retained in memory, but that is unnecessary if the uses are frequent and convergent enough to become embedded in our practices and habits. Admittedly, except for outright assertion, actions leave much room for alternative interpretations and indeterminacy. However, the point of the second and fifth assumptions is that sheer varied usage narrows the alternatives and diminishes the indeterminacy. The thought that interpretation remains wide open is influenced, I suspect, by conflating the question of what someone's commitments are with the question of what commitments we can attribute to that person. The latter question, which is not our present concern, is often hopeless to answer on the spot, and that itself is part of the explanation of persistent, distorted belief.

The third and fourth assumptions are that the procedures and criteria that we constantly apply for evaluative and judgmental purposes are primary candidates for remaining as implicit beliefs. Since they are widely known and used habitually, they lack or lose salience. The procedures are applied readily and casually in everyday situations, tending then to go unnoticed, according to the fourth assumption. The background—what is implicit—contains what is obvious, not worth attending to or noticing and so less available. Implicitness facilitates not only forgetting, but also purposeful overlooking. In the parable of "The Emperor's New Clothes," the boy's cry that the emperor is naked states explicitly what everyone knows. It is because the boy is less attentive than others to social norms and he does not fear being thought a fool or an incompetent that he finds it easy to notice and to express what is obvious.

Nevertheless, appeal to the five assumptions does not seem promising in application to the far-reaching studies on cognitive illusions in social psychology. These studies, alluded to a number of times, demonstrate cognitive faults in belief formation that operate outside of consciousness, and which therefore do not seem to function as covers for incoherence.

For the sake of its vividness and its influence, I will respond to this objection by the use of an example from the most well-known cognitive-dissonance experiment. In that experiment, subjects in a group who received low pay are much more willing to describe a contrived study that they participated in as interesting than are subjects who received high pay (Festinger and Carlsmith 1959). The latter experience no dissonance in correctly calling the study a bore. The subjects in the low-pay group do not suspect that their judgment of the study as interesting or worthwhile is motivated by the low pay they received. (Subsequent research explains the dissonance phenomena in less motivationally loaded [or "hot"] terms. But the observations to follow apply to these alternatives as well.)

There are various ways of explaining the cognitive dissonance phenomenon. A standard view is that the subjects in the low-pay group mitigate the conflict that they encumber in recognizing that their efforts were not worthwhile by judging the study to have been interesting and significant. Another view has it that subjects effectively view themselves from the third-person—they take their own behavior as evidence for the quality of the study in which they participated (Bem 1967). Since they invested a good deal of effort for little financial reward they infer that the study must have been significant. Each of these explanations acquires its natural terminus by revealing the rationality of subjects' behavior or judgment. In the first case, it seems rational both to want to resolve (internal) conflict and to select as the locus for resolution judgments that are more subjective (hence liable) such as one's interest in performing a study. In the second case, the crucial inference is from the evidence of a student's large investment in time and effort for little pay to the conclusion that the study must have interested him. But the conclusion follows only with the assumption that this evidence is known to the student and that he is rational and thus would not want to waste his time and energies. What I argue is that the natural terminus of either explanation in rationality is surrendered when the resolutions are called on to guide further action.

Let us now project the experiment onto realistic circumstances of goals, actions, and feedback. Subjects in the low-pay group are invited back to do further similar tasks. Could the dissonance effects continue to elude their notice, while they repeated a task, if they were cognizant—explicit—about their relevant judgments prior to, as well as subsequent to, the original study? My conjecture is no, though I know of no corroborative studies. Perfect cognitive dissonance resolution, like perfect self-deception, would not be optimal. Imagine that the subjects in the low-pay condition, who judged the study worthwhile, are asked to participate in further studies. They could not easily decline the request, given their own claim that the study was interesting and valuable (with the implication that the study's interest and value is not exhausted in the single participation). Yet, they would likely also have been explicit about the study, describing it to others in detail. Those to whom they spoke would no doubt comment that such a study sounds like a terrible bore. Through ordinary talk and behavior, subjects attest to what they find interesting and worthwhile rather than dull and a waste of time. When a subject examines his belief in the attractions of renewed participation in similar studies in light of these (explicit) avowals, conflict and tensions emerge.

The point I intend through this variation is a general one. Recall that the goal is to answer the objection that the five assumptions above seem impotent in application to the distortion of beliefs uncovered in the cognitive psychological studies. My protest is that these studies are typically one-shot (synchronic, static), whereas distorted beliefs are of long-standing or persistent use.[19] When we think of distorted belief in its natural ongoing environment, the fallacies and biasing that these studies reveal cannot alone account for it, for under dynamic conditions the rationality that we ascribe in order to make sense of subjects' erroneous judgments will become attenuated. The attenuation follows on grounds similar to why in an earlier previous section I claimed that the rationality of self-deception becomes attenuated in continuous environments.

A sadly familiar philosophical reply could be offered to my speculation about the outcome in this variant study. The reply claims that subjects in the study could acknowledge their avowals and still consistently decline to undertake the new study, since those prior avowals did not address the specific features of their low-pay condition. So subjects may decline to repeat the experience without inconsistency, merely citing any number of excuses such as especially pressing business. This reply is an application of a familiar strategy that presumes that avoidance of inconsistency is always available, however much one is explicit.

But there is something suspicious about the reply, as there is about the strategy. The reply assumes the availability of inexhaustible possibilities for evading incoherence. But the question is not whether any strategies could avoid incoherence. The question is whether the beliefs, intentions, and commitments of the subject actually do avoid incoherence. If the role of the above assumptions is to generate commitments that impose a forceful constraint on us, there is much less room for dodging incoherence in actual thought. Given the above five assumptions, it is rare that these incoherences are, or could be, actually evaded. So the reply would substantiate only the accusation that the intrinsic ethics of belief is too weak if it is too weak in practice, which I deny.[20] My claim is that there is no realistic way to avoid inconsistency, not that there is no possible way.

8 Recommending Explicitness Selectively

The most obvious device of explicitness is through written communication or public pronouncement. But very few of the procedures, tests, and criteria that we endorse through our behavior are written down, which suggests that there are serious disvalues to explicitness. Insistence on a written agreement or code, for example, as contrasted to implicit rules or cooperative understandings, is an expression of a lack of trust.

There are other ways in which many of the values of explicitness are complemented by disvalues that counterbalance the recommendation to be explicit. Although explicitness continues to be recommended to promote the test of incoherence and as a barrier to self-deception, it is a circumspect recommendation. There are often good reasons for not being explicit.

Social life, for example, depends on leaving much implicit. If you are confessional about feelings and personal judgments, you surrender privacy, which preserves options and flexibility. To express private opinions is to be bound by them later, particularly through expectations generated in others. (In a related way, you also render yourself more predictable and hence less interesting.) More important, since everyday strains and offenses between persons in social interaction are infrequently settled by admission and apology, we need to allow these incidents to fade away, to be forgotten.

Consider, however, more overtly cognitive or epistemic disvalues of explicitness. Leaving much implicit is generally a way to facilitate memory, communication, and thought. Reasoning goes more smoothly if we can assume transitions rather than state them. Once stated they demand attention and take additional time and effort to comprehend. As an informal test, try to reduce complex questions to avoid committing many-questions fallacies. You will have to subdivide questions to eliminate presuppositions. Since building up shared presuppositions facilitates discourse, the result of explicitness is usually a tiresome prolixity.

The increased vulnerability that explicitness generates is double edged. When one unpacks a loaded term into a series of claims or formulates underlying assumptions, the increased vulnerability may be premature. One subjects oneself to cheap refutation. Putting a point wrong is taken as getting it wrong. Explicitness, while a manifestation of intellectual honesty, is also a burden on it.

Explicitness threatens to dampen diversity of opinion. Some of us are quick to reach conclusions; some of us require much more convincing. From the same evidence, we reach different conclusions. If we see a single headlight moving toward us at night, some of us will judge that it is a motorcycle, others that it is a car with a broken headlight; and some of us will suspend judgment until the vehicle is closer. Yet, we each take our judgments to be supported by the evidence. It is in good part because so much of what is doing the informing is not shared—not explicit—that this variation is possible and not troubling. Because so much is implicit, we have latitude to explain away, and so tolerate, divergence and dissent as based on differences in information or criteria or reasoning without denying that incompatible beliefs are really in conflict. (Consider the havoc that would be wrought by a demand for explicitness on attorneys in courts of law, and note that the lack of such a demand is taken as serving the interest of truth in legal proof.)

Lewis Carroll's (1895) "What the Tortoise Said to Achilles" can be read as a parable about the impossibility of complete explicitness in formal arguments. One cannot demand that inferences, licensed by a logical connective, be reconstructed to express the meaning of that connective as a rule to be added as a premise. For the inferential role of that premise will then itself require expression of a further rule, licensing its use as another premise, launching an infinite regress.

Explicitness is "supererogatory," an exceeding of the normal standards for intellectual honesty. Clarity, for example, is necessary for successful communication. It is compatible with leaving much implicit. When deliberation concludes with a judgment put forward as correct, we represent the procedures by which we decided as open-minded, fair, and impartial. But there is no corresponding conceptual demand to represent oneself as explicit or precise. When it comes to assumptions or presuppositions of an assertion or argument, it could not be a demand, as the example above from Descartes illustrates. Assumptions or presuppositions of a presenter's assertion or argument can be a discovery unavailable to that presenter.

Given all these good reasons to allow assumptions and beliefs to be implicit, explicitness is advantageous only if it is highly selective. But any informed selectivity will be sufficient for the cases central to this chapter. In these cases, explicitness is warranted by manifest challenges to the consistency of one's commitments, as with the example from the *Bible Code*. We know of other, related calls for explicitness, such as where one recognizes oneself as liable to misjudgment or when costs of error are high. Serious argument and debate, but not ordinary communication, require that hidden assumptions be exposed.

The central argument of this and the previous section is that when the beliefs of an individual are seriously distorted that person has special reason to be explicit, which he resists. Although I have tried to give a variety of examples, it may still be suspected that the charge of incoherence is too strong to cover many cases. Simple errors, lack of information, false assumptions, and nonconscious influences are various innocent ways in which believing can become distorted without incorporating any contradiction.

Answering this suspicion is important. The charge of incoherence is the strongest criticism one can make of a set of (purported) beliefs. It implies that they must fail of their own claims to truth, requiring no additional assumptions. Nevertheless, this is the charge leveled in many ordinary cases. This incongruous combination of the strongest criticism—incoherence— applied to unremarkable beliefs that arise through a few central processes of believing match the incongruous combination that is central to this work: Belief is common and yet extremely demanding of evidence or reasons. Throughout I try to soften this incongruity by showing how the combination accords with our practices and self-understanding. I want to provide similar softening for the former incongruity—to show that when we render explicit the details of our criticism of another's belief as distorted, the result is a contradiction.

Consider an example of everyday rumor. Bill says to you, "Jones was arrested for shoplifting." What actually happened was that Jones was standing next to someone who was arrested in a department store, presumably for shoplifting. As the story was passed along, it became transformed into the nasty rumor, which you take Bill to contribute to spreading. Underlying your charge is the following extended thought that you treat as available to Bill:

The belief is hurtful to Jones, and it is the kind of belief that I know is a candidate for distortion, particularly if it is passed along without independent corroboration. Knowing this, I nevertheless did not question the speaker who told me of it, but just accepted it and probably, in part, because I took some pleasure in learning this bit of dirt about Jones. Similarly, I passed it along without checking the story further, though in passing it along I incur responsibility to stand behind its truth. I imply that I am responsible in believing it, yet I have been seriously negligent in not treating it with more doubt.

Although this is very long-winded, it does not venture beyond internal commitments. The thoughts as a whole are in direct contradiction: Bill is affirming and denying of himself adequate reasons; affirming and denying of himself responsible action in regard to believing and asserting.

To put the reasoning abstractly: If one neglects evidence in respect of a belief, then one ignores evidence that one should obtain. So one has reason to believe that the evidence neglected is relevant. If relevant and not yet gathered, it could be either in accord with one's belief or undermining. So one has reason to believe that there is potentially undermining evidence that one has ignored. But then one already has evidence to undermine one's claim to have adequate reasons for one's belief. Since this reasoning applies to ordinary processes of belief-formation, it lends credibility to the proposal that incoherence underlies much blamable or distorted belief, which could be uncovered by explicitness.

9   Full Awareness and Limits on Practicality

The limits on the practical value of explicitness in the improvement of believing goes much further than selectivity, but those limits are illuminated by reference to selectivity. The suggested follow-up study to the cognitive dissonance experiment (section 7 above) was meant to support the claim that the dissonance effects would not continue to elude subjects' notice, while they repeated a task. But the suggestion was not the proposal of a genuine test because of the condition that subjects' were "cognizant—explicit—about their relevant judgments prior to, as well as subsequent to, the original study." Consider the previous section's insistence on the need for explicitness to be selective. The question then is: "How is one supposed to select what to be explicit about?" One cannot be explicit about everything, and to be explicit about just what is relevant to exposing one's own incoherence would require that one already glimpse that incoherence. The requisite explicitness can be directed by a critic, as in Socratic method, but only very indirectly by the self-critic. (For more on this, see chap. 11.)

Without withdrawing from my conclusion that the incoherence test has a wide scope, I do want to put it in an appropriately modest perspective. First, and this is just clarification by tautology, the way our commitments and precedents limit latitude to treat new cases differently is forceful only to the extent that new cases are similar to previous ones. The force will be strong in the cases of distorted beliefs because they are blatantly contrary to judgments reached from one's experience and evidence. But beyond that the force dissipates as is obvious from the legal system. The legal system is systemically bound to adhere to codified laws and precedents, and yet the law continually evolves through new cases that are not settled, though they are to be guided, by precedent and law.

Second, and more important, there is a huge psychological gap between the presence of a set of inconsistent beliefs, stemming from distortive sources, and a person's recognition of them as inconsistent. We do not need to draw on the resources of depth or Freudian psychology for evidence of this gap. Empirical studies on reasoning show a similar wide gap, though of a different kind. In postexperimental interviews of subjects subsequent to the most famous reasoning task (of conditional logic), the interviewer led subjects to expose their own fallacies. Nevertheless, many were not moved to renounce their choice in the study (and neither did it immunize them from failure in related studies): "74 per cent . . . failed to correct their solution after the relevant information had been revealed and evaluated and . . . only 48 per cent . . . succeeded at the end of the interview" (Wason 1977: 123).

The condition of full awareness is a way to abstract from a host of these difficulties, although, as just indicated, the difficulties are not specialized ones. Much belief arises nonconsciously, subject to a myriad of influences. Fortunately, for our purposes of trying to show the further reach of the incoherence test, ordinary full awareness does not require that we become aware of our nonconscious reasons, except when their being nonconscious is our own doing. In these applications, full awareness amounts to little more than an absence of selective inattention, which is a main mechanism of self-deception.

But, as I observed one paragraph back, our normal condition is not one of full awareness. It is naive to think that a demand for explicitness and full awareness will be sufficient to expose to the person his own distorted beliefs. In this regard, the Meletus example from the *Apology* makes the exposure and elimination of distorted belief appear too easy. We should not confuse our knowing that someone's beliefs are distorted with that person's coming to know and appreciate it on self-examination or questioning. The arguments and examples in this chapter show that much distortive belief is the cover for incoherence, and that explicitness could, under full awareness, expose that incoherence. But we do need to rein in ambition: the "could" is not that of a practical, everyday cure or corrective.

4

Evading Evidentialism and Exploiting "Possibility": Strategies of Ignorance, Isolation, and Inflation

In the 1957 film "Twelve Angry Men," at the start of the jury's deliberations a straw poll yields one "not guilty" and eleven "guilty" votes. The lone juror, played by Henry Fonda, concerned that conviction on a murder charge not be hasty, says defensively, ". . . supposing we're wrong." To this another juror responds indignantly, "Supposing we're wrong? Suppose this building should fall down on my head! You can suppose anything."[1]

My sympathies are with the second juror. In fact, throughout roughly the first third of the movie the Fonda character repeatedly appeals to mere suppositions, typically without the least attempt, as he recognizes, to back them up as at all probable.[2] This reasoning fits the popular *argument from ignorance,* a fallacy first labeled by Locke (*Argumentum ad Ignorantiam*)—though I do not adhere to his characterization. (Locke 1975: book IV, ch. 12, section 20). One argues from ignorance when the failure to disprove a claim is taken to be sufficient for establishing either that it should not be rejected, or that it is creditable, or even that it is worthy of belief.

The argument from ignorance is one of three strategies or arguments that seek to circumvent evidential demands. (By stipulation, "strategy," "circumvent," and related words or phrases, as used here, do not imply any devious intent.) Less attention is given here to strategies of *isolation* or *inflation,* however, because the argument from ignorance is the most relevant to the ethics of belief and the most influential. (Also, strategies of isolation are already the subject of an extensive literature, though not so labeled.) Isolation arguments attempt to protect favored beliefs from the reach of criticism by claiming that these beliefs are intelligible only within a specific framework of assumptions and practices. Criticisms outside that framework inevitably fail to reach these beliefs, for failure of sufficient overlap in assumptions or meaning.

Arguments from ignorance and isolation provide handy ways to protect favored beliefs from evidential demands. The protection affects a difficult-to-discern shift of attention away from examining those favored beliefs to broader, usually controversial, issues. Where the broader issues displace critical examination of the focal ones, the protection realizes an *inflationary* strategy. In chapters 1 and 2, I treated as inflationary the extrinsic claims that evidentialism requires foundationalism, voluntarism, or a substantive account of rationality.

Interest in these strategies is both practical and theoretical. Practically, they defend beliefs that oppose scientific method and findings, as well as common sense. Theoretically, these strategies challenge evidentialism.

I   Arguments from Ignorance

1   "Possibility" and Arguments from Ignorance

A subtle example of an argument from ignorance derives from a recent book by C. D. B. Bryan reporting on the 1992 conference at MIT on reports of alien abductions:

> During the days immediately following the conference, I am struck by how my perception of the abduction phenomenon has changed: I no longer think it a joke. This is not to say I now believe UFOs and alien abduction are *real*—"real" in the sense of a reality subject to the physical laws of the universe as we know them—but rather that I feel something very mysterious is going on. And based as much on what has been presented at the conference as on the intelligence, dedication, and sanity of the majority of the presenters, I cannot reject out-of-hand the *possibility* that what is taking place isn't exactly what the abductees are saying is happening to them. And if that is so, the fact that no one has been able to pick up a tailpipe from a UFO does not mean UFOs do not exist. It means only that UFOs might not have tailpipes. As Boston University astronomer Michael Papagiannis insisted, "The absence of evidence is not evidence of absence." (Bryan 1995: 230)

As this example shows, arguments from ignorance come in such varieties that it is easy to overlook not only the nature of the arguments, but that any argument is being offered at all. The writer explicitly denies concluding that alien UFOs are real. In effect, he is denying that the reasoning even constitutes argument. Moreover, if there is a conclusion, it is only for the *possibility* that the abductees story is correct, a judgment so weak that argument seems hardly called for.

Nevertheless, the above reasoning does amount to an argument with forceful implications, and it is an argument from ignorance. Although they have many guises, the fullest arguments from ignorance have the following structure:

(1) No one has disproved (refuted) that *p*.

So, (2) it is possible that *p* is true.

So, (3) there is reason not to reject *p* as false. (Or: *p*'s truth is seriously possible.)

(4) If there is reason not to reject *p* as false, then we should keep our minds open to the investigation of *p*'s truth.

So, (5) we should keep our minds open to the investigation of *p*'s truth.

(6) If we should keep our minds open to the investigation of *p*'s truth, then it is reasonable (permissible) to believe that *p*.

So, (7) it is reasonable (permissible) to believe that *p*.[3]

There are three crucial inferences in this schema. The first is from (1) to (2), and the second is from (2) to (3). Steps (3) to (5) introduce nothing new. (The opening two examples proceed explicitly to step (2) and by implication to step (5).) The final steps from (5) to (7), which are most evidently in conflict with the intrinsic ethics of belief, are the subject of section 3 below. In this and the next section, my main concern is with the step from (1) to (2), with some, but much less, attention to the step from (2) to (3).

It is apparent that this form of argument and any number of variants cannot be valid. Each of the crucial inferences moves from weak claims to considerably stronger conclusions. This appearance needs to be firmed down. But then the task remains of explaining why instances of this form are persuasive and influential. The two parts of that explanation that I focus on are related: ambiguities in uses of "possibility" and pragmatic or conversational expectations. Although I shall take my main example from the previous quote on the alien abduction stories, I shall not be interested in any detailed refutation of it. My point is to expose the fallacies inherent in any argument from ignorance, not especially those in this one.

In practice, and as the prior quote substantiates, arguments from ignorance are rarely presented as starkly as the formal rendition above. They are embedded in accounts that support a hypothesis not merely by noting the absence of refutation, but by offering or suggesting positive reasons or evidence. Still, the abstraction is justified if an argument from ignorance is one strand of reasoning in the account.[4]

The structure as it stands licenses inconsistent beliefs.[5] The argument calls for only one observational or factual claim (1). All the rest are to follow by inference ((4) and (6) are conditionals that express inferences). Let p=The Yankees will win the World Series in 2007, which obviously satisfies premise (1). No one has disproved it. We then derive (7): It is reasonable to believe that the Yankees will win in 2007. But premise (1) is also true if p=The Yankees will not win the World Series in 2007, licensing as well the derivation of the inconsistent belief at step (7).

This inconsistency is to be set aside. Presumably, further restrictions are intended on the content to which arguments from ignorance are to apply, although the only ones I am familiar with, as discussed in section 3 below, do not solve the problem. More pertinent is that there is no inconsistency if we stop at step (3), yet treacherous assumptions remain in the moves from (1) to (3).

There are stronger and weaker readings of "disproved," which recur for "possibility," that are crucial to the persuasiveness of the argument. On the weaker reading, an empirical hypothesis is disproved only if there is either a proof or demonstration of its falsity or specific observations against it. A hypothesis not disproved on the weaker reading is disproved on the stronger reading if it is incompatible with our background beliefs and with readily drawn inferences from them and our evidence.

No one has observed the absence of alien invaders and, let us suppose, there is currently no proof of the impossibility of the alien-abduction stories. (We return to this supposition below.) Does the lack of disproof on the weaker reading imply a lack of disproof on the stronger reading? If the hypothesis is possible in the weak sense of being self-consistent and consistent with current observations is it possible in the stronger sense of being either worthy of investigation or compatible with physical regularities and laws? These alternatives allude to a central distinction between *real, genuine,* or *metaphysical* possibility and *epistemic* possibility (possibility according to one's beliefs or knowledge). However, if the latter is understood as consistency with one's beliefs or knowledge, then a negative answer follows for both alternatives. The argument from ignorance will fail of cogency at its first step, from premise (1) to (2).

In "Twelve Angry Men" the second juror's background beliefs (together with various facts and observations) exclude the (physical) possibility of the building falling down on his head, since that is incompatible with his knowledge of natural laws, the construction of buildings, and just normal goings-on. The second juror knows that it isn't (physically) possible that the building will fall, unless there were great and noticeable disturbances (e.g., a bomb is exploded in the building). But since the crucial background beliefs reflect the regularities or laws governing the world, the second premise is false also if taken to imply a real possibility.[6] Against the reports of the alien abductees is the vast evidence of the established physical laws that would have to be violated if they were correct.[7] Specifically, regular visits of aliens assume possibilities for space travel at velocities that accelerate close to, if not exceeding, the speed of light.

I have so far not questioned the assumption that denies evidence, or significant or decisive evidence, against the alien abduction stories, a denial that is characteristic of arguments from ignorance that seek to establish existential claims (e.g., we are subject to astrological influences, some persons have telekinetic powers, there is life after death). The denial seeks to draw strength from the truism that you cannot observe what does not exist. But it falsely assumes that the only way empirically to establish nonexistence would be through direct (observational) evidence.

We find this misleading focus in the quote above, which ends with the clever turn of phrase that "The absence of evidence is not evidence of absence." This claim is false both in detail and in spirit. One of the most important ways we accumulate warrant for our beliefs is through *"absent" evidence*. If a hypothesis (or belief) is true, then it is expected to have certain effects. Its having these effects confirms it; their absence disconfirms it. But if these effects are expected, their occurrence will typically go unnoticed.[8] For example, driving toward the Holland Tunnel with the radio on, I hear no announcement of a traffic jam. If there were a traffic jam, the radio station would have mentioned it. Since no traffic jam is announced, I just stay on course. My belief that there is no traffic jam is confirmed (without notice or tacitly, as discussed in chap. 6). A memorable illustration of absent-evidence reasoning is the climax of Conan Doyle's Sherlock Holmes story "Silver Blaze." In that story, a dog's not barking is not noticed because it is a mere absence. But for Holmes it is a crucial clue that someone who knew the dog well is the culprit. Holmes's brilliance is his ability to find a clue where no one else finds anything even to notice.

Absent evidence justifies our dismissal of claims that are in stark conflict with massively well-confirmed factual and scientific beliefs (e.g., claims such as the denial that the Holocaust took place as standardly reported). The lack of active reports from credible sources supporting these claims is hardly explicable except on the assumption that there is nothing to report. For the Holocaust, in particular, the long series of closely related events denied is of great interest and importance. If the denials were credible, many historians, of very diverse backgrounds and commitments, would converge on the project of investigating them. Furthermore, the Holocaust is not just one contained event, but rather a history of many, interrelated events with many, readily detectable consequences of different sorts. For the Holocaust deniers to be correct requires an incredible, unprecedented conspiracy of silence or gross incompetence among historians. Even before the detailed evidence supporting the reality of the Holocaust is again brought before public scrutiny, the thundering testimony of absent evidence, which we all share, constitutes more than adequate refutation.

Relying on absent evidence is, then, a great device of economy. We needn't gather it to be entitled to use it. Yet, its workings allow us to ignore denials of background beliefs. Our confidence in such background beliefs sometimes needs bolstering because, when the occasional denial is actually made, we are in an uneasy position. We represent ourselves as in a commanding position of knowledge. Yet the actual specific evidence most of us can point to is scant, since there is little point in retaining it. Worse, though absent evidence is enormously prevalent and forceful, it is easy to overlook because of its constancy.

In the case of claims of alien abductions, there is enormous absent evidence against them. It is not credible that clear evidence would go undetected, if the stories were true. Yet, if even slight genuine clues were discovered favoring the stories, they would be of incalculable interest to diverse investigators and to the public. But at present there are no real stirrings among reputable investigators, only murmers at the extremes. The lack of interest is supported by extensive scientific studies that so far detect no intelligent life outside the earth.

Absent evidence for a hypothesis assumes that, if the hypothesis were correct, its implications would be readily apparent and reported. Specifically, counting the lack of attention among scientists as absent evidence against an empirical hypothesis depends on numerous assumptions such as that enough open-minded investigators are attuned to the consequences of the hypothesis that its predictions would be readily detected. Otherwise the neglect may be due to external influences such as that the hypothesis offends religious or political groups.

In the case of fringe claims, there are, in fact, always scientifically knowledgeable persons with an interest in their verification. The proper way to understand the motivation of these "fringe watchers" is curiosity and a concern that the public not be hoodwinked. There is neither inconsistency nor hypocrisy in investigating or discussing claims that one regards as worthless.

If absent evidence can have the force that I accord it to establish the falsity of existential claims, it will also be capable of establishing their impossibility. After all, if in diverse enough circumstances where a hypothesis ought to have noticeable effects, it does not, the best explanation might be that the hypothesis could not be true. The result appears too strong if we identify all possibility with only formal consistency or consistency with observations, ignoring narrower kinds of possibility, especially physical. But even in the latter case, the result seems too strong if genuine possibility is confused with epistemic possibility, as what we can conceive or seem able to conceive. Whether a hypothesis appears possible often turns on our ability to conceive it true compatible with our evidence. It seems to me that I can readily conceive that the alien abduction stories are true. Science fiction is packed with such conceivabilities.

However, *conceivability* (or the appearance of conceivability) does not establish genuine possibility—that what we take ourselves to conceive is really a way that the world could be; that what we take ourselves to conceive is compatible with physical laws and conceptual necessities. Hilary Putnam (1975, especially 229–235) makes this point vivid, based on his and Saul Kripke's (1972) work: We can conceive that water is not H_2O, even if it is. Yet, nothing could truly be water, however similar its ostensible properties, unless it is H_2O. Analogously, we seem able to begin coherent thoughts: "If my parents were the Rockefellers, then . . .". Although it is imaginable (or seemingly imaginable) that my parents are the Rockefellers, it is not really possible. No child of theirs could be me.[9]

Once the distinction between conceivability and real possibility is drawn, it becomes hard to understand how the two could be confused. One is about us and what we know and believe; the other is about the world (what's really possible in it). Nor is it apparent how a lack of evidence against a possibility can be recast as evidence supporting that possibility. Stephen Yablo rightly wonders, "do I acquire evidence in *favor* of a proposition's possibility, by finding myself *without* evidence against its truth? That would be very strange, to say the least. Among other things it would have the result that there is a necessary limit on how bad my epistemological position can get: the *poorer* my evidence for p's truth, the *better* my evidence for its possibility. . . . Yet the fact is that I can be *completely* in the dark about truth and possibility simultaneously" (1993: 8). In general, we cannot infer from "It is not the case that the evidence shows that p is impossible" to either "p is possible" or "The evidence shows that p is possible." For comparison, observe that from "It is not the case that the evidence shows that John does not believe p" we cannot derive either "John believes p" or "The evidence shows that John believes p."[10]

We have been arguing that the lack of direct disproof or the weak possibility that the alien abduction stories enjoy yields almost nothing further. We can still know that the stories are false, and even that it is not now possible for them to be true, where the latter "possible" is used in its rich, narrow, and ordinary sense. The confusion here is found for much less dramatic claims. In a setting treating of induction, we affirm the possibility of a future event's occurring contrary to well-founded expectations (e.g., the flipped coin will land on its edge). But, unless we are in the grip of skepticism, we will allow both that we can know in advance that the coin will not land on its edge and that it is not possible for it to do so.

However, there is a standard move in opposition to the claim that we know that the alien-abduction stories could not be true because, among other obstacles, they would violate known laws of nature: "just because UFOs and their occupants defy our laws of physics does not mean there are not further laws of physics we have not as yet discovered or do not as yet comprehend" (Bryan 1995: 422). This blank-check assumption attempts to protect the hypothesis of alien visits from the reach of massive undermining background evidence. Yet, in a crucial way it actually weighs it down. However implausible it is to hypothesize alien visits, it is vastly more implausible to claim that they obey new, undetected laws of physics.

The reduction in this quote to bare possibility is disguised overtly ("does not mean"), but also covertly. The suggestions offered appear as specific (contentful) hypotheses ("further laws"). Yet, there is no evidence cited on their behalf.

As a methodological matter, however, why shouldn't we take bare possibility as sufficient for worthiness to investigate, since it would increase the number of candidate hypotheses put forward to explain phenomena, and so decrease the chances of overlooking the correct hypothesis? The suggestion is, however, illusory. It is a banality of the philosophy of science that an unlimited number of hypotheses are strictly compatible with any finite collection of evidence. The banality implies not that for any interesting phenomenon, there are always a vast number of hypotheses worth investigating, but rather that a vast number must be dismissed as a precondition for any serious investigation.

There is a deeper objection to taking the bare possibility that p as a sufficient reason not to disbelieve or reject it. The second juror's implied argument is that if the bare possibility that the defendant did not commit the crime is a reason not to believe that the defendant is guilty, then, by parity, one ought not believe that the building will not soon collapse. But to have reason not to believe something as evident as the latter is to have reason to believe practically nothing. Admitting possibilities as reasons not to disbelieve appears innocent, when it is not realized that these thereby also constitute undermining reasons. And because these possibilities are so cheaply harvested, they would undermine a vast number of innocent beliefs. This is the central wrong and danger with arguments from ignorance. If so weak a notion as not being disproved or being a bare possibility is a sufficient reason to withdraw from disbelief, then reasons or evidence in general lose force.

Once we appreciate the equivocations on "possibility," it is pointless to expend energy on steps (4) and (5) in the original reconstruction. Step (5) asks, in seeming innocence, that we keep an "open mind." But "open mind," as invoked in arguments from ignorance, is the wolf in sheep's clothing, trading on the same ambiguities we found in the use of "possible." In fact, contrary to the usage suggested in premises (4) and (5), "open-minded" should be applied to one's procedures for belief, not to the content of what is believed. When evidence is inconclusive a gap is thought to open for the will to operate. But, as noted in chapters 1 and 2, there is no real gap. The inconclusiveness of the evidence as to whether *p* holds is conclusive that we cannot fully believe (or disbelieve) it. Inquiry remains open. Analogously, what marks an open-minded person is not what he regards as live possibilities. That is a conclusion to be reached. It is the way the conclusion is reached that marks an open-minded person. The open-minded person follows where the evidence leads. If the evidence against alien abductions and against many other supernatural and paranormal conjectures is overwhelming, an open-minded person must reject them.

2   Selective Relevance and Some Pragmatics for "Possibility"

On the analysis I have offered the argument from ignorance is a fallacy. To understand a fallacy requires not just exposing flaws in the reasoning, but explaining its persuasive force, despite the lack of cogency.

In the previous section, we observed that the claim that there is no disproof of the alien abduction stories focuses us on forefront evidence. But in conceding this focus, we do not attend to our background evidence or beliefs that, together with current evidence, may yet be incompatible with *p*.[11] This illusion of focus was a main part of my effort to explain the persuasiveness of the fallacy through noting confusions and ambiguities in uses of "possibility" and related terms. The explanation suggests that our conversational expectations are being exploited. In accepting premise (1) ("not disproved"), we charitably treat the implied "possibility" at its weakest, so premises (1) and (2) seem true. However, in moving from (1) to the explicit assertion of a possibility in (2) or in moving from (2) to (3) ("there is reason . . ."), we are charitable in the opposed direction by taking "possible" as much stronger, so the inference appears warranted.

In a common use of "possible" (and the cognate use of "may") a commercial says that eating Cheerios regularly *may* prevent cancer. The proposed possibility is meant to refer to something stronger (narrower) than physical possibility (Lycan 1994: chap. 8). The commercial is alluding, presumably, to studies that indicate that persons who eat substances like that in Cheerios regularly have a lower risk of certain forms of cancer. But compatibility with these reports is still too weak to differentially favor Cheerios over its competitors. Rather, the commercial's *saying* that Cheerios may prevent cancer comes to suggest or implicate that there is a significant probability that it will, since only then would the contribution distinguish Cheerios from its competitors, and so be informative. However, to simply assert the latter would require empirical backing, which the company cannot marshal (in a commercial anyway) and which would also subject them to legal challenges. So they assert what is too weak to be either differentially informative or risky. But they get their meaning across by suggesting or implicating what is more relevant and informative, without raising either an expectation for backing or a legal threat.

These unearned transitions are promoted both by a lack of explicitness (chap. 3) and by pragmatic expectations.[12] Conversational or pragmatic expectations have the right scope and influence to explain the persuasiveness of arguments from ignorance and many similar fallacies that lead us to tolerate incredible or starkly implausible claims. For conversation is pervasive, natural, and generally successful. The fundamental expectation is after all that the speaker will be cooperative, and so we are reluctant to judge as wildly off a speaker with whom we are conversing. Indeed, as I discuss briefly in chapter 5, since hearers will not accept a speaker's assertion if blatantly wild (untruthful), conversation is tightly shaped so that speakers do not offer strikingly false assertions. Why waste your breath? But if so, the effectiveness of our plausibility assessments, and our competence and ease in making them, are not salient or explicit. On occasions when actually incredible claims are offered to us—like about alien abductions—we are then disposed not to view them as wild.

I want to delve further into the role of a lack of explicitness and pragmatics to help explain the persuasive force of arguments from ignorance, especially their exploitation of the ambiguities of "possibility." A memorable example from Wittgenstein is useful for showing the connection-between slides on "possibility" and a lack of explicitness. In opposing Platonic views of the necessity of logical or mathematical laws, Wittgenstein (1956) asks us what we would think of a tribe that

148. . . . piled the timber in heaps of arbitrary, varying heights and then sold it at a price proportionate to the area covered by the piles?
   And what if they even justified this with the words: "Of course, if you buy more timber, you must pay more"?

149. How could I shew them that—as I should say—you don't really buy more wood if you buy a pile covering a bigger area?—I should, for instance, take a pile which was small by their ideas and, by laying the logs around, change it into a "big" one. This *might* convince them—but perhaps they would say: "Yes, now it's a *lot* of wood and costs more"—and that would be the end of the matter.—We should presumably say in this case: they simply do not mean the same by "a lot of

wood" and "a little wood" as we do; and they have a quite different system of payment from us.

Even if Wittgenstein's description is merely a lengthy way of convincing us that the practice he describes is not contradictory (weak or bare possibility), there is more than a hint that the practice is meant as a serious possibility—that such a tribe really could thrive in some remote region. Barry Stroud casts doubt on whether the description succeeds on the stronger reading. He observes:

> When first presented with these examples it seems that we can understand, and that we can come to know what such people would be like. . . .
>   When we look more closely at the examples, are they really as intelligible as they seemed at first? For instance, consider the people who sell wood at a price proportionate to the area covered by the pile of wood and who defend their doing so in the way described earlier. Surely they would have to believe that a one-by-six-inch board all of a sudden increased in size or quantity when it was turned from resting on its one-inch edge to resting on its six-inch side. And what would the relation between quantity and weight possibly be for such people? A man could buy as much wood as he could possibly lift, only to find, upon dropping it, that he had just lifted more wood than he could possibly lift. (1971: 456)

After further illustration of the dubious intelligibility of this group, Stroud declares, "the initial intelligibility and strength of Wittgenstein's examples derive from their being severely isolated or restricted. We think we can understand and accept them as representing genuine alternatives only because the wider-reaching consequences of counting, calculating, and so forth, in these deviant ways are not brought out explicitly" (1971: 457). Once we render *explicit* the implications of these practices and actions, they cease to be intelligible.

According to the discussion in the previous chapter, explicitness would unmask incoherence. The generalization underlying these practices will imply that the mass or weight of an everyday physical substance varies with the surface area it encompasses. Inevitably this generalization will be incompatible with commitments of members of the tribe through their ordinary practices and activities, as in measurement, which require conservation of matter. By keeping implicit the details of this practice, Wittgenstein ensures that the inconsistencies do not show up. So the lack of contradiction in the description of the tribe is liable to be mistakenly treated as sufficient for its being a serious and real possibility that such a tribe exists.

A second way we are led to jump from weak to strong possibility (constituting a reason not to disbelieve) is grounded in the conversational expectation that speakers will be informative. We take it that what the speaker affirms about a particular, he does not intend to affirm about a much broader class; for if he did intend it, he should make the stronger, more informative assertion as long as this would not introduce prolixity. If you tell me that Tony is an honors student in Mrs. Murphy's class, I infer that you do not know whether all the students in Mrs. Murphy's class are honors students; for if you did know that, you would say so ("Tony is in Mrs. Murphy's class of honors students"). Consequently, in presuming that a speaker is cooperative, we take his affirmation about a particular not to hold, as far as the speaker knows, throughout the broader class. Call this kind of expectation of informativeness *selective relevance* (Adler 1984). This expectation disposes us not to view Wittgenstein's story as establishing only that his tribe is minimally possible, a possibility less secure than monkeys typing out Hamlet, given unlimited time. That possibility applies to almost any self-consistent tale, including ludicrous ones.

The equivocations on "possibility" that we have been exploring stem from two sources, lack of explicitness and pragmatics. The two are related. Consider how the members of Wittgenstein's proposed tribe resemble the children younger than 7, described by Piaget, who fail his "conservation" tests. In a typical Piagetian experiment, two sticks of equal length are aligned. The child is asked whether they are the same size, and he answers "yes." One of the sticks is then moved forward, and the same question is asked. The nonconserving child now answers "no." Wittgenstein's tribe members are also nonconservers—change the area taken up by a pile of wood, and you have more (or less) wood. We are puzzled by Piaget's children, although not nearly as much as we should be by Wittgenstein's tribe of adults. Many of the ordinary activities and judgments of these children would obviously be distorted by a lack of conservation. Do children think that when they crouch, their height or weight is altered?[13]

Other experimenters in child development have conjectured that children younger than 7 fail Piaget's tests partly for pragmatic reasons. The children expect that when the experimenter moves the stick, his manipulation serves a purpose, which is selectively relevant to answering the question he asks as to whether the lengths remain equal in size. The child's answer that the sticks are unequal in length grants selective relevance to the experimenter's action, and thus renders his questions and his conduct cooperative. Otherwise, his moving of the sticks is pointless. The pragmatics of children older than 7 is more sophisticated. They know that some persons perform actions that are noticeably bad for fulfilling their manifest purposes, whether for reasons of fun or inadvertence or indifference.

If this conjecture is correct, then if experimenters cancel the expectation of relevance, the young children should now give the conserving answer as well. In one of a huge number of variations on Piaget's basic design, the children are introduced to a mischievous "teddy" doll who just messes things up. When it is teddy who destroys the alignment, the young children give the more "conserving" answer (Donaldson 1978: chap. 6). The expectation of selective relevance is relaxed because teddy's actions are visibly not purposeful and not directed at the child. Once the expectation is relaxed, conservation seems to exercise a compelling pull and so the illogic formally ascribed is not sustained.

Unlike Wittgenstein, Piaget appears to establish the serious possibility of nonconserving children from an actual demonstration. The transition from taking Piaget's description to be self-consistent to taking it to actually hold is facilitated by the combination of a lack of explicitness and conversational expectations. Once these expectations are cancelled, the experimental design no longer establishes the realistic possibility of nonconservation, even if it does succeed at showing a fault in children's expectations.

The result suggests a conjecture that is applicable to arguments from ignorance generally. The seeming conceivability of an interrelated set of states of affairs (as in the alien abduction stories) is evidence for its genuine possibility only if the conceivability can be sustained on explicitization of the details assumed or required. The hypotheses and claims that we have been considering in this and the previous section, even when weakly possible and not directly disproven, fail this conjecture. The more we articulate the conditions that would have to hold for them to be true, the sooner we come across inconsistency with firm beliefs.

3   William James and Willing to Believe

The most famous argument illustrating, and also defending, the steps from (5) to (7)—from the possibility of a hypothesis to our having a reason to believe it—is William James's argument in "The Will to Believe" (1951). Very briefly, James claimed that if the evidence for a proposition is indeterminate but there are deep personal reasons for believing it—and suspending judgment is effectively no different from disbelieving—then it is permissible (and rational) to come to believe that proposition. The avowed target of James's argument is evidentialism. In examining James's argument I will not rehash chapter 2's topic of whether we can decide to believe.

James assumes that many religious (and ethical) propositions are undecided by the evidence. He thinks that for some people these propositions meet the additional conditions that the questions raised are forced (or nonoptional), and that the matter for decision is "living" and "momentous." By adding these conditions, James restricts the scope of his argument. Still, none of these conditions removes the (alleged) indeterminacy of the evidence. Many potential beliefs will be living and momentous to some people, including belief in the existence of Santa Claus, Zeus, the devil, ghosts, angels, or the earth as the center of the universe. These can each be "forced" in James's sense, if a lack of belief leads one to actions indistinguishable from that of disbelievers. What is to block these and similar unwanted applications of his reasoning?

Yet, James viewed his argument as offered on behalf of an interest in truth. Early on in the essay, James observes that "There are two ways of looking at our duty in the matter of opinion. . . . We must know the truth; and we must avoid error—these are our first and great commandments as would-be knowers. . . ." He then formulates his most basic thesis in terms of gaining or losing truth: "*Our passional nature . . . must decide an option between propositions, whenever it is a genuine option that cannot by its nature be decided on intellectual grounds; for to say, under such circumstances, 'Do not decide, but leave the question open,' is itself a passional decision . . . and is attended with the same risk of losing the truth*" (1951: 95, his emphasis). How is our decision to believe supposed to yield a gain of truth, even if it risks error? James writes: "There are . . . cases where a fact cannot come at all unless a preliminary faith exists in its coming. *And where faith in a fact can help create the fact,* that would be an insane logic which should say that faith running ahead of scientific evidence is the 'lowest kind of immorality'" (1951: 104–105). The analogy here is with trust. James compares the risk of error in willing to believe with the risk of disappointment in trying to be friends with someone or asking someone to marry. The risks of rejection and the benefit of a safer policy of always waiting for the other to take the first step can be more than offset by the expected rewards of extending oneself. However, one is trusting in the hope of reciprocation, perhaps even in order to inspire it. The trust may be well founded, but one can have a trusting attitude while well aware of one's limited chances of success. In contrast, belief's claim to truth applies in the very adoption of the attitude; it does not wait on a future payoff.

James's most crucial condition is that the choice is "forced." This condition has a formal dimension unlike his other conditions, which are overtly personal and prudential. A forced choice is created by exhaustive alternatives. The choice of loving me or hating me is not forced because "your option is avoidable." However, he writes, "if I say, 'Either accept this truth or go without it,' I put on you a forced option, for there is no standing place outside of the alternative" (1951: 89). If you do not "accept this truth" you thereby "go without it," and vice versa. A forced choice is meant to rule out suspension of belief.

James is presumably thinking here of the law of the excluded middle (p or not p). However, even where the alternatives are exhaustive, because of a "complete logical disjunction," injection of belief creates the further alternative of not believing, that is, suspending judgment. But the religious hypothesis James holds is a forced option: "We cannot escape the issue by remaining skeptical and waiting for more light, because, although we do avoid error in that way *if religion be untrue,* we lost the good, if it be true, just as certainly as if we positively choose to disbelieve" (1951: 106). If we fail to believe, and not just if we disbelieve, we do not act as believers. In not acting as believers, in not taking part in religious practices or rituals, we effectively lose any truth that the religion has to offer. The agnostic is no better positioned than the atheist to grasp religious truth, if it is true. If suspension of judgment amounts to disbelief, then either attitude (belief or disbelief) will exceed the evidence. Neither response is settled by the evidence. But we must take one. Since neither option is more rational than the other, James's resolution is that it is open to us to do either.

Obviously, James is drawing an analogy with practical reasoning. In general, when options press themselves on us and call for decision, action is effectively under a "one must act" axiom, and so in the simplest case, if the choice is doing A or doing nothing:

Not-doing A implies (effectively) doing not-A (e.g., not applying to medical school implies [effectively] deciding not to apply to medical school).

It is this axiom that James wants to import into belief. This is the point of his various comparisons with friendship or love, and their call on us to extend trust. Not to decide to extend oneself to another is in practical consequences indistinguishable from deciding not to extend oneself.

The comparison holds up only when options are pressing themselves on us. However, the vast number of acts that we might do or options for action that we might select do not press themselves on us. You are under no pressure to choose between the options of wearing a crown of silver and diamonds or one of platinum and rubies. Similarly, there is no question before you as to whether you should believe that Babe Ruth drank two-fifths of a half-filled glass of water on his thirteenth birthday.

In the relatively few cases, when options do press themselves—for example, the deadline to apply to medical school is imminent—we can still only say that not deciding to apply is *effectively* no different from deciding not to apply. In the case of belief, to hold that there are no effective or practical differences between not believing and disbelieving assumes, prominently, that there is no side-effect on integrity—that disbelieving as an act of choice has no bearing otherwise on oneself as a believer.

But there is a more fundamental way the qualifier "effectively" is necessary. We simply cannot make the alternative of not-believing or suspending judgment go away. When James allows that, if we remain agnostic, "waiting for more light," then "we do avoid error in that way *if religion be untrue*," he is admitting the crucial distinction between claiming (believing) that *p* and not claiming (not believing) that *p*.

Moreover, contrary to the forced choice that James attempts to foist on us, his *"risk of losing the truth"* is a choice to which we regularly resign ourselves. Just think of all the facts that are buried in the past and that would greatly assist our understanding of history. If we cannot ascertain them, we just let them go, resigning ourselves to gaps in our historical understanding. It would surely not serve an interest in truth to "will to believe" those unknown facts. It is a commonplace that we risk error in accepting hypotheses, which always apply beyond our evidence. But taking that risk is not the same as knowingly adopting an attitude (belief) under conditions false to it. To the contrary, the risk is minimized to the extent that belief is in accord with the evidence.

Revealingly, James's argument is triggered not when the evidence is indeterminate, but only when it is *essentially* indeterminate. If a hypothesis is merely in fact undecided by the evidence so far, James grants that we should wait on the further evidence. He means his argument to enter only when the evidence is incapable of deciding an issue. Why should that be a difference that makes a difference? On the view defended here, it isn't. In full awareness, we find no difference between these cases—in both belief is withheld. James's reasoning trades on an illusion discussed in the previous section and in chapter 1. When the evidence is indeterminate a wedge is alleged to open up for the will to shore up the gap, as if certain propositions come to us begging to be believed. But no gap exists if the proper determinant of belief is one's epistemic position.[14]

The criticism of James's argument is that it does not follow out the implications of his own commitments. James knows that the choice between believing and disbelieving is not an excluded middle. Yet, the crux of his argument is that it should be so treated. But you cannot alter a logical truth to harmonize with a practical end.

In fact, James's essay, though it is probably the most famous attack on evidentialism, concedes a good deal to evidentialism. The evidentialism James seems to endorse is actually of the strong kind that I have defended here rather than the weaker, traditional kind that Clifford defended, and which is the explicit target of his attack. In section 2, James writes, "Does it not seem preposterous on the very face of it to talk of our opinions being modifiable at will? . . . Can we, by just willing it, believe that Abraham Lincoln's existence is a myth, and that the portraits of him in McClure's Magazine are all of some one else? . . . We can say any of these things, but we are absolutely impotent to believe them; and of just such things is the whole fabric of the truths that we do believe in made up" (1951: 90). What is the nature of this "can," which dictates that we cannot just will to believe for "the whole fabric of the truths"? It seems evident that it is not the "can" of mere ability, as James's closing statement indicates ("absolutely impotent"). But if it is the conceptual "can," so that the impossibilities stem from the concept of belief, then how could there be any room for the exceptions that James so famously argues for?

II   Isolation and Testability

If you ask yourselves, "How shall we recognize a word that the Lord has not uttered?", this is the answer: When the word spoken by the prophet in the name of the Lord is not fulfilled and does not come true, it is not a word by the Lord.
—Deuteronomy 18: 21–22

4   Testability and Burdens of Proof

In the next two sections, I consider the attempt to isolate beliefs in order to protect them from exposure to criticism. In contemporary civilizations, the attempt at isolation as a practical maneuver faces even more forcefully the difficulty that C. S. Peirce noted for two inferior methods of belief fixation. The *method of tenacity* has the "social impulse against it": "The man who adopts it will find that other men think differently from him. . . . Unless we make ourselves hermits, we shall necessarily influence each other's opinions; so that the problem becomes how to fix belief, not in the individual merely, but in the community." Similarly, the *method of authority* faces the difficulty that "no institution can undertake to regulate opinions upon every subject" (1957: 23–24).

In this section, the isolation strategy considered is the attempt to immunize favored beliefs from the reach of testability, a demand of evidentialism. For our beliefs to reflect the world accurately, we need to allow them to be vulnerable to refutation. Although I shall be promoting testability in opposition to the isolation strategy, that promotion, like the recommendation of explicitness in chapter 3, is circumspect. There are important conditions under which testability should be resisted.

Although the opposition between isolation and testability is the focus of discussion, the harm to testability of isolationist ploys is only one kind of danger. I use the term "isolationism" to suggest erecting barriers to appreciation of a claim's full range of significant implications. In section 3 above, the realistic coherence of Wittgenstein's description of his strange nonconserving tribe was shown to depend on an extremely limited account of their activities. Once we draw out the implications of a tribe of nonconservers in everyday and unavoidable activities, the coherence evaporates. In the previous chapter, I sought to corroborate my claims about the limited rationality of projects of self-deception, including cognitive dissonance and related phenomena, by removing isolationist strictures. Under conditions of ongoing behavior, the potential costs from hiding or obscuring a well-founded belief increase. As a consequence, the rationality of the self-deceptive projects diminish. Both of these examples illustrate ways that isolationist strategies seek to dodge demands of testability, which I now proceed to treat at length.

Karl Popper originally introduced falsifiability as a criterion for demarcating science from nonscience: "it must be possible for an empirical scientific system to be refuted by experience" (1959: 41). Since the spirit of falsifiability is of much broader import than its implied restriction to scientific claims and because I want to distance myself from some of Popper's (anti-inductivist) metaphysics, I prefer to speak of "testability." Testability is a broadened and vaguer kind of falsifiability. A judgment or claim is testable if it has precise implications that can be subject to critical tests. It is a hallmark of intellectual honesty to express one's judgment or claim so as to facilitate testing it. Explicitness furthers testability, because it enlarges the range of beliefs to which new beliefs need to cohere and it limits in advance maneuvering room to evade refutation, subsequent to negative discoveries. However, the benefit of accepting the greater risk is that the credibility of one's own view is accordingly raised, if it survives the risk.

Testability is one of those unavoidable commitments that give explicitness its bite. What renders testability an unavoidable commitment is that, since we care that our beliefs be true, we place them under conditions where they risk exposure as false. However, testability can have this great value only if it is accompanied by barriers to the ever-available routes to evasion.

The requirement of testability is generally accompanied by two others. The potential falsifying instances are specified in advance; and, correlatively, reports of falsification of a hypothesis or theory are not to be responded to through ad hoc protective maneuvers.[15] The underlying purpose of these additional requirements is clearly not restricted to science. They are simply devices to enforce impartiality and to impose external controls, like "double-blind" medical experiments.

In public argument, related meta-criteria weigh in through the structure of *burdens of proof*, alluded to in chapter 3 section 5 above, which dictate who must establish a case, and who must merely defend against a challenge. The onus falls on the violator of our "unavoidable . . . canons of evaluation." So if you appear to treat like cases differently, you carry a burden of showing that the cases differ. Although "burdens of proof" has a legalistic ring, these burdens arise naturally within many practices like those that impose a structure of authority. We are not jolted by the opening of the *Declaration of Independence*, with its forthright admission that political rebels, like the authors, bear the burden of proof: "a decent respect to the opinions of mankind requires that they should declare the causes which impel them to the separation." If the burden were not carried by those who seek to "dissolve the political bands," the state would be denied authority and hence legitimacy.

Burdens of proof help maintain practices not governed by an explicit code (e.g., a legal code). If you are late, you ought to offer an excuse. Repeated excuses, however, shift the burden of proof from someone who refuses to accept an excuse back on to the one offering them. Those to whom the repeated excuses are offered can reject the umpteenth one, relieved now of the demand of politeness or civility that they not reject an excuse without explanation. We use statistical measures, similarly, as meta-criteria to detect biases. If a company with a commitment to impartial hiring appoints a highly disproportionate number of persons who are relatives or close friends of the manager, then we judge its hiring procedures, or its application of those procedures, biased. The statistical assessment is not merely another weight favoring some candidates over others. The burden has shifted, so that we may reject the fairness of the hiring without a duty to delve into the specifics of each case.

The spirit of testability is to accept the burden of supporting a claim at its fullest. It is to place one's reasons and arguments under an independent control or external constraint. Here's an example purposely selected for its familiarity and ethical import. A mother recommends to her son that he share his toys with a friend who is visiting. If the son balks, the mother conjectures that her son would want his friend to share with him if the son were at his friend's house. By offering her recommendation, the mother places determination of whether she is right or wrong outside her control. The mother places it on her son's moral imagination, although undoubtedly the placement is backed by her confidence in the Golden Rule. The mother accepts her burden and discharges it in the strongest way. In an only slightly extended usage, the mother can be said to render her recommendation testable.

5   Dodging Testability

Despite the broad scope and appeal of the spirit of testability, isolationist maneuvers to defy it are an enduring attraction. The simplest isolationist ploy is just to retreat from full belief to a non–truth claiming attitude such as *belief in*. In an avowedly Wittgensteinian vein, Norman Malcolm (1992) inclines toward finding incoherence in one's believing *that* God exists. He prefers belief "in God," which is a commitment only to a set of actions and practices. But, as Plantinga observes, "believing in God is indeed more than accepting the proposition that God exists. But if it is more than that, it is also at least that. One cannot sensibly believe in God and thank him for the mountains without believing that there *is* such a person to be thanked and that he is in some way responsible for the mountains. Nor can one trust in God and commit oneself to him without believing that he exists" (1983: 18).

Retreat from "belief that" is implicit when, for example, ostensibly divergent claims made by science and religion are held not to really conflict: "Science did one thing, religion did another: there was no logical contradiction."[16] If the claims of the Bible and of supernatural religions are not in conflict with those of science over, for example, the origins of the stars and of life, then the corresponding beliefs are not in conflict either. But, if not conflicting, they are not beliefs. Beliefs contrary in content (e.g., species arose through a purposeful act of creation; species evolve through natural selection) are conflicting beliefs.

A famed application of testability outside science is in Antony Flew's (1955) criticism of traditional defenses of theistic beliefs. In the example Flew develops, one explorer, looking with another at a clearing where flowers and weeds are growing, proclaims that a gardener is tending the clearing. After each test to detect the gardener fails, the first explorer seeks to explain away the failure by modifying his hypothesis: "But there is a gardener, invisible, intangible, insensible to electric shocks, a gardener who has no scent and makes no sound, a gardener who comes secretly to look after the garden he loves." Finally, his fellow explorer throws up his hands in exasperation: "But what remains of your original assertion? Just how does what you call an invisible, intangible, eternally elusive gardener differ from an imaginary gardener or even from no gardener at all?" (1955: 96). Without independent support, the qualifications reduce the proposal to a kind of bare possibility (that there is a gardener) that, I argued in section 1, is too weak to count as a genuine reason or evidence.

A less obvious cost of avoidance of testability is to diminish prospects for confirmation. Assumptions that protect one's claims limit the force of one's evidence. In Flew's example, if we had found a gardener's glove in the garden, we would take that as strong confirmation that a gardener had been working at the location. But if we introduce such unsubstantiated protective assumptions as that an invisible gardener was at work, the possibilities for explaining the glove independent of the gardener hypothesis expands accordingly, and so the surprise and confirmatory value of the discovery diminishes. Perhaps, the garden grows gloves, as well as plants?

In an article promoting experiential validation of religious beliefs, Alston (1983) begins by dismissing Flew's dilemma. The Christian beliefs that Alston considers "say that God will manifest Himself in certain ways in our individual or corporate experience. From time to time we find such manifestations in our experience. This provides empirical confirmation for the beliefs in question" (1983: 105). However, if confirmation involves the risk of falsification, then the absence of these manifestations should be disconfirming. But Alston's formulation leaves no room for disconfirmation: "our examples are not decisively disconfirmable by experience. They are markedly unspecific. They do not say *how* God will provide for His people, *when* or *under what conditions* one can expect a particular fruit of the spirit, just *what* Christ is going to do through his church, and what the *timetable* is. These 'somehow-somewhere-somewhen' statements are so formulated that whereas any positive instance will be confirming . . . , there can be no negative instances . . ." (1983: 106; see also Mitchell 1955). Alston's response to the not "really serious challenge" of testability is that although his favored hypothesis is protected from decisive disconfirmation, it is clearly open to confirmation by God's manifestation.

We should expect, however, that Alston's strategy to circumvent testability has serious costs. To diminish testability is to diminish possibilities for confirmation. If we drop Alston's artificial protective devices, all but logically or observationally decisive disconfirmation is readily available. Consider, as Alston does, the hypothesis that there are unicorns. If that hypothesis is unadorned with the "somehow-somewhere-somewhen" qualifier, then it is amply refuted by the absence of positive evidence. It is because we do treat the hypothesis as unadorned that the existence of unicorns is disconfirmed, a result that Alston no doubt endorses. The "somehow-somewhere-somewhen" protective device is self-defeating in another way. The absence of specification of conditions for repeated occurrences reduces opportunities for replication, a crucial check on the acceptance of an experiential or experimental report.

Use of Alston's maneuver in discussion or debate would violate norms of fair argument. Claims should be formulated that do not impede and in fact facilitate criticism, since in argument we seek to learn from others.

If the key step in Alston's isolationalist strategy is the appeal to what is "decisively disconfirmable," then, once again, the culprit is the ambiguity of "possibility," this time in the service of evading falsification.[17] Its service in this role is particularly prominent in Wittgensteinian attempts to isolate beliefs of radically different cultures from criticism of their fundamental assumptions. In Malcolm's influential article, discussed briefly above, he contrasts our belief in the conservation of matter with the beliefs of members of another culture who don't share our view. For them, "sometimes material things do go out of existence." They just vanish. The conception is not "radically incoherent," though it is unlikely. Malcolm remarkably declares: ". . . it does not appear to me that one position is supported by *better evidence* than is the other. Each position is compatible with ordinary experience. On the one hand it is true that familiar objects (watches, wallets, lawn chairs) occasionally disappear without any adequate explanation. On the other hand it happens, perhaps more frequently, that a satisfying explanation of the disappearance is discovered" (1992: 93; compare Wittgenstein 1969: sections 608–612). Contrary to Malcolm's (and Wittgenstein's) implied denial, these hypotheses are testable, and if they were tested, there is little doubt how the results would turn out. We could apply surveillance cameras to a random selection of objects resembling those that have disappeared in what we conjecture to be similar circumstances, in order to detect disappearances. Random samples of the reports of objects claimed to disappear are searched for with great effort, and a significant number of these turn up. The disappearance hypothesis violates laws of conservation while, presumably, proposing no mechanism to explain pure disappearance.

Similarly, under Wittgenstein's influence, in "Understanding a Primitive Society," Peter Winch discusses Azande belief in witchcraft: "The most important way of detecting the influence of witchcraft and of identifying witches is by the revelations of oracles, of which in turn the most important is the 'poison oracle'. . . . At an oracular consultation *benge* [the poison] is administered to a fowl, while a question is asked in a form permitting a yes or no answer. The fowl's death or survival is specified beforehand as giving the answer 'yes' or 'no.' The answer is then checked by administering benge to another fowl and asking the question the other way round. . . . The poison oracle is all-pervasive in Zande life and all steps of any importance in a person's life are settled by reference to it" (1970: 86). Since the practice (as we regard it) is unreliable, there must be times when "the oracle first says 'yes' and then 'no' to the same question." The result is no problem: "This does not convince a Zande of the futility of the whole operation of consulting oracles. . . . Various explanations may be offered, whose possibility. . . is built into the whole network of Zande beliefs and may, therefore, be regarded as belonging to the concept of an oracle. It may be said, for instance, that bad *benge* is being used; that the operator of the oracle is ritually unclean; that the oracle is being itself influenced by witchcraft or sorcery. . . . There are various ways in which the behavior of the fowl under the influence of *benge* may be ingeniously interpreted by those wise in the ways of the poison oracle (1970: 87–88). Winch's account, though avowing that Azande's practices are untestable, actually concedes it from the start. If "various explanations" are offered to explain away putative failure, the Azande presuppose compatibility with observational results as a test of the reliability of their methods.

As Winch recognizes, the success of ordinary Azande practices like planting crops depends on their testability (e.g., p. 103). But once Winch grants that the Azandes do rely on the rudimentary rules of testability, it follows that they grasp the handy ways its value can be cheapened without restriction on protective devices. Since their activities are shaped in response to predictive outcomes, they presume testability in the beliefs informing the predictions. But testability, as I have noted, demands meta-criteria to bar ad hoc attempts to explain falsification away. That Winch's Azande take themselves to have successfully explained away their counterevidence shows that these meta-criteria, like evidentialist-defying incoherence, can easily be evaded, particularly when socially supported and functional. What it does not show is that the Azande do not accept these meta-criteria.

Winch and Malcolm are both concerned, as was Wittgenstein, that to apply the notion of testability to religious or cultural practices would be to misunderstand their purposes. Winch writes: "The chief function of oracles is to reveal the presence of 'mystical' force. . . . The spirit in which oracles are consulted is very unlike that in which scientists make experiments. Oracular revelations are not treated as hypotheses and, since their sense derives from the way they are treated in their context, they therefore *are not* hypotheses. They are not a matter of intellectual interest but the main way in which Azande decide how they should act" (1970: 88). The Azande interest is not theoretical; it does not have to do with control and prediction, but rather guidance and tradition—to "reveal the presence of 'mystical force.'" For Winch, to view these matters otherwise is a "category mistake."

In a similar vein, Malcolm takes science and religion to constitute different "frameworks" with their own distinctive goals. Scientific evidence is appropriate to scientific claims, but not to religious beliefs: "there can be evidence for the particular doctrines of a faith only within the attitude of religious belief" (1992: 101). But why accept the assumption that if a belief is testable, its function must be scientific? The function of a heart is to pump blood. But I can still ask and answer the question of whether the heart would make for a good football. In asking and answering this stupid question ("No"), I in no way deny that the function of a heart is to pump blood. Similarly, however restricted the Azande's purposes are in their use of oracles, these purposes are not denied by asking whether or how their practice works. Applying the notion of testability does not deny that the intended purposes of the practice are other than prediction and control.

Recall from the opening remarks in this section that my objections to isolationist ploys work under the assumption that the isolationist is protecting genuine beliefs. If the Azande's beliefs, say, are not genuine—representational—beliefs, then the objections do not apply.[18] For reasons I have given here and elsewhere, especially chapter 9 below, if these are not genuine beliefs then there are a wide variety of important roles in guiding action, backing assertion, and facilitating inference that they cannot serve.

Contrary to isolationist assumptions, trial-and-error testing and testability are not parochial to scientific inquiries. The attempt to restrain the application of scientific methods is hopeless, because the rudiments of these methods are merely, as Quine claims, "self-conscious common sense" (1960: 3; see also Sellars 1963: 182–183). The isolationist ploy is especially implausible for the beliefs that animate discussion in the ethics of belief. They are precisely beliefs that are rich with diverse, verifiable implications well beyond any one practice. The success or failure of some of their implications should be apparent and noticeable, rather than hidden and ephemeral. If protective assumptions are made without independent support, the strength of a claim is diminished. The end result, as Flew memorably expressed it, is that "A fine brash hypothesis may thus be killed by inches, the death of a thousand qualifications" (1955: 97).

III   Inflation as Distraction

The strategy of inflation deflects focus from a manageable topic to broader issues, not usually germane to the problem at hand or in violation of its presuppositions. Inflationary strategies append ostentatious theses to a doctrine. Criticisms are then directed to these theses, though misconstrued as challenging the doctrine itself. Correspondingly, the objection to inflationary strategies is that they are distractive, introducing irrelevancies. Although I have so far no more than gestured at the target, the examples and discussion to follow provide clarification.

A paradigm inflationary move is ridiculed in a *New Yorker* cartoon, in which a defense lawyer argues his client's innocence on grounds of determinism. (The cartoon is not altogether fanciful, as a standard reading on free will from Clarence Darrow's defense of Leopold and Loeb attests.) The strategy of inflation, as illustrated by this example, begins with an argument that is too strong, given the presuppositions of the proceedings. It would imply that every defendant is innocent.

These defects in the strategy of inflation have to be handled with caution. There is nothing wrong with redirecting attention from a focal question to its assumptions or presuppositions. Often the redirection is progress. But since to question assumptions or presuppositions is to shift discussion, the minimal demand is simply to be explicit about the proposed shift and one's reason for it. If focus is shifted surreptitiously, we are likely to misunderstand what is the topic at hand.

The most convenient of inflationary strategies can be traced to Socrates, however unintended, and it is one we touched on in chapter 3. In the dialogue bearing his name, Meno innocently inquires, "Can you tell me, Socrates, can virtue be taught?" (Plato 1981: 70a). Before Socrates can even begin to answer that question, he insists that he must know (define) what virtue is. Generalizing, the inflationary strategy is to ask "What is F?" for any evaluative or abstract term F used in an assertion. Next, the assumption is made that if the person to whom the question is directed does not have a satisfactory answer to that question, then he cannot be justified in any claim that predicates F. If A claims that "Plants have feelings," and

B declares "That's not true," *A* responds "Well, what do you mean by 'true'"? The strategy is inflationary because we have been surreptitiously shifted to a broader, more tendentious issue, and the shift involves the false assumption that the failure to answer the "What is *F*?" question precludes answering the original one.

We have previously met inflationary moves, most prominently that evidentialism implies foundationalism or, indeed, any substantive account of rationality, morality, or knowledge. Arguments from ignorance are inflationary, tacitly maneuvering us to the issue of skepticism; for if a bare epistemic possibility is a reason in support of a claim, then it is likewise adequate as a reason for doubt. But this is just the key step in radical skeptical arguments.

The same disguised skeptical shift is found in Malcolm's isolationist apologetic. Recall the simple-minded tests that I proposed above to settle the hypothesized differences in belief over the reality of vanishing objects. These rather obvious tests, such as placing a camera to guard various objects, would be a waste, and the proposal to use them would be obtuseness on my part, given the criterion that Malcolm proposes: "Each position is compatible with ordinary experience" (1992: 93). That is, Malcolm invokes the bare possibility standard, which would render any empirical testing worthless.

Consider again Wittgenstein's strange tribe who sell wood by the area taken up. When we try to point out to them that, on their construal, the wood pile is greater when it merely takes up more area, it "[149] . . . *might* convince them—but perhaps they would say: 'Yes, now it's a *lot* of wood and costs more'—and that would be the end of the matter" (1956). The possibility invoked ("perhaps"), which ends discussion, is going to be no more than the consistency of the supposition. Stroud so understands Wittgenstein's positing of the strange tribe: "And surely it is not logically impossible for there to be such people: the example does not contain a hidden contradiction" (1971: 453). But, as earlier noted, when we make this practice and its commitments explicit, a contradiction does arise. If the purpose of proposing the tribe is to deny this contradiction, the proposal is inflationary.

The exploitation of epistemological loopholes is another characteristic inflationary strategy. We know in advance that, in profoundly difficult areas, there will be perplexities and gaps in understanding. Because the scope of these areas is virtually unlimited, it is judicious not to weigh down potentially fruitful inquiries with these perplexities and gaps, since they are not distinctive of, or selectively relevant to, these inquiries.

A frequent form of exploitation of epistemological gaps is through attempts at parity of reasoning or *"tu quoque"* ("You too!") arguments. Early in "The Will to Believe," James reminds us how even scientists with their experiments cannot answer the skeptic: "But if a Pyrrhonistic skeptic asks us *how we know* all this, can our logic find a reply? No! certainly it cannot" (1951: 94). So scientific beliefs are in the same leaky boat with religious and ethical beliefs.

Those influenced by Wittgenstein hold that science and religion, as each constitutes a framework, are both groundless—they neither have nor need grounding. Malcolm writes: "But we should not expect that there might be some sort of rational justification of the framework itself" (1992: 98). The great advances of chemistry count for nought as empirical support of its assumptions. Support according to assumptions of the framework cannot be support for the framework. The proposal is seductive only if we treat it as spatial metaphor, where a self-enclosed world can be held up only by something that is outside that world and so does not share its framework principles.

Another Wittgensteinian *tu quoque* argument claims that religious believers may look on their beliefs as akin to our belief that "material objects exist when none of us perceive them." Although "most people have [not] justified these claims," it is "certain" that "we are all nonetheless entitled to believe these claims" (Gutting 1982: 79–80).[19] In chapter 6, I reject the initial assumption that our belief that material objects exist when none of us perceives them lacks grounds. It is exactly the opposite of the truth, as we all know.

The rejection suggests the fallacy inherent in (inflationary) uses of the *tu quoque*. Abstractly, there is no formal fallacy. If doctrine D is accepted, despite property *r*, then we should not refuse to accept a different doctrine E just because it has property *r*. However, consider how defenders of hypotheses overtly at variance with accepted scientific beliefs actually use this strategy. They identify their claims with the latest, most far-out reaches of scientific thought or speculation (e.g., telepathic ESP with quantum field theory) and then argue that if we accept one theory with far-out consequences, such as a breakdown in causality, we should therefore

accept or at least not reject another. But these *tu quoque* reasonings require a hidden assumption: Doctrine *D* has no additional support that
does not hold of *E*. The fallacy is evident. We accept the far-out claims of
the favored theory only as a tolerable price to pay for a fruitful theory with
massive experimental verification and predictive success. The huge difference in background support blocks this consistency or parity *tu quoque*
reasoning.

The chief fault in inflationary maneuvers is usually their implicit preemptive claim—that the original problems cannot be addressed before we
address the inflationary ones. That claim is always suspect. Mathematics
and logic did not halt with the discovery of various paradoxes, waiting on
their solutions. Research in one field rarely needs to wait on research in another just because the latter is more fundamental. Geologists do not have
to wait until the mysteries of quantum physics are cleared up before they
can advance their own explanations (e.g., continental drift and plate
tectonics).

Despite the failure to defend their preemptive claim, inflationary strategies are often persuasive. The strategies are difficult to reveal because their
claims are expressed in the very terms of the issue under discussion or dispute, which hides the shift in focus to broader issues. The fault we just observed in inflationary maneuvers is nonstandard. The natural form of
disagreement is to deny the truth of a claim, but that is not the primary
fault of inflationary strategies. Their primary fault is the kind of distractive
irrelevance that is comically illustrated by our opening example of a criminal defense founded on determinism. It is a fault that Aristotle commented
on: ". . . an argument which denied that it was better to take a walk after dinner, because of Zeno's argument, would not be a proper argument
for a doctor, because Zeno's argument is of general application" (Aristotle 1984: 172a, 8–10). The failure is a failure to be distinctively or selectively relevant to the claim being made or supported, while pretending
otherwise.

Ultimately, these three kinds of argument—ignorance, isolation, and inflation—are facades, even when sincere. No one believes that ignorance is
sufficient for belief, or concedes the skeptical conclusions that would follow. No one believes that if he jumps from the Eiffel Tower, the possibility
that he will survive is at all a reason to believe that he will survive. No one
treats everyday hypothetico-deductive reasoning as merely a parochial

method of scientists. No one rejects rational argument, analysis, or logic on the ground that it is culturally bound. No one thinks that religious beliefs can just be taken for granted on analogy with our taking for granted such evident beliefs as that there are cows. Representing one's beliefs or thoughts otherwise is pretense, and, if sincere, a case of distraction by abstract reflection or argument. For in full awareness the alleged beliefs cited above cannot really be believed or thought.

5

Testimony: Background Reasons to Accept the Word of Others

1 The Problem of Testimony

You ask a stranger for directions, and he offers them to you. Normally, you believe him. Why should you? You do not know him. You know that people make mistakes and deceive. This in a nutshell is the problem of testimony, at its broadest. It is the problem of why we should accept the word of a speaker. It is a problem for evidentialism, because we openly and regularly accept the assertions of informants and thereby come to hold the corresponding beliefs. We take ourselves to have good reasons for doing so. Do we?

In more detail, the problem of testimony is the discrepancy between two sets of credible claims: (1) (a) We readily accept testimony. A paradigm case is, as noted above, accepting directions from a stranger. (b) Many of our beliefs originate in testimony, and our knowledge would be severely limited if we subtracted from it that portion which originates in testimony. (c) The speaker's word is the hearer's reason to believe the testimony offered. What justifies the resulting belief is the fact that the speaker asserted it and that the hearer trusts the speaker. But, (2) (d) we typically have little or no grounds attesting to the reliability of our informants, for example, that of the stranger who offers directions. Yet (e) we are vulnerable to our informants' reporting falsely, either because they are unreliable or because they are not truthful.

The discrepancy is that (1)(a)–(c) imply far-reaching dependence on the word of others, whereas (2)(d)–(e) signal weak backing. The theses under (1) imply extensive dependence on testimony, and easy acceptance of it. But the theses under (2) imply that we normally have limited evidence for trusting our informants, although we are vulnerable to their false testimony. The discrepancy is thought to expose the fragility of our beliefs and claims to knowledge. Trudy Govier writes: "Trusting another for the truth, we risk being led into error. Perhaps this possibility is responsible for the philosopher's unwillingness to recognize the pivotal role of interpersonal trust in the construction of knowledge: it makes painfully clear the fact that our beliefs are risky and we are vulnerable to error" (1993: 22).

When we accept testimony, we need to trust our informant. But how is knowledge or warranted belief possible on so fragile a basis? Contrasting, ironically, our claims to knowledge with its dependence on the morals of strangers, especially in science, John Hardwig concludes that "the trustworthiness of members of epistemic communities is the ultimate foundation for much of our knowledge" (1991: 694). It is not evidence, or experimentation, or proof, or observation, but trustworthiness on which our knowledge ultimately, and insecurely, rests.

The position I defend is that our acceptance of testimony has strong empirical support. The problem of testimony neglects this support by focusing on the information-seeker (hearer, audience) who must rely on the word of his informant without benefit of knowing him. However, the background, which is out of focus, supplies an enormous, if hardly noticed, critical foundation for the information seeker. The warrant for our *background beliefs* generally, not just those related to testimony, will be addressed in chapter 6.

I do not deny that we frequently meet dishonesty, indifference to truth, and unreliability. Used-car salesmen, advertisers, and gossips are only the most popular examples. Nevertheless, it is an illusion of salience that in communities of robust communication these defections will constitute more than a minuscule portion of the totality of testimony.

The problem of testimony is standardly presented as a contrast between the views of Hume and Reid: "Reid's position is that any assertion is creditworthy until shown otherwise; whereas Hume implies that specific evidence for its reliability is needed" (Stevenson 1993: 433). The Reidian view is favored by those who attempt to defend our acceptance of testimony on a priori grounds. Unlike those who argue that our acceptance of testimony is fragile, these attempts are not threats to evidentialism, which does not hold that evidence alone can serve as reasons. The main criticism of these views in sections 7 and 8 below is for their underestimation of the availability and force of (background) empirical evidence, an underestimation that is at one with the inflated contrast between Hume and Reid.

Assertion or testimony is "creditworthy until shown otherwise," according to Reid. But this recommendation also can be endorsed from a Humean perspective, since it is backed by (background) empirical evidence of the overall reliability of testimony.

In arguing for these claims, I avoid settings in which distortions and failures of testimony do, as a matter of fact, prevail. My excuse is that I am challenging the general thesis that what threatens our beliefs is our dependence on testimony (or trust) itself, not merely the frailty of testimony (or trust) in this or that setting. Consequently, I abstract from the familiar interferences with good testimony such as the suppression of a free press or the instigation of propaganda. A related abstraction is that assertions are assumed to be offered sincerely and meant literally, unless indicated otherwise. Although this simplifying assumption was introduced earlier to govern the whole book, it needs to be prominent in discussions of testimony. In particular, I shall put aside misunderstandings as when a hearer takes literally a remark that was intended ironically or figuratively.

2 Clarifications

A crucial ambiguity infects talk of our dependence on testimony: Are we saying only that the belief *originates* in testimony or that, additionally, it is *sustained* by it? Does the testimony serve not just as the originating, but also as the continuing, ground for belief? In the quote above from Hardwig: Is the trustworthiness of others a foundation for generating knowledge, or a lasting basis for it?[1]

Similar questions arise with respect to an interesting argument of Richard Foley's (1994). Foley argues that if we trust our own beliefs then we ought to trust the beliefs of others, since we rely on others for our own opinions. But Foley's conclusion follows only if "our belief systems are saturated with the opinions of others" (1994: 61) not only in origination, but also as sustaining grounds. The much stronger, sustaining, claim is not credible. Unless one believes that an item of knowledge retains hold of its origins, its "pedigree" (Levi 1980: 1–2), there is no reason to expect that dependence on testimony is a lasting feature of our beliefs or of our knowledge.

Almost any example of the purposeful acquisition of information through testimony disconfirms the "sustaining" claim. I come to believe that it will be sunny today because the weather report says so. But, three hours after that report, it is either confirmed or disconfirmed. If it is confirmed, then the original testimonial report is no longer of value for sustaining my belief. Or consider my learning of a serious crime through hearing of it from a neighbor, for example, the killing of a tourist in Florida. Almost immediately there is verification from many other sources, in particular, newspaper and TV reports. Their convergence corroborates, in familiar ways, the report's accuracy, as well as my reasons for accepting it.

Aside from possibilities for corroboration through other sources, there are many opportunities for subsequent confirmation. If one acts on the testimony and if the success of that action depends on the truth of the report, there is often opportunity for immediate confirmation (or disconfirmation). In an institutional setting like science, where information is acquired purposefully, testable applications of testimony are to be expected and so beliefs acquired through testimony have no lasting dependence on that testimony for its support.[2] But even information that originates in testimony is not always fully sustained by testimony. Extended testimony—a scientific report or a narrative of an event—must display a high degree of coherence, which generates reasons to believe it beyond the word of the informant. A narrative about a mountain expedition, where it is asserted that some newer members suffered shortness of breath, coheres with the fact that there is less oxygen at higher altitudes. The internal coherence lends the narrative credibility beyond the word of the informant.

Although our acceptance of testimony typically amounts to believing it, not all such acceptance yields full belief. As a preliminary, however, what is the "it" that we accept? Minimally, what one accepts by testimony is simply that a sentence or statement is true. The audience need not even understand it. One may accept the word of a native French speaker that "*Londres est jolie*" without knowing what it means or what proposition it expresses (Welbourne 1986: 21). In the usual case, of course, acceptance of testimony is acceptance of more than this; it is acceptance of assertions with meaning or content that the hearer understands. The hearer's acceptance is then an endorsement of that content.

Sometimes the hearer will not accept the speaker's testimony, without taking it to be unwarranted, if, specifically, the hearer is under high *risk* in relying on the speaker's testimony. I am not disrespecting you or doubting your word when, after you tell me that the Mustang is the best car in my price range, I consult *Consumer Reports*. Rather, I risk much greater than usual loss if you are mistaken, and it is common knowledge that consumers are inferior to impartial, easily obtained, professionally based reports on automobile value.

Reliance on testimony is not always acceptance as true, although that is typical, as argued below and assumed elsewhere. But even where it is, the contours of acceptance can be cautious and discriminating without creating friction with the smooth, rapid flow of conversation. Testimony provides a vast source of information for us, though it is much less prominent as a sustaining ground of that information.

3 Knowledge and Trust

The clarifications in the last section were aimed at diminishing the problem of testimony. We are not as dependent on the word of our informant as it appears. In this section, I examine a fertile source for exaggerating the problem of testimony—our need to *trust*. Specifically, I want to question whether where trust is needed, it is to compensate for a lack of knowledge (justification, or adequate reasons).[3]

The reasoning behind a reliance on trust in testimony is this:

(1)   For the most part, it is not feasible to gather specific evidence of the reliability of our informants before accepting their testimony.

(2)   So, if the testimony of others is to account for the extent of the knowledge that we think we have, we must accept, without specific evidence, that our informant is reliable.

(3)   Thus, we ought to accept testimony on trust.

Premise (1) figures prominently in C. A. J. Coady's (1992) objections to Humean views in his pioneering study *Testimony*.[4] The Humean is alleged to hold that specific evidence for the reliability of particular testimony is needed. The answer to the Humean position is supposed to be something along Reidian lines, whereby testimony is prima facie credible until proven otherwise.

The conclusion (3) conflicts with acceptance of testimony as empirically grounded only given two assumptions. First, only if a hearer has specific evidence of the reliability of his informant does he have good reason (or knowledge or justification) to believe him. Second, if the hearer has good reasons, trust is unnecessary. The second assumption is criticized in this section, and it is the burden of this whole chapter to undermine the first.

The opposition between knowledge and trust is readily assumed. Annette Baier writes, "And how do I know that my outstretched hand will be accepted, not treated with suspicion? I do not know, I take on trust, without any hypotheses about the egoism or altruism of the person to whom I extend my hand" (1994: 177; see also Holton 1994: 63). But handshaking, unlike, say, a salute, is a commonly endorsed form of greeting, dishonored only in rare and charged circumstances. So I object both to Baier's opposition of knowledge and trust and to her assumption that knowledge of another's actions is possible only with verification of hypotheses about that person's character, rather than background knowledge about the practice—of handshaking or testimony—in the relevant community.

The alleged opposition between knowledge and trust is not germane if it is merely an expression of inductive skepticism. For then one could equally hold that one only trusts, and so cannot know, that the snow on the ground in February will be melted by May. If we put aside the vulnerability that is the risk of any inductive knowledge, we are still left with vulnerabilities specific to testimony. Trust in informants is distinguished from trust invested in nature because we and our informants are free agents. There is an inescapable level of vulnerability we have to informants' failing us, which we do not have to the failings of our other sources of belief, such as perception, that operate according to physical laws.[5]

Clearly, however, our free will does not exclude knowledge of how we will act. I can know that my mailman will greet me with "Good morning" when we meet, even though he is free to do otherwise. Free will, which yields a special risk in accepting testimony, excludes neither regularities governing nor, as a consequence, knowledge of human behavior. However, I suspect that the possibility that free acts or inductive predictions do not conform to our expectations, however well founded, is operative in the alleged opposition between knowledge and trust. When we focus on the possibility that the mailman will not offer his standard greeting, it seems wrong to affirm "I know that he will say 'Good morning.'" However, although it may be inappropriate to claim to know in advance that he will, if he does offer me his normal greeting, I can still be said to have known that he would do so.[6]

A more glaring source for the alleged opposition between trust and knowledge is that we accept testimony from speakers with whom we are not acquainted. We do not know whether the speaker is trustworthy.

Hardwig writes: "A's good reasons depend on whether B is truthful, or at least being honest in this situation . . . A's reliance on B's testimony must include reliance on B. The reliability of A's belief depends on the reliability of B's character . . . .

In short, A must TRUST B, or A will not believe that B's testimony gives her good reasons to believe p. And B must be TRUSTWORTHY or B's testimony will not in fact give A good reasons to believe p" (1991: 700). This passage implies that trust in testimony is trust in character. But if it is trust in character, it will not usually allow for adequate reasons or knowledge, since, typically, one does not know the character of one's informants.

But *A*'s trust in *B*'s testimony need not be trust in *B*'s character. *A* may trust *B*'s testimony without trusting *B*. Consider scientist *A*, who relies on the research findings of another scientist *B* in setting up an elaborate experiment. *A* discovers that *B* has been claiming originality for work to which his contribution was rather minor. *B* is not trustworthy. But *A* recognizes that *B* will lack motivation to deceive as long as his success is not exposed. So *A* will continue to rely on *B*, while perhaps now lessening the credit he attributes to *B*.[7] What matters to *A* is that *B*'s pronouncements are correct, not that they are derived from a trustworthy character. In fact, as this case illustrates, we are inclined to say not that we trust the scientists who wrote the report, but that we trust that the reports have been accepted only after a thorough refereeing process.

The alleged opposition between knowledge and trust is itself a difficulty for those who promote it. If I need to trust my informant but cannot know that he will testify truly, as they allege, how can knowledge be transmitted through his testimony? The promoters cannot have it both ways—they cannot hold both that knowledge (or good reasons) and trust are in opposition, and that testimony is a main source of our knowledge. The former view should be surrendered. If testimony presumes trust and testimony can transmit knowledge, trust and knowledge (or good reasons) are compatible.

4   Summary and the Problem of Justification

The tenor of our discussion is to diminish the gap between our dependence on testimony and the fragile nature of testimonial trust. Our dependence on the word of the speaker is not as great as suggested, and, more crucially, we as hearers are not as insecure as alleged. These gap-narrowing themes are extended below.

To determine what grounds are generally available to hearers in accepting testimony, I will focus on minimal testimonial settings, where the hearer has no specific information concerning his informant's reliability or trustworthiness. This is the main, but not the only, condition. The costs of error from false testimony are not very high, and seeking or acquiring the information offered through testimony in other ways is costly. Otherwise testimony loses its driving force as a device of economy. I refer to these conditions as the *null setting*, illustrated by the opening example of receiving directions from a stranger.

With reference to the null setting, there are three contrasting positions on whether it is right to accept the informant's testimony:

1. The *neutral* position: that trust or acceptance should be judged on a case by case basis. There is no presumption favoring or disfavoring acceptance of testimony. In null settings one should accept testimony as one should accept any hypothesis, just in case one has adequate evidence that it is true.

2. The *negative-bias* position: that one should always regard the word of another critically. It is suspect, until proved otherwise, because, most prominently, other informants in broadly similar circumstances have been unreliable or dishonest. We need special reason to believe that this informant is not like the others.

3. The *positive-bias* (or *default*) position: that one ought simply to accept a speaker's testimony unless one has special reason against doing so.

The main (and decisive) argument for the default view (3) is that it is a practical necessity, since our need for the information from others is great, yet we have little time or resources for investigation. However, the neutral position would be viable, if we are able on-the-spot to acquire large amounts of specific evidence of a speaker's trustworthiness, through a range of clues.[8] Along these lines the contrast between the neutral (1) and the default view (3) threatens to be blurred. (Since the objections brought against (1) apply more forcefully to (2), which places greater demands on hearers, I do not treat of (2) directly.)

One difficulty for specifying the views so that the contrasts are preserved is that there are actually hardly any genuine null settings where hearers lack any specific information or evidence. As soon as you meet someone, you can make some assessment of his knowledge of the particular matter at hand, say, by the ease of his response. Still, there are settings, like that of asking the stranger for directions, that, even if not truly null, should draw the line between the default and the neutral views. Besides our not knowing the speaker in any personal way, in these settings it is known that errors are not unusual, and these errors would not be readily detectable at the stage of offering and accepting testimony. So, generally, the default view (3) will here call for acceptance, but not the neutral view (1).

If these alternative views are stated precisely enough to sustain the contrast, the facts can decide between them. The correct position is the one that fits our testimonial practices, broadly conceived. Our practices are well shaped by a large amount of experience, so that they will reflect only one of these positions, given the sharpness of the contrast. The way the practice proceeds will also reflect how it ought it proceed, since it is not credible that we would remain so heavily dependent on testimony were it not able to secure for us overwhelmingly useful (true, relevant) information.

Our practice displays an extreme *uniformity* and of a defaultlike type, which you can corroborate from your own experience. If the practice is highly uniform, that confirms the default view and disconfirms the neutral view. By and large, hearers accept speakers' testimony, unless hearers have specific reason to object, and hearers do so, in particular, in null settings (like asking directions), where there is vulnerability to error. When the stranger tells me, in response to my inquiry, to take the number 4 downtown to 14th Street to get to the Union Square, I, as the hearer, will generally do so because I accept his word.

Admittedly, the uniformity that we observe is imperfect, and the behavioral data somewhat equivocal. The default rule is an informal rule acquired tacitly, and it leaves much latitude for violation. The behavioral data are equivocal because when the hearer conforms to the default rule, he may not truly accept the speaker's word. If the hearer is under time pressures, he may have no practical choice but to do what the speaker says, and a hearer can appear to be accepting the speaker's word, but not do so in the privacy of his mind.

Despite these soft-spots in the data, a closer look at our practice still clearly supports the default view. The neutral view (1) must posit a great deal of variation in how we receive testimony, given the wide variation in hearers' experiences and abilities to discern clues about the speaker's reliability or trustworthiness within normal testimonial (conversational) settings.[9] This wide variation is not found. Speakers generally offer their assertions (e.g., directions) without supplying, even briefly, their credentials or reasons. Hearers do not regularly request speakers' credentials. To do otherwise would be rude. Finally, normatively and statistically, speakers expect hearers to take their word. If I am offered directions and do not challenge them, then if the speaker observes me not following his directions, he will be offended ("Why didn't you trust me?"); and if he confronts me, I am shamed.

Our practice favors the third—positive-bias or default—position. We want to understand better why. The *reconciliationist* position that I defend endorses this positive-bias position and claims that it has empirical backing.

5   Entitlement and an A Priori Argument

Tyler Burge (1993) has presented the most persuasive a priori rationale for the positive-bias or default position. In "Content Preservation," Burge finds an *entitlement* to accept testimony in reason's function to maintain and transfer truth. But the entitlement is cautiously formulated. To be entitled to accept is not to be justified in accepting. Nor is it to be able to offer that entitlement as one's reason to accept. It does not imply any degree of reliability for testimony. The entitlement is an easily defeasible norm that only describes our epistemic condition.

Burge defends the "Acceptance Principle":

A person is entitled to accept as true something that is presented as true and that is intelligible to him unless there are stronger reasons not to do so. (1993: 467)

More pointedly, "Truth telling is the norm that can be reasonably presumed in the absence of reasons to attribute violations" (1993: 468). Much of Burge's article is taken up with showing that this principle does not depend essentially on perception or memory as premises (but only as sources for preserving content), which is crucial to the a priori nature of the principle. The heart of his argument is given in the following passage:

We are apriori entitled to accept something that is prima facie intelligible and presented as true. For prima facie intelligible propositional contents prima facie presented as true bear an apriori prima facie conceptual relation to a rational source of true presentations-as-true: Intelligible propositional expressions presuppose rational abilities and entitlement; so intelligible presentations-as-true come prima facie backed by a rational source or resource of reason; and both the content of intelligible propositional presentations-as-true and the prima facie rationality of their source indicate a prima facie source of truth. Intelligible affirmation is the face of reason; reason is a guide to truth. We are apriori prima facie entitled to take intelligible affirmation at face value. (Burge 1993: 472–473; see also 469)

If we broadly accept Burge's argument, it is an advance on, but not a solution to, the problem of testimony. With qualifications to come, it yields the view that we should accept testimony in the null setting. We are right to follow the positive-bias policy. But it does not answer those who claim that accepting testimony is empirically fragile, and it is not sufficient to ground our testimonial practices in common settings.

The entitlement conferred by Burge's Acceptance Principle requires "empirical supplementation" to meet the usual run of specific counterconsiderations (Burge 1997: 23). But the critical point is that from the first-person point of view the range of counterconsiderations vastly expands, unless empirical supplementation is present at the outset. Without empirical backing, even highly implausible possibilities of error become undermining reasons. If the stranger who gives me directions belongs to any reference class that includes people who at some point offered me directions that failed, and if I cannot isolate that failing and show its irrelevance to the present case, then the stranger's membership in that reference class is sufficient to override (defeat) my entitlement. The flimsiest of negative stereotypes—wearing dark socks with white sneakers—can override the a priori entitlement to accept testimony, though dismissing these doubts is characteristic of our ordinary practice.

Neither of these possibilities (suspicions due to membership in a reference class other members of whom have been guilty of false communication; an unreliable, anecdotal negative stereotype) is normally considered serious. But their lack of seriousness is against the background of our shared, empirical knowledge. In divesting his entitlement of empirical impurities, Burge dilutes the power of that entitlement to dismiss these possibilities as negligible.

Burge's argument begins with a contrast between justification and entitlement that explains why he thinks that the positive-bias or default proposal can be defended only on a priori grounds. Justification calls for the articulation of one's reasons. Presumably, these reasons must be accessible to conscious understanding. Burge takes us not to have access to background knowledge of empirical reliability, since we can not uniformly articulate that background knowledge as an argument in defense. But, as argued in the next chapter, the articulation and accessibility requirements are unwarranted.

6 Arguing from Preponderance

There is a recent, popular form of argument, related to Burge's, that seems to be perfectly suited to an a priori justification of the positive-bias position. The premise is that a preponderance of our beliefs must be true, and the conclusion is that a preponderance of testimony, as expressing our beliefs, must therefore be true (or warranted).

A more complex version of this one-step a priori argument is provided by Coady (1992). Hearers assume that they share with speakers many beliefs. These shared beliefs provide overriding reason for a hearer to believe that a speaker's assertion is true. Along these lines, Coady[10] concludes that we have a priori reason to endorse testimony as a source of true beliefs.

The difficulty with Coady's argument is that, even granted the necessity that a preponderance of our beliefs is correct, it does not follow that our assertions are likewise correct. For the preponderance of the former—the broad set of beliefs that we must share—will be, in Donald Davidson's words (which Coady quotes), "too dull, trite or familiar to stand notice"(1984: 200). Since, however, what we assert purports to be informative and relevant, our assertions will not come mainly from this set of obvious and shared beliefs.[11] What we assert comes from our riskier beliefs (Adler, 1994b).

A related argument, mentioned above, is offered by Foley, though his argument is broader than Coady's.[12] If we trust our own opinions and intellectual faculties, then consistency demands that we trust those of others, because "it is reasonable for me to think that my intellectual faculties and my intellectual environment are broadly similar to theirs" (Foley 1994: 63). But Foley does not take account of the special source of our trust in ourselves. When I trust my own beliefs and their sources, my trust is first-personally compelled. The fact that these are my beliefs implies, as we observed in chapter 1, that I regard them as rightly based. But there is no such compulsion from my point of view to regard the beliefs of someone else as rightly based. I can believe that you believe *p*, while I do not. Consistency demands that I regard you as taking the same attitude of reliance and trust toward your beliefs as I take toward mine. But since my attitude is necessitated from a first-person point of view, consistency does not demand that I take the same attitude toward your beliefs.

What if, as a matter of fact, a preponderance of testimony is true? Would that justify our practices? Two ways suggest themselves of moving from preponderance alone to something like the positive-bias position:

1. Since a preponderance of the testimony is true, it is highly probable that any individual piece of testimony is true. So we should accept testimony in proportion to that probability.
2. Since a preponderance of testimony is true, we should just accept all its offerings.

Neither strategy fits well with our practices. Since both take a certain error rate as their basic datum, each would inspire a policy of accepting testimony only as qualified by that error rate, whereas our practice is generally one of simple (unqualified) acceptance. Setting this shortcoming aside, the second strategy is more secure for maximizing truths. Assume that the preponderance of true testimony is 80 percent. The first strategy tells us to "match" the probability—believe 4 of 5, and do not believe 1. In the best case, this strategy rejects every one that is wrong and accepts just those that are correct. But for every 5 judgments, there are 4 other possibilities that, on the first strategy, one might reject. As soon as a user of this strategy rejects one that is correct, he has an incorrect rejection plus the same error rate otherwise as the second strategy, which will definitely get 1 in 5 wrong. So if we adopt the second strategy and accept all the (more correct than not) testimony that comes our way, we will be right more often than if we tried a "matching" strategy like (1).

Nevertheless, (2) is no justification for the acceptance of testimony qua testimony. It applies equally well to guessing the colors of balls in an urn. What is doing the work is not anything specific to testimony or to the nature of assertion. It is, rather, just the workings of statistical logic.

7   The Empirical Background for the Default Position

The main motive for finding an a priori rationale for the positive-bias or default position is that, in null settings, the hearer lacks adequate specific evidence of either the trustworthiness of the speaker or the truth of what he asserts. But this motivation loses its grip if we have enormous background evidence supportive of compliance with the default rule.

This background evidence (our background beliefs) consists of knowledge in four interrelated areas. Besides the easy, but limited and variable, on-the-spot ways of detecting a speaker's major lack of reliability or trustworthiness, we have knowledge of the massive success of the practice, of constraints to speak reliably and truthfully, of the teachings of the institutions and community of our informants, and of how the world works (and lots of other facts about it). We also have patterns of reasoning and assessment that inform our testimonial acceptance without special effort or attention (and so in conformity with the point of the default rule). Let us treat these in more detail.

First, and most obvious, we have enormous evidence, from our earliest years, of reliable testimony in its basic role of conveying information—the weather, the time, directions, location of items, scores in games, schedules, names, phone numbers, and so on. Much of this information we are able to verify directly simply by acting on it. Since these verifications obtain in diverse settings (different informants under different conditions), there is an extremely high degree of confirmation for the natural generalization to the reliability of testimony and the trustworthiness of informants overall. In brief, testimonial practice is regularly successful, and that provides it with continual confirmation. (This conclusion will be developed below and in chapter 6.)

Of course, there is the occasional lie or deception, and, more often, the innocent error: Those who give (complex) directions, to recall our ongoing example, omit to remark on potential interruptions or special conditions or confuse routes, or their interest in being helpful leads them to overestimate their knowledge, and so on.

The extent of these cases is easily exaggerated because false or misleading testimony is far more salient than the vast, but routine, accurate testimony. When we are spoken to falsely, we suffer the costs of accepting another's word. Naturally, we then tend to think of ourselves as foolish, and the default and trust we extended appears as gullibility. Because our dependence on trust and truthfulness is far-reaching, when it is violated the whole communicational fabric seems very fragile. The result is that the possibility that new testimony will be defective is inflated. We fail to treat such cases as minor exceptions to the normally good quality of testimony.

Much of what we hear and read is dominated by our social and intellectual interests, rather than purely informational ones. Testimony in these ubiquitous settings is less susceptible to checking. But even where testimony is not subject to any simple verification, there are powerful sources of indirect checking. Consider the vast amount of information students absorb from textbooks. They cannot verify most of this information, and even where they can, it is only through further testimony—teachers and other textbooks. (Schmitt 1999). However, since these will be extended passages, there is a demand of coherence that provides a check on sharp deviations from accuracy. Moreover, convergence with the testimony of other sources constitutes corroboration, to the extent that these sources are independent.

Second, additional to the constraint of coherence just noted, we know that there are powerful institutional and social constraints on us to speak truthfully and reliably—most prominently, reputation.[13] The strength of these constraints varies according to such factors as sensitivity to the detection of deception or error, the expected costs to the informant once an error is detected, and the rapidity and extent of communication about these findings. (Contrast: science, newspapers, business, everyday conversation, gossip.) This knowledge provides a further reason that many ordinary testimonial settings are still far from null, even where we do not know the speaker personally. Previously I noted our dependence on textbooks. But it is misleading to assimilate the pronouncements of a textbook or other forms of public media as to the occurrence of, say, a historical event with that of an ordinary stranger. Only the former is subject to stringent constraints on false or deceptive reporting. These sources are continually checked by professional readers and scholars, and their future standing depends on maintaining a good reputation. Testimony that falls under these constraints is not sustained purely or even mainly on the word of the informant, even in origination.

These constraints are particularly powerful in professional science with its intensely competitive system. Discovering errors in others' work is a source of publication; the more notable the claims, the more the glory. Recall the quick and decisive disposal of claims to have generated "cold fusion." (Intense competition also, of course, motivates defection—cheating, misleading reports, hasty publication. But the strength of these restraints, including the demands of replication and peer review, is attested to by how rare and limited are the defections.)

Although everyone recognizes the checks on testimony that are supplied by peer review and replication, some critics emphasize weaknesses in peer-review systems, especially difficulties of replication, due to limited interest and obstacles to financing. Those critics fail to appreciate, however, the unobtrusive and practically cost-free implicit replication that is a by-product of new research building on old. Once it is allowed that fraud and error are rapidly identifiable in intense areas of research, the uncovering of fraud is increasingly likely over time so long as an informant's results are, as is standard, part of a larger research project. The greater the role in research, the more rapid the likely exposure of error or fraud, without requiring either strong motivation to replicate or additional resources solely for replication purposes.[14] (Plagiarism and subtler ways of securing undeserved credit are not at issue. These do not introduce false or unreliable data.)

Restraints inherent in the practice of science lessen the need for trust in individual character, as discussed earlier. Similar though much weaker systemic restraints also operate in politics. Can we believe that a politician in office will stick, even if only roughly, to his or her program or policies? Given the extent of media scrutiny, politicians' actions are regularly checked against their pronouncements. The only significant latitude is to offer those pronouncements with sufficient vagueness to evade tight verification. But, additionally, politicians who hope to stay in office are beholden not just to their constituents but to financial and political support sustained by their positions. These dependencies preclude a casual attitude toward avowed positions, as well as the evasion of politically identifiable positions.

Third, we have a good deal of knowledge of teaching and learning in regard to testimony in our community. Because the learning is so rudimentary to social life the relevant "community" is extremely broad. We learn that our informants are by and large competent about their factual reports. Much of this competence follows simply from shared, reliable sources of belief such as perception, memory, reasoning, and testimony.[15]

There are fundamental values that are widely accepted and taught, especially honesty and concern for others. In the case of testimony, these values are easily accepted as one's own because of the obvious advantage of receiving accurate information. Endorsement of these values does not comport well with self-interested exceptions. If honesty is not taught as deserved by all, then it cannot be endorsed on grounds of consent or the Golden Rule. Since we want our beliefs to be true, we want others to speak to us truthfully. We should do the same for them. Since they have the same reason we have to speak truthfully, they have reason to be truthful too.

Truthfulness is fundamental to linguistic communication, not merely an enhancer of it (Grice 1989; Lewis 1983: "Languages and Language"). Truthfulness governs conversational exchange, allowing assertion to serve its function. Defection from it can come only in small doses, since otherwise it would undermine the trust that the defector requires. Lying and deceiving (evading, misleading) are typically much more trouble and riskier than being honest. One has to calculate the lie or deception that will succeed; given repeated interaction, it must be remembered and supplemented, if an occasion threatens to expose it. Absent a strong motive, dishonesty is also puzzling, for, as Burge observes, "Lying for the fun of it is a form of craziness" (1993: 474).

Competence in conversational practice is sufficient for discerning that the speaker's assertion is proper only if he knows it (Williamson 1996). Hearers then need assurance only that their informants recognize their duties, take them seriously as binding on their performance, and know whether they are in a position to fulfill those duties. Since this assurance is just assurance that one's informant is a decent citizen, no specific knowledge of one's informant is needed. Ordinary decency is something we reasonably presume in myriad, everyday social interactions.

Fourth, we have background knowledge that ground judgments of *prior plausibility* because testimony, to be minimally acceptable, must not be dissonant with the hearer's beliefs. When testimony is low in prior plausibility, we are reluctant simply to accept it. Prior plausibility assessments provide one explanation for why the child's credulity as compared to the adult's does not reside in one's following the default rule but not the other. Rather, the child has a much more limited knowledge and understanding of when the default is properly suspended or weakened because, in particular, he has a much narrower basis in experience to instantly generate prior plausibility assessments of speakers.

Prior-plausibility judgments are at the heart of Hume's argument against reports of miracles, as expounded in "Of Miracles," the locus for the Humean view of testimony. Hume famously concluded: "The plain consequence is . . . 'That no testimony is sufficient to establish a miracle, unless the testimony be of such a kind, that its falsehood would be more miraculous, than the fact, which it endeavors to establish . . .'" (1977: 77). Specifically, a miracle would imply a violation of (what we know to be) a law of nature. But we know in advance that a law of nature is accepted only on the basis of enormous evidence; so the testimony for the miracle begins with extremely low prior plausibility.

Nothing in this reasoning commits a Humean to the claim that we ought not to accept testimony without first acquiring specific evidence of the reliability of our informant. All he requires is that there be a mutually recognized overriding of the default, even if we restrict ourselves to the implausible (or Hume's "marvellous"). The implausible conflicts with shared, well-founded understandings or "common sense." It stretches credulity beyond the unusual, improbable, or rare. (Indeed, given enough trials, some unusual, improbable, or rare events are bound to occur.) There is a (mutually recognized) suspension of the default rule if someone asserts "I grew up in New York City and never heard a 'dirty' word." Miracles, as Hume understood them, are even more extreme in prior implausibility, since they conflict with well-attested laws of nature. There is mutual recognition that the default rule is overridden.

Although prior-plausibility judgments are not burdens on thought, it is a resource that we do not avail ourselves of to its fullest. When a pronouncement is not starkly implausible, we are disposed toward trusting our informant and accepting it, a trust in accord with our defense of the default rule. Many years ago there was a rumor that a basketball star (Jerry Lucas of The New York Knicks) had memorized the entire Manhattan phone book. Given what we know of human self-interest and limits, however, it is not credible that anyone would want to devote that much time and study to so worthless an accomplishment, even conceding its feasibility. Estimating conservatively, if the Manhattan phone book contained 1,000,000 listings and the basketball star memorized each one in 30 seconds, the time he would need to memorize the whole book is 8333 hours or around a year of nonstop memorization. We can reject this rumor on a moment's reflection, though strangely, for this and many other extravagant pronouncements, many do not bother with the moment's reflection.

The lesson to be derived from such cases is not a general withdrawal from trust, since, in small doses, they confirm its value. As noted previously, occasions in which we recognize that we have been duped or gulled lead to an overreaction in which a general attitude of trust is regarded as naive. But our credulity could not position us to be suckers for false or deceptive testimony without the well-founded expectation of truthfulness and reliability that are ripe for exploitation. The lesson is the importance of knowing *when* not to be trusting, a lesson about trust similar to the one about explicitness offered in the closing sections of chapter 3.

Prior-plausibility judgments do not burden thought when properly operating merely as filters on the admission of testimony. They can tell us easily what is grossly unlikely, and thus warn us off expending energy in assessment. Consequently, those to whom we listen—or their words—are automatically prescreened. Since we by and large ignore or dismiss wild stories, speakers would be foolish to waste their breath trying to get us to accept the grossly implausible on their word alone.

As a final resource that accompanies us in any testimonial setting, our testimonial practices work largely under conditions that risk detection of error (or falsification). If testimony often failed, it would be noticed and communicated, even if less assuredly, and our reliance would either decrease or become more qualified. Our maintenance of the default rule reflects a resilient history of overwhelmingly reliable testimony.[16] This final resource of implicit absent evidence reasoning returns us to our first—the evidence we have of overall reliability and trustworthiness of communication. This evidence should now appear wholly unsurprising given the other resources, especially the constraints on us to speak truthfully and the fundamental role of truthfulness in underwriting a rich practice of informational exchange through testimony.

8   The Default Rule: A Closer Look

Is the enormous amount of background evidence that supports compliance with the default rule sufficient to justify default-accepted testimony? The issue is complex. Besides our background evidence, there are practical and ethical grounds that support compliance with the default rule.[17]

The practical constraints that underlie the default rule or positive-bias position are pervasive and constant; they are not demands peculiar to particular settings. Our normal epistemic position is that we need large amounts of diverse information (the news, the weather, history, local events, timetables, proper attire to a party, gossip), but we are extremely limited in time and resources. It is seldom feasible to gather all of this diverse information ourselves. We know, however, that there are others who are in a much better position to acquire and to evaluate this information, and who are willing to share it with us. It would then be irrational for us not to take advantage of the natural *division of epistemic labor.*[18] If we did not, we would waste resources and learn less.

Default reasoning generally has the following structure: If [condition], then Do [act], Unless [special circumstance or overriding command] (Bach 1984). If the condition is met, then the act is done. Satisfaction of the "unless" clause need not be checked in advance. It is an option to intervene; if it is not exercised, the act or routine goes ahead regardless. Since there is no waiting on whether the "unless" clause is satisfied, enormous efficiency can be achieved. For example, your computer works on the "default" to save a file to the drive you are working on. You have the option of intervening to specify a different drive. But if you do not intervene the "save" command proceeds. It needn't wait on your action and you are not regularly burdened to select a drive.

The default rule actually functions as a *presumption* that our informants are being cooperative. A presumption is a procedurally demanded bias (for trust, rather than for either neutrality or distrust) made ahead of time. Presumptions, such as that a defendant is innocent at the start of a trial, are made to advance an activity or procedure in the absence of evidence (Ullmann-Margalit 1983). There is no corresponding judgment (that the defendant is innocent). Presumptions are procedural matters, not counting as reasons for the truth of what is presumed.

The default rule also has a grip on us ethically.[19] As noted earlier, when a hearer does not conform to it, he recognizes that he has wronged the speaker, however minor, and he will be ashamed if confronted by the speaker whose word he has noticeably not taken. Part of the default rule's pull is inherited from social norms of civility and courtesy. It would be rude to ask a host of a dinner party if you should bring your own comfortable chair or good-quality salt. It is, then, a mistake to treat the hold of testimony on us as purely evidential. Angus Ross is correct when he objects to the view that "the words of others are . . . a species of natural [as opposed to conventional] sign. They have a claim on our judgment only in so far as we have reason to regard them as evidence of the existence of the state of affairs they purport to report" (Ross 1986: 69). Still, these two sources do not detract from the force of our background beliefs on acceptance under the default rule. The presumption extended via the default rule renders us as hearers extremely vulnerable to speakers' false testimony to an extent that exceeds other social relations.[20] The default rule is not posted on bulletin boards, and we are not explicitly taught it. We do not learn it merely as we learn other implicit rules, such as the rules of pick-up basketball games.

We would not continue to abide by the default rule, given the vulnerability it subjects us to, if it lacked a gripping rationale that we can learn and appreciate. The practical economies secured by the default rule are respected because we have good reason to expect that the benefits are not purchased at the cost of incurring serious error. The central pillar of that rationale can reside only in our background knowledge.

The default rule is a cooperative arrangement, and so viewed it is credible that the ethical dimension of the default rule also has an epistemic dimension. We know that cooperative arrangements are well explained as resolutions of (repeated) conflictual (non-zero-sum) situations. Testimonial situations allow modeling as repeated Prisoner's Dilemmas at least, presumably, in their origins (when testimony is more functional and local, and so defection more readily detected). These resolutions arise only with evidence of cooperation by others. Cooperators seek to supply other "players" with evidence that they will notice the cooperators' acts and intentions. The noticing is facilitated if one's cooperative acts stem from stable dispositions and habits, and it would be less facilitated if dependent on the uncertainties of individual case-by-case cost-benefit analysis.[21]

These resolutions can be finely shaped and tuned, and this applies to the presumption of trust in testimony, which is responsive, even if only loosely, to prior outcomes. The presumption of trust is not purely procedural, like the presumption of innocence governing criminal trials. Rather, it is subtly contoured by experience. We draw all manner of distinctions between classes of potential informants. Car salespersons are not as trustworthy (within their role) as librarians; professional journals are more reliable than the popular press; *Consumer Reports* is better than your neighbor for deciding whether a particular type of car is worth buying. These distinctions influence our responses to equally sincere testimony, yet in no case need there be a breakdown in communication. Similarly, we readily distinguish between conversational settings as to whether the norm of truthfulness is in full force. Social occasions usually relax the norm in the interests of harmony, as well as to encourage tact and politeness. On controversial matters, the speaker's assertion is not default-accepted (whether this is to say that the default is overridden or that it does not apply I leave open).

Outside these special occasions, our acceptance of ordinary testimony normally assumes under the default rule that:

were the speaker not to (believe that he) know(s) that *p*, he would not assert that *p*.

This assumption dominates over almost any reason that you attribute to the informant as the reason he knows. Take a very ordinary case. I see you reading the sports section of the newspaper. I ask you how the Yankees did last night. You say that they won 5 to 4, and I believe you. If you do know it, then I come to know it. But now imagine that the Yankees' game finished too late for the score to make your edition of the paper. Instead, you heard the score over the radio. So you still know that they won 5 to 4. Do I? The answer is clearly "yes," even though you do not know for the reason I attribute to you. After all, I asked you what the score was, not what the score was for the reason that I attributed to you. When you tell me that they won 5 to 4, although I reasonably believe that your answer is due to what you learned in the newspaper, you are also implicitly giving me assurance that your word can be counted on. Given that you are trustworthy, if you did not (believe yourself to) know, you would not offer the report. So when you do report, my acceptance of it is backed by the weightier reason that you are to be trusted in this matter.[22]

The limits of the ethical grip, as far as the grounds for the assertion accepted via the default rule, are highlighted through the difference between the hearer and the *overhearer*. Someone who overhears a speaker's directions feels no ethical compulsion to accept them as does the hearer. Suppose someone overhears Sally providing Harry with directions to Battery Park City ("Take the no. 2 or 3 downtown express to Chambers St. and change for the no. 1 or 9 local to the last stop"). If Sally knows these directions, then the overhearer who relies on them will be held to know as well as the hearer.[23] If knowledge is transmitted to the overhearer, then a strong ethical tie is not required, even if it serves as part of the overhearer's support for accepting the speaker's word. The result favors an affirmative answer to the opening question of this section: Our background evidence is sufficient to default-accept a speaker's testimony in roughly null circumstances, though the sufficiency depends on epistemic facets of both practical constraints and ethical bonds of civility and trust.

9 Conclusion: The Problem of Testimony Deflated

The problem of testimony with which we started exaggerates our vulnerability. Were we as vulnerable as it alleges, it would be a vulnerability that we would feel. Yet our first-person view is that we naturally and regularly accept testimony, and we take ourselves to do so for good reason. It would be remarkable if this attitude turned out to be some product of wishful thinking or cognitive dissonance rather than the well-earned confidence of competent, experienced listeners.

When an informant makes an assertion to a hearer, the hearer operates on the reasonable inference that the best explanation of why the speaker asserts it is that she believes what she asserts responsibly, and that she intends that the hearer shall believe it too.

The conclusions we have reached, especially that our empirical backing for the acceptance of testimony is massive, run contrary to the standard presentation of the Hume-Reid dichotomy. The reductivist-Humean is held to maintain that "at no stage can one justify a belief *merely* because someone has told one so, even if one has no evidence against it or against the informant's reliability" (Stevenson 1993: 437). This proposed condition is hardly ever satisfied. It only seems to be satisfiable, and the Humean and Reidian doctrines only seem to be in sharp opposition, if we construe evidence narrowly so that all evidence that a speaker is reliable can be only specific evidence of the reliability of that speaker. For it is only such specific evidence that we normally cannot readily obtain.

On the view I am defending, our normal situation is both Humean and Reidian. We both have an enormous grounding for accepting a piece of testimony and do not first investigate its credibility. We ought to reject the following natural reasoning:

Since it is normally infeasible to gather evidence as to the reliability of our informants, if we are to rely on testimony, we must do so without evidence to trust them. But the empiricist view demands that the hearer have specific evidence before accepting the assertion of an informant. Consequently, either accepting testimony is generally unwarranted, or we should reject the empiricist view.

The arguments above are directed against the opening statement in this reasoning. Lack of evidence as to the reliability of one's informant is compatible with overwhelming, effortlessly obtained evidence to accept the informant's assertion according to the positive-bias or default rule.

The claim (or accusation) that an empirical view is reductionist can be taken in one of two ways:

1. A reductivist about testimony holds either the neutral or the negative-bias position. We are not warranted in accepting the testimony of others unless we have specific evidence of their reliability. Warrant then follows from reliability. Testimony itself no longer has an independent role in warrant.

2. A reductivist about testimony holds that the pattern of inference in accepting testimony is just another inductive pattern, where testimony has no independent place.

My argument rejects (1) and casts doubt on whether anyone, Hume in particular, endorsed it. Judgment on (2) is more complex. The pattern of inference in testimony is not unique to testimony. But the background beliefs, as well as the default extension of trust, invoked by these patterns give prominence to constraints, values, and norms, such as truthfulness, that are distinctive of the practice of testimony.[24]

A last word about (2) and reductionism. In this chapter, my main target has been the thesis that since our knowledge and beliefs arise largely through testimony, they are fragile because dependent on trust or character. But consider now the starting assumption that so much of our knowledge or beliefs does arise through testimony. This assumption is also suspect, unless we moderate it in accord with the obvious fact that testimony is not an ultimate source of knowledge. Every chain of testimony must start from—be grounded in—knowledge obtained in other ways: perception, memory, reasoning, and so on.[25] In this regard, we are all reductivists.

Of the five conditions I set out in the opening paragraphs as generating the problem of testimony, the culprits are tendentious readings of (c)–(e):

(c) The speaker's word is the hearer's reason to believe the testimony offered. What justifies the resulting belief is the fact that the speaker asserted it and that the hearer trusts the speaker.

(d) We typically have little or no grounds attesting to the reliability of our informants.

(e)   We are vulnerable to our informants' reporting falsely, either because they are unreliable or because they are not truthful, both of which often occur.

Each of these is subject to distortion by those who use them to oppose evidentialism or to promote trust as the foundation of knowledge or belief.

The word of the informant is only the most salient ground for believing what the informant asserts, because it is the most specific. The wrong use of (c) is to infer that it states the only or even the most important reason to believe the speaker. In (d) the false suggestion is that the limited grounds we have as to the reliability of our informants are all the grounds we have relevant to whether we should accept our informant's testimony. The difficulty in (e) is the term "often." If the background is the vast amount of testimony regularly offered, then false testimony is fairly rare, even if it is especially striking and vivid when it is noticed.

Once we reject the portrayal of testimony as relying on the fragile thread of trust, we find the problem of testimony to be exaggerated. Our background beliefs supply enormous empirical support for the acceptance of testimony. No additional specific evidence concerning the informant is necessary to warrant the acceptance. We need and ought to extend trust to our informants, and we have excellent reason to do so.

10   Afterword: The Belief-Assertion Parallel

Although this chapter concentrated on denying that testimony is a fragile source of belief, an underlying purpose is to further the belief-assertion parallel. The central claim was that there is an empirical pillar for the default rule that a hearer is to accept a speaker's assertion, unless he has specific reason to challenge him. An implication of the default rule, as I construe it, is a surprising asymmetry: The hearer has the burden of backing a challenge to the speaker's assertion, not conversely. This is surprising because it is the speaker who, in offering his assertion, enters a strong claim (to the truth of what he asserts). Nevertheless, the speaker is not burdened to present his reasons. Rather, the burden falls on the hearer. So, for example, here is a fragment of an ordinary exchange:

Harry (the hearer):   How do I get to Eastern Parkway?
Sally (the speaker):   You take the number 2 downtown to Brooklyn.

Harry will accept what Sally says, unless he has specific reason to object:

Harry: Excuse me, but I thought that the number 2 runs express, and Eastern Parkway is a local stop.

The asymmetry is built in to the assertion exchange. Standardly, even when there is no explicit inquiry by the hearer, the purport of the speaker's assertion is to inform the hearer, which suggests that it is information that is valuable to the hearer. In these circumstances, it would be impolite for the hearer to just question (challenge) the speaker's response without explanation. For to ask the speaker for information is for the hearer to ascribe to the speaker authority or competence on his conversational contribution. That authority or competence is denied if the speaker's contribution is not accepted without justification.

However, it bears repeating that we cannot read the default rule or asymmetry directly off behavior. Couldn't Harry just ask Sally, "How do you know?"[26] and couldn't Sally just accept the challenge? This and other deviations do occur. Aside from explaining them as expected in our actual nonideal circumstances, there is latitude to sift ("massage") the data of conversation. Challenges may be accepted without backing, simply because the speaker regards the backing as evident. Sometimes a hearer's "how do you know?" is not truly a challenge to the speaker, but merely an expression of interest or curiosity. The hearer wants to understand how the speaker knows without doubting that he does. Other times the speaker will accept the challenge (for free) simply because the speaker wants the excuse to present his reasons.

Appeal to our practices in support of our endorsement of the default rule only denies that deviation could be a frequent occurrence or a regular policy. Occasional deviance from the default rule is expected, since it is a tacit rule governing a huge number of diverse interactions among free agents. When we seek to draw out the parallel for belief, the analogous default asymmetry is, though, particularly worrisome. For then propositions should not be first entertained for evaluative purposes, and subsequent to that evaluation believed or not. This is the pattern for hypotheses, but not the ordinary propositions that enter our minds through normal routes. These propositions are, to follow the parallel strictly, simply to be accepted by default. The burden falls on not believing, rather than believing, even though it is believing that enters the claim (to truth). Now it turns out that there is empirical evidence favoring this "Spinozistic" as contrasted to the more antecedently plausible "Cartesian" view (Gilbert 1991, 1993).

Of course, what strikes anyone as off about the Spinozistic view is that to merely accept whatever propositions come one's way *could* have the consequence that we hold a huge number of false beliefs, whether through assertion or other routes. I emphasize the "could" because the sticking point for this blunt objection is that the Spinozistic view need not be off, but instead quite reasonable and even beneficial, if the possibility proposed is very far from what is actually expected to obtain.

The hold on us of the default rule for testimony depends in large part on the fact that the assertions we are offered are dominantly true. Further, this fact is not mere happenstance, but intimately bound up with our having a robust practice of testimony and assertion.

Our vulnerability under the default rule loses its sting if it is easily overruled and if testimony is massively correct (or true enough). If so, why regularly expend effort to evaluate it? Granted, you will sometimes accept what is false, but that will be the unusual case, and you will surely lose vastly more valuable information if you adopt this skeptical attitude generally. Additionally, we typically cannot well evaluate testimony on our own, particularly where we have limited time and resources.

It is obvious enough how the parallel with belief is supposed to go. Default belief in propositions that enter our minds would be a disaster were those propositions not a highly select group. The systems or processes (perceptual, memory, reasoning, testimony) that provide the bulk of the input to our belief-mechanisms are by and large reliable. Where these processes have weaknesses or shortcomings we can come to learn of them, as we do for testimony, and fine-tune the default rule accordingly (e.g., we do not default accept memory reports on events during infancy). Even when beliefs are accepted fairly automatically and routinely, they are implicitly screened for minimal plausibility, especially by testing against our well-founded background beliefs. Our faculties of imagination do not just generate propositions at will for us to entertain. It thus makes sense that there is a default asymmetry favoring believing over not believing, as we default favor accepting a speaker's assertions over case-by-case evaluation. Since our mechanisms of acceptance are themselves subject to continuous monitoring through our actions, we are poised to become more guarded were this happy circumstance to change significantly. So we can be confident that we are not at serious risk of acquiring a stream of false beliefs, which is the natural objection to credulity and the Spinozistic view.

6

Tacit Confirmation and the Regress

1 Basic Beliefs as a Challenge to Evidentialism

Evidentialism claims that our beliefs ought to be held for adequate reasons. However, if reasons are beliefs, then to avoid circularity or else an infinite regress of reasons, it seems that there must be some beliefs that are held for no reasons at all. Avoidance of this regress, as we observed in chapter 1, motivates the *foundationalist* claim that there is a category of beliefs that provide the grounds for justifying or inferring most other beliefs and that these are held without reasons—that is, *basic beliefs*.[1]

Typically, basic beliefs—such as that I now see a blue screen in front of me—are characterized either as self-justified beliefs or else as beliefs justified but not by further beliefs. Consequently, there is an obvious conflict between evidentialism and the claim that there are basic beliefs. If evidentialism is consistent, then evidentialism cannot imply or require foundationalism, as alleged by prominent anti-evidentialist and extrinsic theorists.

In this chapter I uphold evidentialism by denying that there are basic beliefs. One job ascribed to basic beliefs—to provide a foundation—is accomplished by our vast collection of *well-founded background beliefs,* which played a major role in the defense of testimonial beliefs in chapter 5. These are overwhelmingly evident, usually long-standing, widely shared and variously implicated beliefs, including that there are cows; that ants do not study the calculus; that Santa Claus is not real; and that objects do not disappear when not perceived.[2]

But these background beliefs cannot do the philosophical work of basic beliefs precisely because they are well founded, and well founded because massively *confirmed*. The confirmation is tacit, a by-product of many everyday activities. Far from assimilating background beliefs to basic beliefs as either self-justifying or otherwise held without further reasons, background beliefs are the most extensively grounded of our beliefs.

2   Empirical Support for Our Background Beliefs: Tacit Confirmation

On the contemporary hypothetico-deductive model, a hypothesis is tested by deriving predictions from it. The model, as standardly presented, is this:

$H \& A \rightarrow e$.

If e, then H is confirmed.

If not-e, then H or A is disconfirmed.

"H" stands for a hypothesis, "e" for evidence, "A" for auxiliary assumptions, and "$\rightarrow$" for entailment. Predictions are derived from hypotheses only as mediated by a host of (auxiliary) assumptions.[3] The auxiliary assumptions describe features that must be controlled in order for the focal hypothesis H to be falsified, if e is false. To test the hypothesis that "Ants are attracted to sugar water," one might place a drop of sugar water at one end of an ant farm, away from where the ants are gathered, and cover the drop with some dirt. Later, one observes whether the ants have burrowed a tunnel to the sugar water. If so, the hypothesis is confirmed. If not, either the hypothesis or one of the auxiliary assumptions—including that the drop was large and near enough for the ants to sense, that the water does not evaporate quickly, that the ants are hungry—is disconfirmed.

But there is a glaring asymmetry between confirmation and disconfirmation in this presentation. The auxiliary assumptions A are not included in the second statement—if e, then H is confirmed—as they are in the third. They should be. The auxiliary assumptions (A)—such as that the drop was large and near enough for the ants to sense—are *tacitly confirmed* (Adler 1990). Confirmation of a hypothesis obtains when the hypothesis (successfully) risks being falsified. Since the auxiliary assumptions are included in the third statement, they risk falsification. If the prediction is verified, the auxiliary assumptions are confirmed as well.

For an everyday example: If I recall a canoe trip with a friend, and I want to be told the name of the rental service that we used, I would call the friend and ask him whether he remembered it. In asking, I take for granted that the trip took place. But in calling, I risk his failing to recall the trip, which subjects to falsification what I take for granted. Of course, one reason he might not recall the trip is simply that his memory failed him. But another might be a failure of my memory. So in calling the friend I risk undermining my own belief. The result of the questioning is that I may be led to doubt either that I took the canoe trip at all or that I took it with this friend. Since these background beliefs risk falsification, if they are not falsified they are confirmed, however unintended, effortless, and minor.

Absent evidence, discussed in chapter 4, provides tacit confirmation for many background beliefs. Were cows to cease to exist, the consequences would be noticeable in many different ways (e.g., milk shortages). Since no such loud and dire consequences are noticed, we continue to know that there are cows, even when we live nowhere near a farm. Through such unremarkable activities as finding milk on the grocery shelf, we gain ongoing absent evidence that tacitly confirms the belief that there are cows.

The above model of confirmation derives from Quine's (1980) famed critique of the previously predominant model in which, roughly, A is absent. But, in his original article, Quine expressed the implications of his critique in overly broad terms. He wrote, "Any statement can be held true come what may . . . Conversely, by the same token, no statement is immune from revision" (1980: 43). Tacit confirmation requires that tests not occur in isolation, but it does not require that each test of a hypothesis is a test of the totality of scientific beliefs ("holism").[4] Some, but not all and not the same, background beliefs are held to play the role of auxiliary assumptions in virtually every prediction.

Tacit confirmation also does not require that "no statement is immune from revision." We need to distinguish, as Quine does not, between falsification and revision. Falsification is what the above model is about: As a matter of logic, any statement essentially involved in deducing a prediction risks falsification should the prediction fail.[5] Revision, which presupposes falsification, enters the further claim that if we assign the value "false" (falsified) to a statement previously accepted (as true) then we can follow through with all related alterations of truth-value to yield a new, coherent, and simple system.

Against the backdrop of this distinction, Quine's claims for revision go too far. In his evocative image, our corpus of knowledge or beliefs is likened to rebuilding a ship—"*Neurath's Boat*"—while remaining afloat. What Quine should have acknowledged is that we are not guaranteed to succeed with revision. Moreover, the threat of failure in revision rests not with the abandonment of basic logical principles alone. If we falsify certain background beliefs like that the universe exists or that there is no all-powerful Evil Genius bent on deceiving us, which are empirical and contingent, we also might not know how to form a new, coherent, and simple system. For to assign "false" to beliefs that receive massive tacit confirmation is to undermine our reliance on any evidence or experience for inference.

Because of its continuing and varied occurrence, tacit confirmation is highly discriminating or contrastive. Consider a background belief such as that there are ducks. We will have tacitly tested it not only against its denial (that there are no ducks), but against competitors, such as that the duck-looking creatures we see floating on the pond are only robot-ducks. Given the wide variety of conditions under which we draw predictions and expectations that assume that there are ducks—that bread tossed into the pond will be eaten; that ducklings will soon be born; that the immediately surrounding park land will be fouled—the tacit confirmation that we have for the existence of ducks would disconfirm rivals. For well-integrated, action-guiding background beliefs, it is reasonable to expect that they survive testing against most any rival.

The proverbial problem of the underdetermination of hypotheses by evidence would then arise only with respect to rivals concocted to evade falsification. The underdetermination problem is that there is an unlimited number of hypotheses consistent with any finite collection of data. It follows that hypothesis testing can go forward only if vast numbers of hypotheses are ignored without testing or effort. In the case of our background beliefs, ignoring competitors is easy and secure, since they are at the fringes of credibility. Try even to formulate a competing hypothesis to, say, "Cows produce milk," which is both consistent with our ordinary data and not a product of contrivance ("Cows have produced milk up to the year 2050, or it is after 2050, and they produce lemonade")[6]

Tacit confirmation for a hypothesis obtains only under a host of assumptions.[7] Only lawlike, as contrasted to accidental, generalizations are susceptible to confirmation (Goodman 1983: part III). We have enormous evidence that background generalizations (e.g., perception is reliable) are lawlike (support counterfactual judgments) because they receive tacit confirmation under widely varying circumstances.

Hypotheses also are confirmed only when they genuinely risk falsification.[8] If a person believes that there are blue diamonds on Pluto, his activities do not involve, even inadvertently, tests of that belief. If certain auxiliary assumptions are exempted from the possibility of revision through very vague formulations or ad hoc hypotheses, they risk nothing and thus receive no tacit confirmation.[9] Similarly, merely long-standing practices, such as astrology, do not receive tacit confirmation since their continuance has nothing to do with successful testing. Or, if scientists do not investigate a hypothesis because of, say, distaste for its political implications, that fact is not (absent) evidence confirming that the hypothesis lacks credibility.

Even if a belief were actually needed to derive a prediction, its credibility is unaltered if a negative outcome of that prediction is irrelevant to its acceptance. Our intuitive picture of motion holds that if a solid object tied to a string is swung in a circle and then released, the object will continue on in the circular path, though ever more loosely as its energy dissipates, until it drops. Despite how often we must have actually viewed this experiment or similar ones, our understanding obscures from us that the expectations we project from that understanding regularly fail—the solid object heads off on a tangent (di Sessa 1982; McCloskey 1983).

However, there is an obvious objection to the tacit confirmation model applied to our background beliefs or practices. Since our background beliefs are what we have most reason to believe, they are the poorest candidates for rejection, given a failed prediction. The reply is that there are a vast number of occasions in which background beliefs, particularly as to the reliability of underlying sources, play a role in forming expectations, guiding actions, and generating predictions. If a variety of errors were to occur frequently, we would exhaust the auxilliary assumptions that could be blamed, until our doubts began to converge on the basic sources as having failed us. So they are at risk, and they do continually gather tacit confirmation.

Tacit confirmation, in sum, typically occurs effortlessly and is hardly noticed. It applies to an enormous range of beliefs—our background beliefs, in particular. Although in any particular case tacit confirmation of a background belief is negligible, the cumulative confirmation of such individually negligible risks of falsification can be massive.

3   The "Too Sophisticated" Objection

A central assumption in my appeal to tacit confirmation as a response to the infinite regress argument will be that the fruits of tacit confirmation are available to us. There are standard objections to evidentialism or "internalist" accounts of justification and knowledge that can be construed as objections to this central assumption. I need to defuse these objections in order to proceed with the response to the regress argument.

The objections cluster around the charge that reasons or evidence are notions *too sophisticated* to justify beliefs that arise without inference through perception, memory, testimony, or simple reasoning. These give rise to beliefs automatically, in the main, and often nonconsciously. Thus there is no opportunity for reasoned argument from, say, data given to the senses, the assumption of normal conditions, and the belief that perception is reliable to the conclusion that the resulting perceptual belief is veridical. Moreover, the crucial belief for effecting the inference—that perception is reliable—is not one that is held, or even can be held, by many, whose perceptual beliefs are by and large perfectly well founded.[10] Children continually form perceptual beliefs, though they cannot conceptualize, let alone articulate, an argument that we are justified in forming these beliefs because perception is reliable. The too-sophisticated objection applied to tacit confirmation claims that its fruits are not available to us as reasons.

At the core of my reply to the too-sophisticated objection is that it construes the notion of having a reason in an inflationary way, to invoke the classification of chapter 4. It implies that only explicit beliefs can serve as reasons, by way of arguments in which they are premises and the conclusion is a new belief.[11] Shamelessly, those who support this objection then complain that the evidentialist's requirement of reasons is too demanding.

We must distinguish reasons for action that explain an organism's behavior from that organism's reasons. We can say that when a simple organism orients toward light through a tropistic response, the source of the light in such-and-such position (e.g., above) provides a reason for the organism's moving toward that position (e.g., upward). But it is not the organism's reason for moving toward that position. That the reason that explains the organism's behavior is not the organism's own reason is evident when the tropistic response is elicited in a way that does not serve the organism's goal (e.g., to feed). Nevertheless, the organism still displays the response (Dretske 1991: 93–95). Not so for our perceptual practices. They are sensitive to alterations in circumstances to which we respond intelligently (flexibly), so to as reach our objective, for example, when we continuously shift our visual attention while driving.

In developing this initial response to the too-sophisticated objection, I begin with the practice of assertion or conversation. Like perception, our assertional or testimonial practices work under conditions that risk falsification. Since these practices are massively successful, the belief that they are reliable achieves overwhelming tacit confirmation.

Consider an instance: When asked how I know that the Yankees beat the Mets in last night's game, I answer that Tom told me. But to the further challenge—"Why should you trust Tom?"—I respond, as would be typical, "Why shouldn't I? He's not lied or misled me before." The response alludes to the normal (default) appropriateness of trusting a speaker on ordinary matters. The appropriateness points to our largely successful communicative practice, which resides in its tacit confirmation. So this implicit appeal to tacit confirmation does not require any conceptualization of that notion. There is nothing sophisticated, let alone too sophisticated, in this exchange.

As this example shows, the too-sophisticated objection is on strikingly infertile territory in challenging evidentialism through testimony. The overworked starting observation goes through: Like perception, memory, and simple reasoning, acceptance of testimony under normal conditions is mainly automatic and by default. But almost immediately their argument from this observation to the too-sophisticated objection falters. What is transmitted is grasped as an intelligible contribution. Hearers do not just come to believe that the sounds "The book is on the table" were made by the speaker. With no less automaticity, they come to understand what the speaker meant, even when that requires complex inferences (such as to compare what is said to near-by alternatives that might have been asserted instead).

Moreover, as we have observed in chapters 1 and 5, an assertion is accepted as true only under the expectation that it expresses what the speaker believes and that the speaker has adequate reasons for his belief. (We know that the groundwork of pragmatics begins, in fact, prelinguistically.)[12] One's assertion can be irrelevant, but it cannot be treated as an assertion—a conveyor of truth—unless it is taken as backed by adequate reasons. If so, the default rule dictates that the hearer ought to accept this speaker's word, and so, contrary to the too-sophisticated objection, children's thoughts and judgments are infused with reason-backed "ought"s and "ought not"s.

When children are pressed to explain their improper behavior, they may say, if appropriate, something like "Jane told me to." This seems a characteristic remark of an early Piaget-Kohlberg stage of moral development—a simple appeal to authority. But the child is offering it not just to explain his action, but to justify it, and adults so understand it. If a parent thinks that what the child did was wrong, so that it is no help that Jane told him, the parent will offer a pat sarcastic response: "Would you jump off the bridge if Jane told you?" The critical point of this question would be lost if the child did not recognize the appropriateness of justifying his action and the limited value of appeals to authority to provide that justification. The parent assumes that the child is competent with the distinction, highlighted in the *Euthyphro,* between "Doing *A* is right because *X* says it is right" and "*X* says that doing *A* is right because it is right." The child's competence with this distinction does not presuppose that he can conceptualize what he is engaged in as, say, restricting appeals to authority.[13]

So far I have addressed those parts of the too-sophisticated objection that claim that reasons apply only where there is correlative reasoning, and that the automaticity of the acquisition of new beliefs implies the absence of backing by reasons. I turn now to the claim that for anything to be a reason it must correspond to an explicit belief, one that is available to the believer for reflection and various roles. I shall concede to the too-sophisticated objection that this requirement is too strong. But the concession is minor. What we want to capture about the reason relation is twofold: first, that the reason relation is a support-as-true relation, characteristically between propositions, and second, that it is not a purely external fact about the agent, but something within his grasp.[14] We can capture these features without explicit belief, even if explicit beliefs and deliberative argument best model these relations.

Think of how we interpret one another via a *principle of charity.*[15] Our initial and rapid interpretation of a speaker's assertion is to make it, or the speaker's asserting it, appear reasonable, especially in the case of figurative usage. But it is unlikely that most of us would simply endorse the principle of charity understood as implying that we interpret others to believe what we do or that what they say is mostly true, to take familiar renditions. We lack the belief, and may avow disbelief, that the principle of charity governs conversation; yet it plays a reasoned (belieflike) role in our (automatic) interpretations of one another.

The rejection of automaticity as in opposition to an internal grasp of one's reasons casts doubt on a requirement that reasons must be explicit beliefs. Consider intelligent skills like typing.[16] Looking now at my keyboard in order to construct this example, I recognize (and come to know) that the "A" key is one row above and six keys to the left of the "M" key.[17] But I hardly have any explicit knowledge of the layout of the keyboard, so I would not have been able to make a confident determination of relative position by memory or reflection. Yet, I can touch-type fairly well, and I would immediately (without looking) hit the "M" key after the "A," if typing the word "amoral."[18] Even though I would not assent to it, I have reason to believe that my right-hand index finger should go down next on the "M" after hitting the "A" key with my left-hand pinky finger.

Presumably, when I first learned to type I did have that explicit belief. But in improving my typing, in rendering it a skill, that explicit belief is lost as a hindrance. The relative position of the "A" and "M" keys is embodied in dispositions and skills affecting use. It would be a worthless burden on memory storage to retain it, when it is of more value if absorbed into automatic responses. Yet, it is so stored because regarded as true, the crucial mark of belief. Learning to type takes place within a structure of intelligent responses to errors, understood as incorrect (and not merely behavioral shaping by reward and punishment).

The example also brings out a strikingly dubious consequence of the too-sophisticated objection. If I could make best use of a belief in guiding action by embedding it in a set of skills, a consequence of which is that I lose the explicit belief, then, according to the too-sophisticated objection, the beliefs that result from application of these (now improved) skills are no longer believed for good reasons.

A requirement more far-reaching than automaticity and explicit beliefs is that an internal grasp of a reason requires a correct understanding of it. The rudiments of this requirement I stated and began to challenge in chapter 3, and here I extend that challenge. To borrow from Pascal, belief can have its reasons that reason knows not. The requirement would identify the person for whom a belief is a reason with the conscious self at a particular moment for whom it is recognized and applied. But we sometimes have reasons for a belief that our "on-line" self misunderstands.[19] An earlier example was of a person who exclaims to a friend, "The *Mona Lisa* is beautiful." But he finds himself stymied by the friend's challenge to explain what "beauty" means. As a consequence, he is pressured to withdraw his observation and avow that he no longer holds the belief. Still, it persists and justifiably so. More pertinently, few of us can clearly articulate the role of absent evidence, discussed above and in chapter 5. Nevertheless, we each implicitly appeal to absent evidence to justify many background beliefs—for example, there are cows, when we do not perceive them—if the arguments in this chapter are at all on target.

The too-sophisticated objection has been repeatedly shown to inflate the notion of reasons. But, in one respect, it commits the opposite error—it deflates the demands of belief. Those who raise the too-sophisticated objection are suspiciously quiet on the question of the nature of the belief that is the outcome of routine processes of belief-formation. In these cases, the outcomes are generally full beliefs.

Without a place for a backing by reasons (and so a judgment of rightness, even if implicit), we would not so readily acquire full beliefs. In particular, and as discussed further in chapters 8 and 10, to maintain a full belief on awareness of it is to enter a commitment. When Tommy is wondering whether his mother is at work and he spies her slippers in the den, he will withhold judgment that she is at work, until he checks further. But were he to come to fully believe that she is in her office, and then subsequently spy her slippers, he will not reopen inquiry as to where she is. Instead, he will just assume that when she left, she uncharacteristically did not put her slippers away. Tommy's full belief is playing the sophisticated role of a commitment that overrules many countervailing indications.

Empirical work is, in fact, convincing that even young children act and judge within a normative dimension (correct-incorrect; right-wrong) that involves full beliefs.[20] If a child can comply with a rule, then he is competent with a very sophisticated reason, though primarily a reason to act (Raz 1990: chap. 1). If the rule is that batters in baseball keep their order throughout the game, a player cannot insist on batting sooner because his parents are watching and they have to leave early. All could agree that this is a good reason for him to bat earlier, but it is overruled, not merely outweighed, by the batting-order rule.

The position I am developing is that a creature could not have full beliefs without available reasoned-backing. Tacit confirmation is the only plausible source of such backing.[21] This is a claim with empirical, if speculative, import. Let us assume that psychologists are able to identify behavior that corresponds to full, as opposed to degrees of, belief and distinguish between acting (believing) according to the fact that one's perceptual processes, say, are reliable and acting (believing) in compliance with one's competence (or belief) that one's perceptual processes are reliable. The empirical conjecture is that full belief and competence go together. The empirical question is whether we ever find the former without the latter. If not, then it is plausible that they are interdependent. We will then have empirically refuted alleged conceptual objections —that the interdependence claim is circular and that a normative grasp of the reliability of perception is impossible for a creature who is unable to articulate justificatory arguments. Since if the conjecture is confirmed, it would actually be the case that full belief does not arise without the competence, it is obviously possible for it to do so.

The broad theme of this section has been that our belief-practices are sophisticated in their logic, but not, as the too-sophisticated objection maintains, in their presupposed psychology. Tacit confirmation extends to our background beliefs, even if it accrues unintentionally, where the ideal model is of intentional hypothesis-testing and control of variables. Similarly, reasons can provide internal support for beliefs, effortlessly, even though the ideal model is that of argument—rational agents giving reasons to one another on behalf of their claims.

4   Tacit Confirmation and the Endless Chain of Reasons

Now that we know how tacit confirmation arises (section 2) and that it provides a background of reasons for us (section 3), I turn directly to the infinite regress argument. Tacit confirmation is crucial to my attempt to defuse the regress problem as a problem for evidentialism. The problem is that if a belief is to be justified, there must be some further (different) belief that justifies it; otherwise there is circularity. However, that further belief can have justificatory force only if it is itself justified. So, in order to be a justifier, a belief must be justified by another belief, which itself must be justified. But an infinite chain cannot provide a justification, since it can never be completed.

My response to the regress problem is addressed to the specific allegation that evidentialism requires foundationalism—the view that there are (basic) beliefs that can justify others without being justified themselves—in order to stop the regress.[22] In a recent book, Nicholas Wolterstorff observes that the evidentialist "demand for universal justification poses insuperable problems," and he quotes approvingly the following explanation: "if one demands a justification for *everything,* one must also demand a justification for the knowledge to which one has referred back the views initially requiring foundation. This leads to a situation with three alternatives, all of which appear unacceptable . . . 1. an *infinite regress,* which seems to arise from the necessity to go further and further back in the search for foundations . . ." (1996: 68, quoting Albert 1985: 18). The other two alternatives are circularity or arbitrarily breaking off the demands for justification.[23] Foundationalism is recommended as the only way to avoid these three unpalatable alternatives.

But were evidentialism to require foundationalism, evidentialism would be self-refuting, since the essence of foundationalism is that some beliefs are exempt from the demand for (noncircular) reason-backing. So the alleged dependency is really a way to deny evidentialism. It also has the consequence that our understanding of our own justificatory practices—of giving, receiving, accepting, and challenging reasons—is misunderstanding. For our first-person judgments in concrete cases is that we have good reasons for our so-called basic beliefs, including our simple perceptual beliefs (e.g., that there seems to me to be a blue screen in front of me).

These first-person judgments are a primary reason for why we are not actually obliged to respond to the claimed dependency of evidentialism on foundationalism, just as we were not actually obliged, as noted in chapter 2, to respond to the claimed dependency of evidentialism on voluntarism. The grounds for, and the claims of, evidentialism are so innocent of substantive epistemological commitments that it is not credible on its surface that it is tied to so tendentious a doctrine as foundationalism.[24] Nevertheless, in arguing against the alleged dependency and the path to it via the regress problem, we clarify the nondemanding nature of evidentialism.

In beginning to respond to the regress problem, I focus on perceptual beliefs, since that is the standard way to pose the problem. Immediate perceptual beliefs—for example, that there appears to be a black cat on the stoop—are the best candidates for beliefs that can justify others, though they themselves are not justified. Take an ordinary case. I come to fully believe that my neighbor's minivan just pulled into her driveway because I see *that* it is there (I register it as a minivan).[25] My "seeing that" justifies the forefront belief that the minivan is in the driveway only because it is supported by my background belief that, roughly, my visual processes and judgments are reliable in these circumstances.

I argued in the previous section that this background belief is, in turn, justified because it is tacitly confirmed.[26] I regularly use my vision successfully. Were it to suffer serious errors or weaknesses relevant to the current judgment, I surely would notice. But I do not. So I am justified in believing that these sources are reliable because they are tacitly confirmed, and it is their tacit confirmation that shapes my competence as a participant in practices of acquiring and modifying beliefs.

The extensive tacit confirmation for our present epistemic (e.g., perceptual) practices swamps even the specifics that are normally invoked in giving reasons. If asked how I know that the van is there, the answer might be "Because I saw it turn into the driveway around noon." But this characteristic kind of response is misleading in the prominence it accords to the specifics of the case. Given the overwhelming reliability of our perceptual practices within their normal circumstances of use, over time it becomes more and more pointless to hold on to the specifics of how one obtained a belief, presuming that one does not value these specifics in themselves. Thus, given tacit confirmation, beliefs can be, and typically are, well founded for us without our retaining the specifics of how we acquired them.[27]

Tacit confirmation is justificatory because of its method. The chain of tacit confirmation is *endless* (the history of trial and error learning). But I secure its justificatory force as part of my competence in practices that garner and depend on tacit confirmation, not by tracing out and verifying each step in the chain.

The endless history of tacit confirmation is a history in which we are less and less epistemically dependent on the truth of earlier links. Even where some links are failures—there is no real tacit confirmation—we standardly have good reasons to believe that these do not reverberate, since presumably they are subsequently corrected for.[28] Within this self-correcting system, some background beliefs, those that are less interdependent with others, may be false (e.g., that the sun revolves around the earth), and yet reliance on the practice is overwhelmingly conducive to acquiring true beliefs. Justification is from the "top down"—from our present practices, whose workings are shaped by a history of largely successful uses. It is not, as with causal regresses (crucial to "Cosmological Arguments"), from the "bottom up" (the energy for a recent causal interaction can be derived only from that imparted at the start of the causal chain).[29]

Within the framework of the regress problem, the justificatory force of tacit confirmation may, however, be disputed in two ways. I did not address these criticisms earlier because they arise naturally only within the regress framework.

The first objection is that what is certain is not confirmable. The objection rests on the *asymmetrical* structure of knowledge central to the regress problem and the foundationalist response. Ernest Sosa writes: "There is a nonsymmetric relation of physical support such that any two floors of a building are tied by that relation: one of them supports (or at least helps support) the other. And there is, moreover, a part with a special status: the foundation, which is supported by none of the floors while supporting them all" (1999: 5). If the asymmetric support is determined by comparative certainty, then, according to this objection, background beliefs, since they are as certain (foundational) as any of our beliefs, would not themselves be tacitly confirmable.

The asymmetry assumption that Sosa describes is incorporated into Wittgenstein's (1969) proposal at 250 in *On Certainty* of groundless beliefs: "My having two hands is, in normal circumstances, as certain as anything that I could produce in evidence for it.

That is why I am not in a position to take the sight of my hand as evidence for it." So almost immediately after 250 at 253, we have Wittgenstein's answer to the infinite regress problem:[30] "At the foundation of well-founded belief lies belief that is not founded." Wittgenstein accepts the foundationalist picture of the structure of knowledge, even as he rejects its characterization of the ground floor.

At 148 Wittgenstein observes: "Why do I not satisfy myself that I have two feet when I want to get up from a chair? There is no why. I simply don't. This is how I act." Normally, we are not called on to justify such beliefs as these. We just find ourselves believing them.

The alternative story for why I do not "satisfy" myself that I have two feet is evident. Empirical support for it is overwhelming. All who have two mobile feet have excellent reason to believe that they do by virtue of the decisive evidence from seeing, feeling, and moving them, as well as tacit confirmation for the reliability of processes by which we acquire this evidence. Our attitude is that it is just pointless to request reasons, since the belief that one has two feet is manifestly well founded.[31]

We are distracted from appreciating this numbingly obvious account, owing to a confusion generated by the asymmetry of justification picture. The picture confuses differences in our attitude (our degree of certainty) and differences in support (confirmation or a right to be sure).[32] Confirmation is survival of risk, not change in degree of confidence. If we are faithful to this distinction, there is no difficulty in what is more certain being confirmed by what is less certain. Even if p (e.g., I have two feet) is more certain than q (e.g., In two seconds, my right foot will intentionally move forward), when q is a genuine prediction from p (together with auxiliary assumptions) it can confirm p.[33] This first objection—that what is certain is not confirmable—fails. As long as our certainty does not control the world, prediction is always risk.

The second objection to treating our basic sources or epistemic practices as tacitly confirmed is that it involves circular reasoning.[34] For tacit confirmation to occur, there needs to be verification of the outcome of a test or prediction. But verification of the outcome inevitably makes use of these sources or practices. A version of this objection is clearly stated by William Alston: "The basic trouble . . . is that it is blatantly circular. We have to use PP [perceptual practice] to determine that the predictions we make on the basis of perceptual beliefs often turn out to be correct, and to determine that there is a large measure of agreement in perceptual beliefs" (1983, 118; see also 121). Elsewhere Alston refers to this problem as that of "epistemic circularity."[35]

Consider the following exchange as an illustration of straightforward circularity:

S: Michael Jordan will be in Brooklyn at 2 P.M.
H: How do you know?
S: My crystal ball told me.
H: Well, let's check that you are right.
S: OK, I'll ask again at 2. Yep, the crystal ball says that Jordan is in Brooklyn.

This is a preposterous response, since no independent check is made. There is no real risk of falsification: It is not Michael Jordan's presence or absence from Brooklyn that is testing the belief, but only the same believer-dependent source.

Risk is necessary for tacit confirmation. The reliability of perception is assumed when, in my previous example, I verify that the neighbor's minivan just pulled into the driveway. To check, I peek into my neighbor's garage soon after and sure enough the minivan is there. I've assumed that perception is reliable, but it does not foreclose falsification—the minivan might not have been in her garage, as I could have discovered. (Imagine that unbeknownst to me there is a back door. The van just went through it, and the door closed. I would observe, when I peaked into the garage, no van there, and so prima facie disconfirm the belief.) Given that my belief in the reliability of perception does not control verification of my particular perceptual judgment, straightforward circularity is avoided. Since the risk of falsification remains, the reliability of perception can be presupposed and yet garner further tacit confirmation.[36] In the above dialogue, risk is foreclosed because we look to the alleged verificational source (asking the crystal ball again) to learn whether the prediction is borne out.

There is a technical hitch, however. If you know that perception is reliable, then does not that imply that any particular prediction (or most of them) will be borne out? Normally, yes. However, we are capable of stepping back from our belief that perception is reliable to inquire as to its basis. At those moments, when we view them as subject to tacit confirmation, we bracket our knowledge or full belief in them, to treat them as akin to hypotheses. Perception has been reliable, and we now find that it continues to be so in the present case. To reject this claim would be as if to reject the banality that our best-supported theories can be, and have turned out to be, mistaken. The reliability of my vision and memory in judging that my neighbor's minivan pulled into the driveway is not the same reliability that is presumed in walking up and closely checking it. These checks can then further tacitly confirm the reliability assumed in forming the judgment.

5   Traditional Responses to the Regress

Unlike the tacit confirmation or justified practice view, traditional responses to the regress problem overreact to the regress by rejecting its credible assumptions. "Coherentism" saddles itself with the regress picture of belief as a system, inviting the question of how the system is attached to the world. Its basic move is to reject the ban on circularity, which is an intuitive one and in accord with conditions for confirmation.[37] Foundationalists claim that certain beliefs are self-evident or self-justifying, which either violates the ban on circularity or just posits exemption from the demand that reasons be well founded, a posit in discord with the very starting point for distinguishing warranted from unwarranted beliefs. Wittgenstein's groundless beliefs are externally founded in a stance we take, dependent on our history and related facts, which, again, is just to reject the demand that the stopping point of justification is itself noncircularly good reasons.[38]

Each of these traditional responses to the regress problem weakens its own claim to provide an answer, when it rejects just one of the regress's assumptions. The typical form of argument is by elimination: Nothing else works to block the regress, so you should accept my way, even if it means rejecting such-and-such intuitive assumption. Arguments by elimination are shady in philosophy because of their assumption that all alternatives (and their implications) are laid out. But in this case the elimination form is particularly shady because its answer to the problem is simply to reject an intuitive assumption—either that justification is noncircular or that its stopping points are nonarbitrary.

The very different externalist response of "reliabilism" also rejects an intuitive assumption—that justification can be transmitted only through what is justified. On reliabilist views,[39] questions of warrant or justification for our beliefs are directed to the processes leading to the formation of beliefs (and, on some views, that our belief-formation mechanisms are functioning properly). Reliabilists favor themselves when they select such sources as perception, memory, testimony, or simple reasoning as their paradigms, for these are processes that we know to be largely reliable. But, from the point of view of any agent ascribed reliabilist-knowledge, there is no basis to favor perception over, say, tea leaf readings or crystal balls. In either case we have the same conditionals: *If* the tea leaf readings are reliable, then such-and-such belief is warranted; *if* perception is reliable, then such-and-such belief is warranted.[40] Reliabilism severs the connection, at the heart of the demand for justification, between believing and intellectual responsibility.

Of course, the reliabilist's central externalist assumptions are correct: To have justified belief or knowledge does not require one to show that one is justified or knows, and there is a difference between taking oneself to be justified and really being justified, as successfully fulfilling all one's epistemic duties or responsibilities. But acceptance of these assumptions does not go so far as to yield purely externalist analyses of fundamental epistemic notions like knowledge or justification.

In fact, the suggested sharp contrast between internalist and externalist views blurs when we look at detailed cases. It is difficult to imagine that anyone would genuinely maintain a full belief without being in a position to judge herself to have good reasons to do so. It is also difficult to imagine that a reliable process like perception would regularly issue in full beliefs and yet remain outside an agent's grasp in the very weak sense defended in section 3 above.

In one of the most famous passages in the *Investigations,* Wittgenstein expresses dissatisfaction with standard philosophical methodology as applied to meaning. We insist on finding what is common to all games, dismissing the evidence of an irreducible diversity. The insistence assumes exactly what Wittgenstein (1953) calls into question, at 66: "Don't say: 'There *must* be something common, or they would not be called "games"'—but *look and see* whether there is anything common to all." This advice captures exactly my complaint about responses to the infinite regress problem, Wittgenstein's included. The felt sense that there must be stopping points to justifying that are distinct from the everyday acts of offering and challenging reasons drives us to indifference toward particular cases. We are distracted, and we do not really "look and see." We are antecedently convinced that we must reach a groundless endpoint. So we needn't look at our actual judgments.

The tacit-confirmation account accepts a ban on circularity and agrees that what is reason-conferring does itself stand on reasons. There can be no problem of connection to the world, since the stopping points are the products of an extensive history of testing against the world. Exercising competence in these practices cannot float free of the world, since our competence is shaped by the world. If one does not acquiesce to the regress problem, one will refuse to inflate justification into anything beyond everyday observation, argument, or confirmation that draws strength from a vast background of well-founded beliefs.

One root of the regress picture is the common misinterpretations of an unending chain of justification as requiring an unending chain of justifying, an infinite doing. The reasons we need for the justification of other (and previous) reasons do not always or typically require the performance of a further test. There is, rather, an unending and pointless-to-trace trail of tacit confirmation.

On the tacit confirmation view, the endless chain of justification enters when we reach reasons that are a proper stopping point for justifying a belief. A chain of endlessly grounded reasons—which is all that is implied by the combination of noncircularity and reasons as grounded—does not entail an infinite regress of acts of grounding (testing, justifying). Justification does not demand justifying; and reasoned backing does not require reasoning, as noted earlier. The chain of reasons can comply with norms "all the way down" (Brandom 1994: 41) because it is tacit confirmation "all the way down."

6   Conversation and Regress

As corroboration of our response to the regress problem, let us revert to the parallel with assertion. Conversationally, the infinite regress argument amounts to asking "how do you know?" whenever an assertion is made. Since the answer takes the form of offering further assertions (reasons), we have a regress of challenges. But there is no conversational entitlement to these challenges. Robert Brandom rightly denies that challenges have a free ride: "challenges have no privileged status: their entitlement is on the table along with that of what they challenge. Tracing the provenance of the entitlement of a claim through chains of justification and communication is appropriate only where an actual conflict has arisen, where two prima facie entitlements conflict. There is no point fixed in advance where demands for justification or demonstration of entitlement come to an end, but there are enough places where such demands *can* end that there need be no *global* threat of debilitating regress" (1994: 178). Brandom's succinct response, however, requires an addendum. As he states in the quotation's opening, challenges "have no privileged status." But if their status is equal to that of the original assertion challenged, then the regress problem does seem to capture a constant "entitlement." Claims (assertions) always require justification; challenges are merely calls for it. However, the regress is blocked if challenges bear the burden of proof. I have argued that they do in consequence of the default asymmetry, which, as emphasized in section 10 of the previous chapter, is a facet of the default rule for testimony. The asymmetry places a burden on challenges to overrule the default presumption.

A moment's reflection shows why the price of withdrawing the default would be a widespread withdrawal from assertion. Much of what speakers

usefully assert to hearers are beliefs for which we typically do not know of
the specific reasons backing them, beyond the vaguest hints:

Harry: When did Columbus sail to America?
Sally: 1492.
Harry: How do you know?
Sally: I'm not sure—I suppose I read it in some history text or some
teacher told me or maybe a friend.

Obviously, if the demand on ordinary speakers like Sally is for a more precise and informative accounting without sacrifice in truthfulness, speakers
would become extremely hesitant to supply hearers with the information
that they seek, as is now the easygoing practice.

   For ordinary speakers to have to retain their reasons or evidence, when
they serve no further purpose than that of backing their assertions, would
be an enormous burden and it would deny to speakers a minimal authority—that their word is good enough. However, the implied denial that
challenges have a free ride does not signal a retreat from evidentialism.
Challenges demand the presentation of reasons. If a hearer is not entitled
to challenge the speaker for his reasons, it does not follow that the speaker
lacks them. Quite the contrary: It is because the hearer is entitled to presume that the speaker has those reasons that the default rule maintains its
hold and that its hold has an epistemic dimension (testimony as a source of
knowledge). In chapter 5, we observed that the acceptance of testimony is
governed by an instance of the following conditional:

Were the speaker not to (believe that he) know(s) that p, he would not assert that p.

When this holds, the specific account of why the informant holds the belief
(expressed in his assertion) is no longer germane to accepting it. The hearer
already believes that whatever the speaker's reasons, they will be
adequate.

   But if a challenge to an assertion is appropriate, then it imposes a constraint on the speaker in defending his assertion. The speaker cannot appeal to the bland fact that he has good reasons.[41] The speaker must
produce specific reasons that meet the challenge either by refuting it or
clarifying how he knows that the assertion is true. Imagine that Sally responds to Harry's request for directions to City Hall by telling him to take
the number 2 or 3 express downtown to Chambers Street. Harry can chal-

lenge her assertion by asking, "Isn't Chambers Street a local stop?" Sally cannot respond with a default-type answer, "But if I didn't know it, I would not have asserted what I did." The response is empty as an answer to the challenge. If the request for justification is appropriate it already overrules so bland an appeal. The appropriate answer is a specific reason, for example "I just checked the map. Chambers is an express stop"; though it need not be that specific—"Look, I've been riding the subways for years, and I'm sure that Chambers is an express stop."

Given the subtleties and looseness of our behavior in complying with the default rules, we can readily misunderstand our epistemic position in the testimonial exchange. If a speaker both accepts a challenge (for free) and follows the rule that challenges require the production of specific reasons, the speaker will take a large range of his assertions to be asserted improperly, since he will lack those specific reasons. If the challenge is to what is actually a mutually accepted assertion, then the speaker, in accepting it, misleads himself; for the challenger represents himself, in casting his challenge, as not accepting the speaker's assertion at face value (e.g., that the speaker knows the time by hearing it on the radio). So free challenges cast the misleading impression that reliance on our background assumptions and beliefs is inadequate.

The move from assertion to belief is mediated by reference to the purpose of assertion as the transmission of informative truths. In the standard case, the hearer is accepting the speaker's assertion as true. The default rule renders the hearer extremely vulnerable to the speaker's faulty testimony. Yet, we by and large comply with the default rule, even though it is not an explicitly taught or codified rule. We would not adhere to it merely as habit, as argued extensively in chapter 5. Whatever the practicalities that underlie the default rule, there must also be background evidence of successful workings, so that we willingly and un-self-consciously comply with it.

7 Puzzling Assimilations and the Ordinarily Uncriticizable

In closing, I want to emphasize a cost in rejecting the tacit confirmation view, additional to that raised by our assertional practices. The tacit confirmation view provides an explanation of a puzzling claim noted earlier. The puzzling claim is that the dullest of background beliefs—that there is an earth, or that material objects exist when none of us perceives them, to repeat the example noted in chapter 4—lack justifying grounds. I will not repeat the rationale offered for this puzzling claim, except to remind you that it has to do with responding to the regress picture by insisting there just has to be a foundational layer, which, by virtue of being at bottom, cannot itself be justified.

Of the reasons to be puzzled by this claim, I want to focus on its defiance of your own judgment and so as well, presumably, of those who enter such claims. You judge that not only are these beliefs justified, but that there could hardly be beliefs better justified. Moreover, if you deny these common-sensical judgments, you will likely also have to reject the related common-sensical judgment, offered by most persons, theist and nontheist alike, that the justification of a fundamental personal belief like "There is an all-good god" or "There is life after death" or "The universe is value-less" is highly problematic, and so to be distinguished from the above background beliefs and numerous others like them. As noted in chapter 4, the mileage to be gained by claiming that background beliefs are not justified is to assimilate them to beliefs like the fundamental personal ones, and then to argue, by parity, that if we are not going to reject the former—indeed, that we are going to maintain them tenaciously—then we are similarly entitled to do so for the latter.

In reminding you that this conception is defiantly at odds with your ordinary judgments, I do not here, or elsewhere, treat our ordinary judgments as sacrosanct. But the possibility of widespread error does not preempt taking widespread agreement as a datum. Were we to be in error in our judgment here, we would suffer a far-reaching misunderstanding of the nature of reasons. That is not credible. It is our reliance on reasons that overwhelmingly explains so much of the accuracy of our judgments and the success of our actions. We could not be so wrong about reasons, and yet so overall correct in our judgments and successful in our actions.

A specific form of the (inflationary) argument, which I just hinted at, is that the existence of god is in no worse shape epistemically than the existence of *other minds*. Traditionally, our knowledge of other minds has been defended by an argument from analogy—I (we) infer from others' similarity in looks and behavior to myself (ourselves) that they have minds, as I know I do. The argument has been subject to forceful objections. Defenses of the argument from analogy have been developed, as well as other types of defenses. But let us suppose that we remain in a quandary about it.

Nevertheless, it is evident that I will claim that my belief that others have minds is overwhelmingly tacitly confirmed.[42]

This claim does not dampen the philosophical quest, since it is a response available to us only given our modest ambitions. When I claim that the existence of other minds is tacitly confirmed, the key implication is that you would not in ordinary argument and discussion criticize someone who implied that he believed that there were other minds. Were you to ask him, out of curiosity, how he knows it, he would allude to its massive confirmation. Within any ordinary exchange, you will find nothing to fault in this reply, as you might if he had instead explained that it makes him happier to so think that these animated, complex humanoid creatures have minds, rather than being cleverly programmed but mindless robots. Perversity aside, you would take his response as effectively uncriticizable, even if it finds critics, just as we noticed in chapter 3 that what is truly unbelievable will find believers.

The tacit confirmation view supports our ordinary discriminations—beliefs that there are other minds or that there is an external world achieve enormous tacit confirmation, unlike beliefs that people are basically good or that god loves us. If you reject the tacit confirmation view, you must provide an alternative account of the vast epistemic divide between these background beliefs (e.g., there are other minds; there is an external world) and the forefront ones (e.g., people are basically good). If not, you must acquiesce to the former's assimilation to the latter as groundless, foundational assumptions, a result that is highly implausible and by your own lights.

APPENDIX: BACKGROUND BELIEFS, STABILITY, AND OBEDIENCE TO AUTHORITY

Because we have firm background beliefs, our worldview is stable. Our resistance to giving them up is a rightful product of tacit confirmation. So it is the stability of the world that ultimately explains the stability of our worldviews. Our knowledge of these background beliefs and the stability they ensure is powerful evidence of our grasp of the workings of tacit confirmation, even if unarticulated. (And so they are further evidence against the too-sophisticated objection in section 4 above.)

Our worldview implies, to speak figuratively, that crazy things do not happen. The worst serial killers in prison do not come close to matching those in seemingly realistic movies and books like *Silence of the Lambs;* nor is it credible that a divorce involving children could resolve itself so neatly, in accord with the audience's objective and sympathetic view, as in *Kramer vs. Kramer,* even conceding that both films are based on real-life cases. Think of a compounding of very ordinary, dull, unlikely possibilities—a stranger you pass on the way to work in New York City, you find at your breakfast table two days later, where he asks you to pass the salt, recites the Hare Krishna, and then leaves. With extremely high confidence, I expect that nothing like this or an unlimited number of other similarly way-out-of-the-ordinary possibilities has ever happened to you. Merely the restrictions on normal human motivation and interests, as Hume emphasized, rather than any conceptual, physical, or logical barriers seem sufficient to reduce the credibility of this scenario to near null. Truth is stranger than fiction only in its occupying so minuscule a portion of the possible worlds, despite numerous opportunities for their realization.

The stability of our worldviews is not (preposterously) in opposition to the new, the rare, the unusual, the improbable, or the unexpected. In 1999, Lance Armstrong won the Tour de France, despite having been diagnosed in 1996 with an especially lethal form of testicular cancer that had spread to his abdomen, lungs, and brain. The stability claim is rather that consistency with our background beliefs reflects very narrow bounds within which such "miracles" must fit.

It is for this reason that I am confident of the far-reaching speculations of chapter 3 that much distorted belief is the cover of incoherence. The person has within his grasp various inconsistencies, but evades or hides from them through distraction, self-deception, or garden-variety inattention. Distorted beliefs (or distorted belief-formation) are bound to conflict with the agent's background beliefs; and these will all be within the agent's grasp.

Tacit confirmation helps to explain the stability of our beliefs, their resistance to being dislodged. We are susceptible to only limited manipulation of our beliefs. Our background beliefs are rarely revised, and then only modestly. Although people can be convinced to buy "pet rocks," they cannot be convinced to enroll their pet rocks in adult education programs. (You cannot fool any of the people, any of the time, any which way.)[43] But, at least in the realm of values, this claim is challenged by Stanley Milgram's (1974) famous studies on obedience to authority. In Milgram's studies, experimenters are able to coax subjects to defy their fundamental beliefs and values that they should not cause gratuitous pain in others. However, I question the inferences Milgram draws from his studies that in realistic, if uncommon, circumstances ordinary persons will violate, and so surrender, fundamental, background beliefs and values in deference to respected authorities. Milgram's inferences assume a degree of malleability of our background beliefs that is neither antecedently credible nor sustained by the evidence.

In Milgram's study, many ordinary individuals were led to administer what they took to be high levels of electric shocks to "learners" in an experimental study. The learners were actually confederates of the experimenter, who ordered the apparent shocks. A pillar of Milgram's explanation of his findings is that we invest great—too great—authority in the experimenter, so that ultimately we transfer responsibility for our actions to the experimenter (1974: 175).

Milgram's study depends on inducing subjects to believe that they are shocking the confederates, when they actually are not. The experiment was carefully designed to be realistic. Subsequent interviews, before and after debriefing, attest to the fact that subjects were indeed deceived (1974: 171–174). In the film of the experiment, subjects are observed visibly sweating and emotionally distraught, when cajoled into giving high levels of shock.[44]

Nevertheless, I deny that the subjects' belief that their setting is real is just another variable for the experimenter to control, where success in control is adequately verified by questionnaires and postexperimental interviews. It is difficult to accept that the subjects were not still influenced by their very well-confirmed belief that highly risky and harmful studies on ordinary persons do not take place in the contemporary United States. (Formally, of course, this belief is confirmed, not refuted, by Milgram's own study.) The regulations binding experimenters to productive, non-harmful research is strong. Subjects know that scientists seek funding, and that their research is overseen by the university, government agencies, and peers. Other subjects will have gone through the same research. Were any-one harmed, reporters would rush to uncover and expose a story of great moment and appeal. Finally, people who appear decent and hold responsible positions of authority in open, long-standing, democratic societies generally are decent. They do not encourage infliction of pain and damage on others, where it is not directly and obviously related, as with dentistry, to removing greater harms.

For these reasons, I defend the conjecture that there is a subtle unreality about the setting for subjects. Milgram's inferences require, though, that subjects are wholly taken in by the settings: That the shocks that they supply for wrong answers are really harmful. To deny this assumption is not, however, to affirm that subjects did not take the experiment seriously. Milgram varied the experiment in a large number of ways, such as in allowing subjects to select the level of shock or to alter proximity to the "learning" or to the experimenter, which significantly affected the degree of compliance. These results are inexplicable unless subjects take the experiment and setting seriously. Moreover, when asked about it afterward, subjects declined the face-saving suggestion that they did not believe that they were really giving shocks.

Nevertheless, my conjecture stands. When the subjects denied that they suspected fakery, they were focused on finding telltale signs of illusion, rather than on a more pervasive, below-the-surface, deception.

Milgram was sensitive to facets of this objection. The study took place at Yale University, a well-respected institution, unlikely to tolerate harmful experiments. So he arranged to have the experiment replicated in a number of ordinary locations in Bridgeport, away from the university in New Haven. Although the results are still highly significant, there is a marked decrease in compliance (from 65 to 48 percent) at the Bridgeport location, which Milgram too quickly dismisses (1974: 69 and 60–61, table 3). For subjects do not alter their judgments that the setting was realistic, in accord with the decrease in their rate of compliance. My conjecture explains the higher compliance rate of subjects at Yale as due to their lessened underlying belief that the scenario was as it appeared.

Crucial to the importance Milgram attaches to his studies is that they can be generalized to help explain the extended barbarity of Nazi Germany. Ordinary persons came to defy their most basic values when, Milgram suggests, conditions and conditioning similar to those in his study were instituted.

Milgram readily admits to a number of disanalogies between his experimental setting and Nazi Germany (1974: 175–178). He downplays these differences, however, as mere differences in degree. But the difference between a one-hour experiment and a decade of barbarity in Nazi Germany is not just a difference in length of time. To cite one pertinent and underrated disparity, in the latter case, though not the former, one also has to suppress the myriad sources that would expose what was going on.

For his generalization to hold, Milgram's subjects must believe that they are really shocking the "learners," as citizens of Nazi Germany believed that Jews were really being sent to concentration camps. Differences in actual external circumstances (what is really going on) are supposed to be neutralized, however, by the construction of the experimental setting. But subjects' very willingness to obey the experimenter's orders itself is facilitated by their belief that there are strong barriers to serious and sustained ethical, legal, or scientific violations' taking place in our society, without exposure and censure. This well-confirmed belief, which the citizens of Nazi Germany did not share, is a yawning gap between the experimental setting and what it is supposed to model.

The temptation to accept Milgram's generalization begins with the following thought: "Were any of us to be subject to commands and conditions similar to those projected in Milgram's studies, then we would have behaved as his subjects did."[45] Given that Milgram did create an internally realistic scenario, then, focusing only on that scenario rather than on the external circumstances that permitted it, we naturally assume that the antecedent of the highlighted conditional is easily satisfied. But it is not at all a realistic or near-by possibility that systematic harm is ordered on innocents in contemporary democratic societies, under the ruse of science, and yet our social world either overlooks it or conspires not to give censure or to even take notice.

Milgram's scenario invites us to assume that external circumstances (e.g., of a free press) conspire to not interfere with the goings on in the laboratory and so, by projection, do not interfere with the real goings on that the experiment is meant to model. Granted that assumption, the possibility envisaged by the experiment seems to be confirmed as realistic, through the study's findings. But the fallacy here, which is a version of one discussed in chapter 4, is to conclude that we can detach the claimed realism for the experimental setting from its dependence on the opening assumption that the contrived external circumstances are just right.

The suspicion voiced in the previous two paragraphs about the tempting reasoning toward Milgram's generalization extends to an obvious alternative hypothesis for explaining the discrepancy in compliance between Yale and Bridgeport. More in line with Milgram's own view, the hypothesis is that the greater prestige of Yale encouraged subjects to be more obedient. But the stark contrast between these hypotheses blurs when we factor out the reasoning just criticized.

The "prestige" hypothesis favors Milgram's view only if the fact of prestige is separated from its basis. (Analogously, the authority we invest in experimenters displays vulnerability to dangerous manipulation only if the authority is treated as independent of desert or merit.) Because the crucial variable is the prestige, the conclusion is that persons can be influenced without much difficulty to perform horrid acts by virtue of prestige alone. But Yale's prestige is earned, and what has to be shown is that it is a realistic possibility that such prestige (or its appearance) could be achieved, almost totally either without desert or instead, with desert that does not generate expectations that future behavior will remain ethical. Yet, it is implausible that seriously deviant and harmful experimentation could proceed at a well-known and well-established university, given the wide range of activities that it undertakes and the myriad sources reporting on those activities, over the stretch of time required to earn the prestige. If the crucial variable is not prestige alone, but well-earned prestige, then this alternative hypothesis is no longer a sharp competitor to our own. For the well-earned prestige of Yale is good reason (for subjects) not to wholly believe that experiments of the kind Milgram pretends to be performing are taking place.

Although empirical questions remain open, I stand by the conjecture that denies the complete believability of the setting in the Milgram studies and affirms an element of pretense. There is no incompatibility between this conjecture and Milgram's claim that subjects do bend their own beliefs and values because of the authority invested in the experimenter and the scientific enterprise. My claim postulates a very hazy sense of unreality, not an articulated thought that the setting is illusory. The postulation is untroubled by subjects' overt distress when confronted by the confederate writhing in pain, after the subject pressed the button labeled to indicate a high degree of shock. We all can experience such distress in reading novels, or watching movies or plays, even when we know that the scenes are not real.[46]

The central clash between my conjecture and Milgram's claim is with his generalization of it outside the laboratory. Milgram must downplay the forceful justification subjects have for their confidence in the authority and beneficence of local scientists and their governing institutions, in extrapolating to situations like Nazi Germany. Were the subjects' investment in authority by itself sufficient, the experimenter might just have ordered high shocks from the start. But the study requires that subjects be nudged along to ever greater shocks by carefully timed increments in the experimenter's requests (Ross 1988; see also Flanagan 1991: 293–298). Subjects had to be moved gradually along a slippery slope, whose psychological and ethical workings are not at all confined to the ascription of authority. Subjects are trying to make good on their own prior complicity with applying shocks at lower levels, and this attempt is threatened whenever they would break off from obedience. Whatever is wrong with shocking at stage $n+1$ will be only marginally less wrong at the prior stage n.

The need for these subtle alterations attests to the extreme difficulty of getting persons to abandon their background beliefs and values. Focusing on the experimental setup alone, we lose sight of all the isolating conditions that its operation depends on. These conditions are rarely realizable in the messy world outside the laboratory. Outside the laboratory, it is difficult to monitor the incremental steps on a slippery slope to ensure that citizens lose their ability to judge that a serious change in severity of treatment has occurred. But though these conditions are not salient to us, they figure in our background beliefs about how our social world works.

It is a mistake to think of the isolation from varied detection, or the use of incremental steps, as merely controls to test Milgram's specific hypothesis, and then to detach the hypothesis from these controls. For the interest in Milgram's specific hypothesis turns on how close we are to circumstances in which it would operate. But the realism of those circumstances depends on the conditions of control. When these conditions are factored in, the threat that made Milgram's studies so exciting diminishes. It is one thing for us to renege on our basic values in extreme and unusual circumstances; it is another for this to occur when the conditions of our social world are not badly ruptured. It is this latter claim that I do not believe Milgram's studies warrant. If as carefully and thoughtfully designed (and replicated) a study as Milgram's does not succeed in nullifying our background beliefs, then it is unlikely that the attempt can fully succeed. We are not highly malleable, because our background beliefs are not, and our background beliefs are extensive. They extend far beyond the excruciatingly dull ones (there are cows; monkeys do not study the calculus). They extend to more subtle, complex, and valuative ones, like the belief that normal citizens in our advanced, democratic community, governed by the rule of law and informed by an active, free press, do not inflict severe harm on other innocent members of the community at the behest of legitimate authorities or scientists.

7

Three Paradoxes of Belief

Many of my claims about belief have been supported by their fit with assertion—the everyday activity of sincerely saying (writing, uttering) a declarative sentence. The parallel between assertion and belief provides a unifying thread among three well-known paradoxes of belief: Moore's, the Lottery, and the Preface. The heart of that parallel is that both are *transparent* to the content of what is asserted or fully believed. Application to these three paradoxes tests out two related and central methodologies of this work: the appeal to assertion as the expression of belief and the appeal to our first-person judgments in testing the coherence of believing.

1   Transparency and Moore's Paradox

Recall that the transparency of belief amounts to this: When one attends to one's belief that p, one takes it to be the case that p. Partial belief or degrees of belief are not transparent. In being only "very sure" that p, one cannot see the world according to that content, but only as filtered through one's attitude.

Moore's Paradox was invoked to support my main criticisms of extrinsic approaches, particularly in chapter 1. Moore's Paradox is that assertions of the following form are heard as contradictory, although the contained sentences are consistent:

(1) p, but I do not believe that p.[1]

For example, it's raining, but I do not believe that it's raining.

In chapter 1, we also noted that Moore's Paradox applies to knowledge as well:

(2) p, but I do not know that p.

We inferred that in assertion the speaker represents himself as knowing what he asserts, or, more strongly, that the truth condition for proper assertion is that one knows what one asserts.[2] We have treated this result as firming down the demand for "sufficient [or adequate] reasons." Full belief requires reasons sufficient for knowledge.[3]

I will approach the explanation for the heard inconsistency of (1) by attending to the stronger version (2). The explanation here, though similar to the one offered in chapter 1, is simpler, owing to the present appeal to transparency. The formal argument for a contradiction in the assertion of (2) proceeds as follows (using "K" for "knows" and suppressing references to the asserter):[4]

$K(p, \text{but} \sim Kp)$	(Asserting implies knowledge)
Kp and $K \sim Kp$	(K distributes over conjunction)
Kp	(conjunction elimination)
$K \sim Kp$	(conjunction elimination)
$\sim Kp$	(factiveness of K)
Kp and $\sim Kp$	(conjunction introduction)

The proof is a bit misleading. It suggests the need for step by step mental reasoning according to natural deduction rules. The best evidence against this suggestion is Moore's Paradox itself. Take the move to the second step. It would be Moore's-Paradoxical to assert "*p* and *q*, but either I do not know *p* or I do not know *q*." Similarly, for the next, it is Moore's-Paradoxical to assert "*p* and *q*, but I do not know that *q*." The denial of any of the above steps cannot be thought while thinking of what the first conjunct (or a previous step) expresses ("I believe that *p*"). (Shoemaker 1996: 74–93).

For simplicity, the proof is offered without constant reference to the person who asserts (2). But this too is misleading. It overlooks a crucial feature of Moore's Paradox—that it is essentially first-personal.[5] As has frequently been observed, there is no Moore's Paradox in asserting (in the third-person)

It's raining, but Jones does not know (believe) that it is raining.

The proof above does not go through in a case where, say, the smartest student in the class asserts that

Hume awoke Kant from his dogmatic slumbers, but the smartest student in the class does not know (believe) it.

This is not Moore's-Paradoxical. The description "the smartest student in the class" does not refer essentially to the asserter, who need not recognize that he is speaking about himself.

How exactly does Moore's Paradox for knowledge (2) resolve the original Moore's Paradox for belief (1)? The easy, but unilluminating, way is by entailment. Given that one properly asserts p only if one knows it, we have the following derivation from the assertion of (1) with all steps but the crucial ones suppressed:

$K(p$ and $\sim Bp)$
Kp and $K \sim Bp$
Kp
Bp (knowledge implies belief)
$K \sim Bp$
$\sim Bp$ (factiveness of K)
Bp and $\sim Bp$.

So we derive a self-contradiction for belief parallel to the one for knowledge from the assertion of (1). This derivation is a way to explain (and exhibit) the heard contradiction in the assertion of (1).[6]

This easy way of getting from the explanation of Moore's Paradox for knowledge to one for belief assumes that assertion is backed by knowledge and that knowledge implies belief. Both of these assumptions have been questioned, although for very different reasons. But there is a stronger motive to put these assumptions aside and focus on the original Moore's Paradox (1), without explicit appeal to the knowledge-assertion connection. For neither proof is sound if p is false. But, obviously, Moore's Paradox applies to the assertion of false sentences.

When we focus on (1) without explicit appeal to the knowledge-assertion connection, that connection still provides us with a crucial insight. The transparency of belief implies an analogue of the crucial feature of knowledge—it is factive (Kiparsky and Kiparsky 1971). The key step in either of the above derivations is the appeal to knowledge as a factive, an expression governing a sentence, which implies the truth of the contained sentence. The paradigm factive is "knows": If Jim knows that Plato is Bill's favorite philosopher then it follows that Plato is Bill's favorite philosopher. All the other assumptions about knowledge, for example, distribution over conjunction, are independently plausible and required by any formal analysis. (However, other accounts, like the one offered in chapter 1, require additional assumptions, e.g., $Bp \rightarrow BBp$. See Shoemaker 1996: section V.)

Belief is, of course, not factive. It can be true that X believes that p when p is false. What is to be explained, however, is the heard contradiction in asserting (1). We hear such an assertion as a contradiction, which reflects what would be a contradiction in the agent's own thought. Transparency implies that, from the agent's own point of view, when he attends to his belief that p, he takes it to be the case that p. Thus, from the first-person point of view, belief is treated as factive, licensing the move from $B\sim Bp$ to $\sim Bp$, which directly contradicts Bp. The agent cannot believe of himself that he believes both that p and that he does not believe that p.

The first-person factiveness or transparency of belief implies that when one attends to a set of one's beliefs $Bp_1, \ldots, Bp_n$, then from one's point of view at that time, the following is true: $p_1, \ldots, p_n$. That is, for each Bp_i to be true, from one's point of view, is for all of them to be true from one's point of view, since the point of view is simply that of a single fully aware consciousness.

This implication of transparency follows from the parallel with assertion. What we assert when we express our belief that p, is simply p not our attitude toward it. When we express a partial belief, we offer a qualified assertion (not merely the assertion of a qualified proposition) like "I am pretty sure that p."

The parallel takes us to the main arguments below. To assert a set of statements $p_1, \ldots, p_n$ is no different from asserting their conjunction. Any one of the statements that one asserts is available with any other. So if there is an inconsistency in asserting each of $p_1, \ldots, p_n$, that is no different from asserting the contradiction $p_1 \& \ldots \& p_n$. But a contradiction is not something that can be asserted—presented as true.

This might be questioned, because surely one can assert what amounts to a contradiction or inconsistency, when one does not recognize it as such. However, it is just this possibility that is eliminated in the very formulation of all three paradoxes. The inconsistency is purely formal—not dependent on additional assumptions.[7] All involve the joint presentation of a set of statements and the negation of it, so no recognition problem arises. All that is assumed is that no one can assert the negation of a set of statements without conceiving that it and those statements cannot hold simultaneously.[8]

2   The Pseudo–Moore's Paradox

The force of transparency for the two other paradoxes will be introduced by considering a traditionally second form of Moore's Paradox, which is much less often discussed:

(3)   *p,* but I believe that not-*p.*

Recall, by contrast, the basic and weaker:

(1)   *p,* but I do not believe that *p.*

Contrary to what might be assumed, solutions to (1) do not transfer to (3). A natural claim to make about Moore's Paradox is that the assertion is heard as contradictory because its second conjunct denies the presupposition of assertion that the speaker believes what he asserts.[9] But although this holds for (1), it does not hold for (3).

In his analysis of Moore's Paradox, Sydney Shoemaker also derives a self-contradiction from (1), though more complex than mine. But he cannot derive a similar self-contradiction when he turns to a version (3). What follows is only that "the subject has inconsistent beliefs—that she both believes that *p* and believes that not-*p* . . . while it is logically impossible for someone to truly believe the content *p and I do not believe that p*, there is not the same case for its being logically impossible for someone to truly believe the content *I believe that p, but not p*" (Shoemaker 1996: 87; with stylistic variations). What is puzzling about this result is that (3) entails (1), given that disbelief implies nonbelief (lack of belief):

If *X* believes that not *p* then it is not the case that *X* believes that *p.* (*X* believes (not-*p*) implies not-(*X* believes *p*))

(The converse obviously fails.) Of course, what is at issue is not the logical relation between (1) and (3), but the relation between the beliefs in each of them. Still, given that disbelief implies lack of belief, the break here is disturbing. As the above proof shows, the sentence expressing that one believes (1) entails a self-contradiction. Why doesn't Shoemaker's analysis yield the contradiction for the assertion of (3) that it does for the assertion of (1), given that (3) is a logically stronger proposition than (1)? Even where awareness of the entailments hold (i.e., "I believe not-*p*" entails "I do not believe *p*"; "I do not believe *p*" entails "It is not the case that I believe *p*"), Shoemaker can not derive for (3) the contradiction that he derives for the weaker (1). Transitivity should carry over from the content of those beliefs to the beliefs that their contents are true. But it does not seem to on Shoemaker's analysis.

The resolution to this puzzle is that when the thought underlying (3) is properly expressed, then asserting it, unlike asserting (1) or (2), generates no paradox at all. What (3) is meant to express becomes more like the assertion "John is very rich, but he is not very rich" (meant literally). The content of the assertion, not just the asserting of it, is a contradiction.[10]

Since assertion expresses belief, the second conjunct of (3) is not expressing the belief that not-p. The proper formulation for what the second conjunct is intended to report would be to assert just its content (not-p). To express the belief that p, I just assert it; I do not assert that "I believe that p," which is heard as a weaker claim.[11] Correspondingly, the qualifier "I believe that . . ." in the second conjunct of (3) should be dropped, so that we are left simply with "not-p."

Thus the proper reformulation of (3) to express the corresponding belief is:

(3′) p, but not-p.

Of course, this yields no paradox, since it is an out-and-out contradiction. (1) and (2) are paradoxical (to assert) because, although neither of these is a contradiction, the assertion of either is heard as a contradiction. But (3′) itself, and not just its assertion, is a contradiction.

3   The Impotence of Rejecting the Conjunction Rule

My results for Moore's Paradox bear on the Lottery and the Preface Paradoxes, though we have special interest here and later (chapter 11) in the Preface Paradox. I begin with the Lottery Paradox (Kyburg 1961: 197). Its first premise is that the criterion for the acceptance of a hypothesis is purely probabilistic:

Accept h when its probability on the evidence is greater than, say, .95.

Second, imagine that there is a fair lottery with 1000 tickets. You have one ticket t_{123}. The probability that you will lose the lottery with that ticket is .999, which is significantly more than .95. (Clearly, no matter how high the threshold for acceptance [below 1], a suitably larger lottery could be constructed.) So you accept the statement that you will lose the lottery.

But now for each of the other 999 tickets, the probability that each of them will lose is also .999. So each of these satisfies the condition for acceptance. If you had bought all the tickets in the lottery, you would accept that each ticket will lose. The third premise is the conjunction rule:

(**CR**) $\text{Acc}(q_1), \ldots, \text{Acc}(q_n) \rightarrow \text{Acc}(q_1 \,\&\, \ldots \,\&\, q_n)$.

By the first premise, we accept, for each of the 1000 tickets, the statement that it will lose; the third premise (CR) is just that the conjunction of those 1000 statements is likewise accepted. It follows that we have accepted that all the tickets will lose. But it is impossible for every ticket to lose, if it is a fair lottery.

The Preface Paradox is so-called in reference to a typical disclaimer that occurs in prefaces to books (Makinson 1964). The author of a nonfictional work writes something like "Remaining errors in the book are my own." The author is justified in making this assertion—given the numerous statements in the book, he is bound to have made some error. He may even know of other authors, whom he regards as exceeding him in care, research, and competence, who have produced works with errors. The author thereby presupposes that "at least one statement in this book is false." Call this the *preface-assertion*. However, for each statement in the book, the author believes that it is true. But now the total set of statements in the book, which includes the preface-assertion, is inconsistent. As standardly presented, the Preface Paradox has the form of "w-inconsistency." All instances of a generalization are true, but not the generalization itself.

There are striking similarities between the Preface and Lottery Paradoxes, but there is one crucial disanalogy. We cannot just reject the claim that one believes or accepts that each statement is true, as we could in the case of the Lottery, where the grounds are purely probabilistic.[12] In the Preface Paradox, for each statement in the book, we can imagine that one accepts or believes it on adequate evidential grounds. The grounds are not purely probabilistic.[13]

The main similarity is that a contradiction emerges only through appeal to the conjunction rule (CR). The result can then be taken as a reason to reject the rule. This rejection is supported on various independently plausible grounds, in particular the claim that a conjunction will be less probable, except in degenerate cases, than the probability of each of the individual conjuncts (Kyburg 1970). Nevertheless, I will argue, on the basis of transparency of belief, that a contradiction emerges even without the conjunction rule. So rejecting it cannot solve the problem.

Besides transparency, the argument assumes that acceptance as true issues in (full) belief.[14] This assumption is generally endorsed as a premise in the Lottery Paradox. We understand acceptance in a standard way as capturing the judgment that sufficient positive evidence has been found in support of a hypothesis to warrant our endorsing it as true. To endorse it as true is to (fully) believe it. (The Preface Paradox is often formulated directly in terms of belief.)

Moore's Paradox confirms this assumption. To accept that p is to judge p true and to detach p from the evidence supporting it. One is then warranted in asserting that p. So if acceptance is sufficient for assertibility, a proposal to allow acceptance without full belief would generate an instance of (1), that is, to assert that one accepts p, and to deny that one believes it.

In the Preface Paradox, the following is held to capture the rational, though inconsistent, set of beliefs:

(4) $Acc(p_1), \ldots, Acc(p_n), Acc(not\text{-}(p_1 \& \ldots \& p_n))$, where $p_1, \ldots, p_n$ are all the statements in the book.

The set of accepted statements is inconsistent—they cannot all be true. But it is urged that the author's excellent reasons or evidence to believe the preface-assertion ($not\text{-}(p_1 \& \ldots \& p_n)$) show that the author is "being rational though inconsistent" (Makinson 1964: 207).

If it is rational to accept an inconsistent set of statements, and if rationality does not exclude full awareness of the inconsistency, then the person ought to be able to recognize this inconsistency among his beliefs. But, to return to a claim of chapter 1, it seems incoherent to hold, as it would be incoherent to assert, that each of a set of one's beliefs is true including the belief that at least one of them is not.

Nonetheless, we should not yet take our stand here. Those who are not troubled by (4) either deny any incoherence in it (or its assertion) or else claim that any incoherence we find applies only to small subsets of belief. They take the Preface Paradox itself to argue that the inconsistency in (4) must be tolerated, since such an inconsistency will hold for most any substantial set of beliefs.

If the conjunction rule (CR) is rejected, the claim is that we do not derive the following from (4):

(5) $Acc(p_1 \& \ldots \& p_n \& not\text{-}(p_1 \& \ldots \& p_n))$.

For those who solve the problem by rejecting (CR), only (5), not (4), is intolerable. For the content of (5) is a contradiction, and thus to affirm (5) would be to accept or believe a contradiction.

The main objection should now be evident: Given the assumption that acceptance issues in full belief, each statement of the form Acc(. . .) in (4) is understood as full belief. But then, given transparency, from the first-person point of view we detach from (4) each of its references to acceptance (Acc) and so to belief as well, yielding

(6) $p_1, \ldots, p_n,$ not-$(p_1 \& \ldots \& p_n)$.

(6) is logically equivalent to the contradiction:

(7) $p_1 \& \ldots \& p_n \&$ not-$(p_1 \& \ldots \& p_n)$.

(6) is overtly inconsistent—the inconsistency is explicit in its logical form, as discussed above, so there is no further call for the recognition of the inconsistency. Rejection of the conjunction rule (CR) is simply irrelevant. (6) is derived from (4) without appeal to (CR).

4 A Positive Proposal

If solutions that reject the conjunction rule fail, how should we resolve the Preface and Lottery Paradoxes? Concentrating on the Preface, the resolution I favor denies that the preface-assertion, not-$(p_1 \& \ldots \& p_n)$, is fully believed by the author.[15] Further, although the author assigns the preface-assertion a high subjective probability (corresponding to a high objective chance of error), it is not, evidence against any of the p_i. The author's attitude toward the preface-assertion is roughly the same as for solutions to the Lottery Paradox, which hold that the individual statements attesting to one's losing the lottery with a single ticket are not accepted (fully believed), but only assigned a high degree of probability.[16] The following three related points extend the parallel (between the preface-assertion and the assertion that one will lose the lottery with a single ticket) and so support the positive proposal.

First, one does not know that one will lose the lottery with a particular ticket. Where one knows that one will lose, betting in a lottery is not just financially irrational, but crazy, almost literally throwing money away.[17] Similarly, the author does not know his book contains an error. If he did, he could not fully believe each statement in it.

Second, if one does win the lottery, one is very much surprised. A highly improbable statement has turned out to be true. But there is no resistance to accepting this result—highly improbable events often occur; over a long enough series of trials, some almost definitely will occur; and sometimes, as in a fair lottery, at least one must occur. This response (of nonresistance) is in contrast to our response when an evidentially very well-supported statement turns out to be false. We resist the discovery, precisely for its conflict with strong evidence.

Our reaction to the discovery of the truth of the preface-assertion follows the former, not the latter response. Imagine that a video tape is discovered of the historical event that the book in question is about. The tape corroborates every statement in the author's book.[18] The author's reaction is akin to that of one who wins a lottery. He is surprised at the occurrence of a highly improbable event. But he is not resistant to it (and not simply because he is pleased). Accepting the veracity of the tape does not conflict with his grounds for the preface-assertion. In the lottery, the holder of the ticket can admit in advance that he might win the lottery, even while being almost sure that he will lose. So too the author. While affirming the preface-assertion, he can daydream that a video will be discovered verifying each and every claim in his book. Thus he cannot (and does not) accept or fully believe (or take himself to be in a position to know) the preface-assertion.

Third, the falsity of the preface-assertion, like the falsity of losing the lottery with a single ticket, does not instigate epistemic self-correction or learning. If, despite high improbability, one wins the lottery, one learns nothing so far as one's assessment goes. Even if you won the previous lottery with one chance in a thousand, the next time you purchase a single lottery ticket in a thousand-ticket lottery, you should assign the same probability—.999—that you will lose. Correspondingly, if one's preface-assertion is shown to be false, as with the discovery of the video, one does not take oneself to have learned that one's grounds for the preface-assertion were inadequate. The same fallibility and complexity will exist in the next case (say, the next nonfictional book the author publishes).

There is an obvious objection to my argument: The Preface Paradox begins with the claim that the author does *assert* that *remaining errors* in his book are his own. My response is that we do not take this assertion literally. The disclaimer "remaining errors" has a conditional ring to it, corresponding to the common formulations: "If there are remaining errors . . . " or "Any remaining errors. . . ."

Moreover, we also assert such things as "I'll lose the lottery." Since assertion represents the speaker as knowing what he asserts, the latter assertion, if treated literally, represents the speaker as knowing that he will lose the lottery (with a single ticket). But that is blatantly false, although such assertions are ordinarily accepted. (Were there a challenge, one would retreat: "OK, I suppose, if you want to be a stickler, I don't know that I'll lose, but I'm still extremely sure.") Instead, there is a tacit, cooperative weakening in our understanding of such assertions. It is mutually known that this is a gamble. It is also mutually salient that many such assertions will be offered. So to lessen the burden on conversation that would be engendered by extensive qualification, we understand the assertion that one will lose the lottery as implicitly qualified to something like "*I am almost sure that* [or, very probably] I'll lose the lottery." Audience-qualification of seemingly unqualified assertions occurs in many other cases, for example, fiction: If *S* says to *H*, "Cookie-monster is obese," *S* intends that *H* should understand that *S* meant by his assertion "In the *Sesame Street* TV show, Cookie-monster is obese." *S* would rightly take *H* to misunderstand him if *H* was critical of *S* by saying "But there's no such thing as Cookie-monster!"

Once we know that there are such cooperative simplifications, we can expect them to occur elsewhere when we can achieve economies without misleading. The asserting of the preface-assertion is, after all, not understood as purely informative, but it is also heard as a mutually recognized expression of modesty. We permit it to be a slight overstatement, as a form of simplification, but also to facilitate expressions of modesty. It would be difficult to express modesty in such terms as "I am almost sure that there are errors in this book," for these formulations appear simply to represent an exact state of mind and thus do not permit self-effacement over one's achievements.[19]

5   The Assertion Parallel and the Pseudo–Preface Paradox

The results in the previous section corroborate our view of the preface-assertion. It is not truly asserted, but rather is understood only as implicitly qualified (a "guarded assertion") corresponding to the author's only partially believing it. Those results depended on our ongoing parallel with assertion. For S to assert that p is for S to express her belief that p. We invoked this parallel in application to Moore's Paradox, although for our purposes all we need is that satisfaction of the conditions on assertion implies belief.[20]

Earlier we contrasted the genuine Moore's Paradox (1) (or (2)) with the pseudo–Moore's Paradox (3) that is often viewed as merely a variant of it. The discrepancy we found is that (3) is stronger than (1), yet a contradiction arises (in thought) only from the assertion of (1). Our resolution is that (3) is just a contradiction, its real meaning hidden by the pragmatics of asserting "I believe that . . .".

We can find a parallel to this discrepancy for the Preface Paradox, but now there is a reversal. What is asserted as the Preface Paradox is a generalization of the pseudo–Moore's Paradox:

(8) $p_1, \ldots, p_n$ but I believe that not-$(p_1 \& \ldots \& p_n)$.

(Let us hold on to the "I believe that . . ." for illustrative purposes.) The Preface Paradox is not, however, standardly presented in the weaker form of a generalized Moore's Paradox:

(9) $p_1, \ldots, p_n$, but I do not believe $(p_1 \& \ldots \& p_n)$.

Why do we accept so readily the Preface Paradox in the stronger form of (8), when we would not accept (9) were we even afforded the opportunity? The discrepancy reveals the misleading nature of the standard presentations.

Imagine that the speaker S asserts each of $p_1, \ldots, p_n$. H then asks "Are you sure that $p_1, \ldots, p_n$?" S, recognizing that he has asserted a mouthful, affirms modestly, "Well, yes, but I suppose I may have been wrong somewhere." My suggestion, drawing on the previous section and in corroboration of a main thesis, is that H can accept this latter assertion (and so (8) on a nonliteral reading) because he implicitly qualifies it. S is almost sure that one of his assertions is wrong. But he does not flat-out assert it—he does not take himself to be in a position to know it.

It follows further that S's grounds for his modest affirmation (of the preface-assertion) cannot be evidence against any of $p_1, \ldots, p_n$. For these are not then surrendered (withdrawn) as assertions.

6   Evidence and the Generality Constraints

The standard presentation of the Preface Paradox treats it as a vivid illustration of a problem that arises for any very large or complex set of beliefs.

The problem is that as the number of beliefs accepted increases, it becomes more likely that at least one of them is false. The total set of these beliefs, including that at least one of them is false, is inconsistent (i.e., (4)).

This presentation tacitly imposes two crucial constraints on solutions—the *conclusion-generality* constraint and the *evidence-generality* constraint. The conclusion-generality constraint is that one does not easily reject a set of well-founded beliefs. It is this constraint that is thought to be violated by the move from inconsistency (4) to suspension of judgment about individual beliefs. However, although our solution to the Preface Paradox rejects (4), it does not run afoul of this constraint, a claim that will be reinforced in the discussion of the second constraint.

The evidence-generality constraint is that the grounds for the preface-assertion must (fully) support that assertion by virtue of some very general feature (like being a complex set of beliefs), not by virtue of problems specific to a particular set of beliefs. The evidence-generality constraint appears to be easily met in the usual presentations. The basis for the preface-assertion is just our fallibility together with the complexity of the set of beliefs in the author's text.

The preface-assertion holds of any complex set of beliefs, and it is taken as "strong evidence" that there is some error in the author's book (Foley 1993: 165). However, if fallibility and complexity were evidence for accepting the preface-assertion, then, on the solution here proposed, we ought to suspend judgment on the individual statements in the book. Evidence that one of a set of beliefs is false is (trivially) part of the total evidence on which acceptance of each individual belief is based. So including such evidence in our reasons for judgment would block acceptance of those individual beliefs.

Take one of many natural examples. Each of a large set of statistical data seems to have been honestly collected; yet, on viewing the totality, we find that the data are just too good (the curves too smooth), given expected interferences and errors. Once we come to accept that the data collected are tainted—that the curves are *too* smooth—we no longer accept the individual data points as correct.

What differentiates such examples from the Preface Paradox as originally formulated? In the case just presented, the undermining observation is supported by background evidence to the effect that expected interferences and random errors in data collection preclude an exact fit with simple equations. Evidence has a built-in specificity owing to its content and the physical relation between the evidence and what it is evidence for. Being evidence for (or against) a complex set of beliefs is almost never evidence for that set of beliefs because of its complexity. The evidence arises from what the set of beliefs is about, not from facts about them as beliefs (namely, that they are complex).

It might be thought that the inherent specificity of evidence is to no avail, since we can virtually stipulate evidence that satisfies the evidence-generality constraint. Simply imagine that the author of the book is "well aware" that "there is independent inductive evidence of a very strong kind that virtually all substantial factual books that have been written contain some false claims" (Priest 1998: 411). But if there is strong evidence—for example, there is some universal defect that arises in the writing of most, if not all, factual books—and if, in consequence, we suspend judgment on the individual statements in a particular book, then there is no violation of the conclusion-generality constraint, any more than when the "too good" data are, nevertheless, deemed accurate. We are not easily or cheaply skeptical. Rather, we have made an astonishing empirical discovery.

More plausibly, the purported strong inductive evidence is that, in each of many randomly sampled factual texts examined, some error is found. But, once we take seriously the existence of such evidence, further assumptions need to be substantiated in order to confirm the startling conclusion that all factual works are infected with error. We need to show, for example, that these errors do not indicate patterns that could be corrected in subsequent works. As soon as we detect any patterns or common faults, either we have a basis for correction (progressive diminution of errors) or, if not, we can reject the details of the individual works without violation of the conclusion-generality constraint, as noted in the previous paragraph.

If, however, no such pattern or common fault is posited so as to meet the evidence-generality constraint, we are drawn back to the view that the grounds are no more than complexity and fallibility, which, I already argued (and will extend the argument in chapter 10), is not evidence for accepting the preface-assertion. Accordingly, again, we are not compelled to suspend judgment on the individual statements. In short, if your grounds for the preface-assertion meet the evidence-generality constraint, then there is no violation of the conclusion-generality constraint. Either the skepticism is an empirically well-founded result independent of Preface-Paradox concerns, or else the grounds support only the high probability of the preface-assertion and therefore do not constitute evidence against the individual statements.

The claim that the rejection of (4) would lead directly to a sweeping skepticism is almost exactly the opposite of the truth. So far we have made good on half of that claim, that is, rejection of (4), because the inconsistency does not carry over to most any other complex set of beliefs (and so does not violate the conclusion-generality constraint). Now let us make good on the other half—it is actually the view being criticized that lends itself to the too-easy skeptical result. For what is the key step in familiar skeptical arguments? It is to take fallibility as an undermining reason. As noted in chapter 4, it is to take the formal consistency of the evidence, with the denial of the belief based on that evidence, as a reason not to hold a belief. But to endorse the view that there is some reason not to believe that *p* is to imply that there is some reason to doubt that *p,* so one can no longer fully believe it.

The skeptical import of this reason to reject (CR) is evident in the resulting retreat from appeal to conclusive reasons or knowledge (for which (CR) holds): "A knowledge *claim* is not the same as knowledge. What we have to work with in the real world are knowledge claims, reasonable beliefs. To have warrant for a number of knowledge claims is not at all to have warrant for the corresponding conjunctive knowledge claim" (Kyburg 1997: 125; see also 115). But to retreat from knowledge to knowledge claims is to deny entitlement to detachment from our own attitudes toward the way things are. For if the move from "*X* claims that *X* knows that *p*" to "*X* knows that *p*" cannot be warranted, the original claim cannot be satisfied.[21]

7   First-Person Methodology

The methodology of this chapter has been relentlessly first-personal, a methodology advocated in this work from the start. The key move from the inconsistency of a set of accepted (believed) propositions (4) to the outright contradiction in (6) depends on our recognition that the latter is how the former appears from the agent's point of view. The Lottery and the Preface Paradoxes (and, more overtly, Moore's Paradox) concern the coherence of an individual's set of beliefs. If a set of beliefs is coherent, then the believer can recognize himself as holding those beliefs (abstracting from any psychological interferences triggered by the recognition).

My approach to the Lottery and Preface Paradoxes is, then, independently motivated. Without reference to those paradoxes, I defend the transparency claim, and then apply it to them. In contrast, the standard solutions to the Lottery and Preface Paradoxes depend on those paradoxes to generate reasons for adopting their proposed strategies—for example, their rejection of (CR).

In the opening section to this chapter, I observed that the steps in the proof of Moore's Paradox (as entailing a contradiction) would be first-personally endorsed. One cannot assert p and assert q, and, while aware of those assertions, not assent to p & q. Here is another obstacle to rejection of the conjunction principle. What, however, is standardly claimed, particularly in reflection on the Preface Paradox, is that for a small number of conjuncts this "adjunction" principle holds, but not when there are many.

Our reflective judgments are equivocal. If one is asked why she endorses the adjunction rule, the explanation would be to the effect that if p is true and q is true, then, of course, their conjunction is true. The explanation makes no allusion to size (the number of conjuncts). The endorsement and the explanation accords with our practice as teachers—this is a standard way of generating the first line of the truth-table for "&," and it could do so only if it is in accord with a presentation unrestricted by the number of conjuncts. However, we also judge that we are fallible, and that this fallibility enters seriously only with a complex set of beliefs.

So, as just indicated, those who reject adjunction are well motivated. Most prominently, in practice, adjunction imposes (computational) complexities that are ill suited to "bounded" reasoners.[22] I have not addressed these reasons, and I hardly think they should be rejected. Rather, we need a reconciliation. The obvious one is to distinguish between the demands of the concept of belief, revealed in first-personal awareness, and the demands of believers. My position throughout concerns the former.

Those who take the boundedness view conceive the Preface Paradox as an argument to show that inconsistent beliefs are a constant condition. Thus, following on the conclusion-generality constraint, they hold that if consistency is imposed as a condition on belief, we will immediately be obliged to surrender most of what we believe. But those who take this view have not made good on this claim, because they have conflated two cases.

The Preface Paradox is one, and we have already denied that the preface-assertion is fully believed. The other kind of case is that of the familiar examples of inconsistency maintained through categorization. As in my earlier example, when I was told of a journal that accepts 10 percent of its submissions I thought that it does not have high standards, though when told that a journal rejects 9 out of 10 submissions, I thought that it does have high standards. The crucial difference between these cases is that in one kind of case the inconsistency is recognized, but not in the other.

This first-person methodology is not standard. Not only does my solution to the Preface Paradox differ from standard ones; my understanding of that Paradox differs as well. The standard methodology takes the perspective of rationality, claiming that we need to accept (4) because it is rational for us to tolerate inconsistency, rather than resign ourselves to a sweeping skepticism (violating the conclusion-generality constraint). Instead of taking the primary question to be "What is it rational to believe?" the first-person approach takes the primary question to be: What can the agent believe? We cannot believe (4), since treated transparently, it is an out-and-out contradiction. That (conceptual) unbelievability signals an incoherence, explicitly represented by (6).

The conclusions we have reached accord with transparency. In the original Preface Paradox, the author looks past the fact of his believing each statement in his book to the statements (content) themselves. He asserts them. But he does not similarly look through his attitude toward the preface-assertion to the preface-assertion itself. Rather, he can properly understand the thought that there is an error in his book only by recognizing that he has a high degree of partial belief in the content of that thought. The author cannot, first-personally, look just to the content of his attitude. He can see it only nontransparently, as mediated by that attitude.

8

Constraints on Us to Fully Believe

1   An Example and a Challenge to Evidentialism

In Jane Austen's *Pride and Prejudice* Elizabeth is indignant at Darcy because years earlier he treated his ward Wickham unjustly. Although previous behavior by Darcy had disposed Elizabeth to think ill of him, her pivotal evidence against Darcy comes from the ward himself. Her judgment is solidified hearing only one side of the story. Yet, the very admirable Elizabeth is not one for hasty judgments. Although she scolds herself for the judgment on later discoveries, when we take a participant's rather than a reader's point of view we sympathize with the conclusion that she drew in the circumstances.

The events illustrate that our social world, institutions, and practices restrict our freedom to withhold belief (suspend judgment). Elizabeth has a good basis for judgment—Wickham's testimony and its coherence with her negative "first impressions" of Darcy. As the default view of testimony prescribes (chapter 5), so long as Elizabeth had no special reason to question the ward's testimony, she ought to accept it. Although Austen means to teach us the danger of "first impressions" or prejudgment, we could not maintain our affection for Elizabeth were we not to resonate with her judgment of Darcy, even while we know it is erroneous and resistant to contrary indications.

Of course, from Elizabeth's retrospective point of view, as from the reader's god's-eye view, it is natural to think that there is a special reason to question Wickham's testimony:[1] either Wickham's own involvement, even if Elizabeth has no reason to think that he had motive to lie, or a caution to hear either "both sides of the story" or to withhold judgment based only on "first impressions." But neither alternative is workable as a generalized directive—one has special reason to question testimony, if the speaker has a personal stake in that to which he is testifying; or, one should listen to "both sides of the story" or not go by first impressions before reaching judgment—too much good information would be sacrificed if we followed either directive.

The example from *Pride and Prejudice* is meant to illustrate the challenge posed by *constraints* on us to form (full) beliefs and that such constraints are a feature of many of our belief-forming practices.[2] We cannot wholesale or largely opt out of these practices, and to participate in them restricts us from forming the whole range of degrees of belief. The participation presupposes full belief—Elizabeth can neither sympathize with the ward nor engage her own disapproval of Darcy without a full belief that he treated the ward ill.

Obviously, constraints on us to form full beliefs raise a problem for evidentialism. If we can form beliefs fully with limited inquiry, then, perhaps, the claims of belief are satisfied by less than conclusive reasons or knowledge, or else, we rarely satisfy those claims. Evidentialism is troubled if nonevidential influences on belief override evidential ones and do not require cloaking.

Moreover, the very limited inquiry under which such beliefs are formed is only one facet of the problem. The phenomenon of constraints on action due to our social practices is a banality. There is little choice but to be a member of a social community; and, whatever social community it is, it will have rules, duties, and practices, however informal, from many of which we cannot opt out. This phenomenon poses no conceptual problem or conflict, since the aim to comply with rules provides a reason for action.

Constraints on belief-formation, however, do raise conceptual problems because belief and assertion enter claims that deny restrictions unrelated to the truth of the belief. If belief-formation is affected by constraints on us to believe fully, the range of degrees of belief that one may form is greatly reduced, before any evidence is discerned. This chapter develops a challenge to evidentialism by exhibiting patterns of everyday, seemingly undistorted belief-formation, like that described above, responsive to nonevidential factors.

2   A Sketchy Background on Constraints

Constraints on belief-formation are restrictions against a lack of full belief (suspension of judgment). A prevalent reaction to evidentialism is that it is too demanding, and this reaction dovetails with the workings of constraints. We need beliefs across a wide spectrum of domains, and we cannot expect there to be strong, let alone conclusive, evidence for all or even many of them. We will be returning to this intuitive reaction a number of times.

In conversation, speakers present their assertion as true. So in forming their assertion, like their belief, they commit themselves to responsivity to all the options that the world offers. But in wanting to contribute to a conversation, one must conform to the situational demands to be brief and to maintain interest, and these serve to limit the expressions one may use. You cannot expect to express the subtle complexities of your views on euthanasia, if you want to participate in the excited argument in the neighborhood bar or dinner party. But since your assertions are presented by you as your belief and taken by others as your position, the social situation itself will affect in turn the shape of your beliefs in this area, given mild assumptions such as that you care to keep the trust of other participants.

A long tradition in social psychology emphasizes situational determinants of behavior and the influence of these determinants on belief. In a classic of "attribution theory," H. H. Kelley observes that it is crucial to the importance of the cognitive-dissonance phenomenon that a subject have an "illusion of freedom"; he can be induced "to feel he has total freedom to express himself when in fact he has none" (1967: 226). The cognitive-dissonance experiments—briefly discussed in chapter 3 above—reinforce a sense of freedom, with the experimenter telling the subject "It's up to you to decide what you want to do" (1967: 227). Kelley goes on to note that the whole setup involves "much pressure and constraint which is exerted so diffusely that the subject's attention is never called to its presence" (1967: 228; see also Nisbett and Wilson 1977: 239; and Ross 1988).

Currently, observations like Kelley's are assimilated to "nonconscious" influences on belief. But the constraints on us to form full beliefs need not operate as surreptitious determinants of our attitudes and beliefs. It is important for the challenges they raise to evidentialism that the constraints we point to are not the distortive influences of ideology, ego defenses, or deep-seated prejudices. The constraints are not specific to individuals. They are a feature of institutional and social practices.[3] The constraints are forceful because the possibilities for restructuring these practices are very limited.

There are literary and philosophical traditions that appreciate the hold on us of social conventions and rules, which represent constraints of a narrower and more evident form than those that are our focus. Moliere's *The Misanthrope* mocks the pretenses of Alceste in disavowing the gracious deceptions and comforting lies of social life (Shklar 1984: chapter 2). By contrast, Plato represents Socrates, particularly in the early dialogues, as one who admirably defies conventional pieties. At the close of his legal defense in the *Apology,* for example, Socrates rejects appeals to pity: "Perhaps one of you might be angry as he recalls that when he himself stood trial on a less dangerous charge, he begged and implored the jury with many tears, that he brought his children and many of his friends and family into court to arouse as much pity as he could, but that I do none of these things, even though I may seem to be running the ultimate risk" (Plato 1981: 34c). Is such purity viable? If you are defending a plan for a system of national health insurance, for example, could you resist telling a few "horror" stories about those who suffered for lack of adequate coverage? You might judge that these stories are typical, and so directly in point. But what if, instead, you judge that the horror stories are few and isolated? They amount to no more than the unfortunate consequences of almost any significant large-scale policy—effectively, they are merely anecdotal evidence. Your argument really rests on bland statistics, and it is no weaker for that. But to be persuasive, your arguments need to be heard. They are much less likely to be given a hearing if they are dominated by statistics, without the compensating enticement of poignant stories.

To take the heroic Socratic route consistently would be a self-indulgent attempt to avoid "dirty hands" at all costs (Stocker 1990: part I). Even Socrates fails in the attempt. For he uses the lawyer's trick of specifying the appeal that he will refuse to offer, and thereby effectively offering it. Socrates mentions his wife and children, something that knowingly garners pity, given that he is threatened by the "ultimate risk." Moreover, by mentioning them, as he denigrates appeals to pity, he disarms the jury from criticizing him for it. (A final touch of Socratic irony is that his denial that he will appeal to pity is appropriate in his legal proof, since Socrates does bear the burden of justifying his deviation from standard legal defenses.)

Compromise with constraints need not be wholesale surrender of principle, as Socrates suggests. The appeal to pity is a means of disposing the audience to fair reception of the argument (though it is still to "dirty" one's hands, since it is expected to cast a more favorable glow on the argument than strictly deserved). Realistically, such compromise is unavoidable. Socrates' contrary actions work only for the isolated case, and even there, not cleanly. The possibility of compromise is further evidence that the constraints on us toward forming full belief are not helpfully viewed as nonconscious forces on belief, even if that is how they typically operate. They are situationally and socially determined antecedent limits on both suspension of judgment (adopting only a degree of belief) and extended inquiry.

The limits apply to a practice, like public argument, overall, and the force of the constraints depend crucially on their not binding us in each instance of that practice—the possibility is open to opt out in any particular case (e.g., not participating in some debates in our vicinity or offering only heavily qualified opinions). If we have that option, we are unlikely to notice the constraints, and so reinforce our stance that our freedom is unlimited, a central theme of the empirical studies noted above.

Our discussion of constraints on believing is strewn with claims as to what *must* or *cannot* be done. You cannot express your complex views in terms of degrees of belief, but must express them as full beliefs. Fundamental roles in our lives must be played by full beliefs, yet these roles cannot wait on completion of optimal and successful inquiry. We can now better appreciate that the necessity alluded to in this chapter is neither the conceptual necessity that dominated the main arguments for evidentialism nor any social or psychological compulsion. The unavoidability is never a barrier to responding to reasons. One can try to negotiate the constraints. One must express one's opinions, but if one's views are very complex, one seeks forums that tolerate more expansive and nuanced argument. My claim is that one cannot regularly opt out when one does not find such sophisticated forums. The strength of this "cannot" is the strength of demands on us to participate in many social, intellectual practices, and of our impotence to shape them.

3   The Argument for Constraints on Reactive Attitude Beliefs

In this section, I argue for constraints on emotion-laden responses to the actions of others toward us, what Peter Strawson refers to as our *reactive attitudes*. These include resentment, gratitude, or indignation, which Strawson characterizes as "natural human reactions to the good or ill will or indifference of others towards us, as displayed in *their* attitudes and actions" (1982: 67). Reactive attitude judgments imply beliefs. If Joe resents Marcia's interrupting him when he is speaking, then Joe believes that Marcia rudely (and so, wrongly) interrupted him.

An outline of the argument for constraints on reactive-attitude beliefs is this: (1) Our reactive attitudes involve judgments of the actions of others (the *"actor"*) toward us and judgments that involve us (the *"reactor"*), even if only vicariously. So a necessary condition for the formation of our reactive attitudes is that we have beliefs about the reasons or intentions that inform the action of others and about the appropriateness of our responses. (2) More specifically, the nature of these judgments requires not just that we have these beliefs, but that we have them as full, nonepistemically qualified beliefs. But (3) there are serious practical restraints that normally limit the evidence that agents in these situations have available to them in advance of judgment. Yet, (4) in order for social life to continue recognizably as it is, we must form reactive attitudes in a large number of the situations in which they are elicited (and these include, prominently, cases falling under premise (3)). So, (5) insofar as we are able, we must often form full beliefs with limited investigation, rather than proportioning (downward) toward degrees of belief. My opening example from *Pride and Prejudice* is meant to illustrate this argument.

The first premise (1) concerns the beliefs implied by the judgments that express our reactive attitudes.[4] The (negative) reactive attitudes imply judgments that attribute responsibility to the actor, not merely causally, but for fault or liability. Specifically, the reactor denies that the actor's behavior is excusable, as when an offensive joke is told in a social group. The reactor judges that the joke is either in poor taste or designed to specially offend some members of the group. So the actor must have recognized (perhaps, intended) that the joke would offend. The actor did not have a particularly bad day and has no other excuse (e.g., severe domestic problems) that, if discovered later, would lead the reactor to regret his harsh judgment. If, instead, the actor did suffer one of these excuses, it would not entail that the joke was not offensive. Quite the contrary, it would make clear why an excuse was needed. But the excuse defeats the inference from an offense committed to a negative judgment of character or a high degree of blameworthiness.

According to premise (2), the nature of these judgments requires not just that we have these beliefs, but that we have them as full beliefs. In principle, and opposed to this most suspect premise, there appear to be a number of ways to sustain such judgments without the corresponding degree of certainty. We might suitably qualify the judgment (instead of judging that p, judge only that, say, it is almost certain that p). As already indicated in section I, this initially credible proposal is not viable.

The wide variety of reactive attitude judgments we are focusing on implies a culpability on the part of the actor for a wrongdoing. Especially, but not solely, when these judgments are moral judgments, the reactor is duty-bound to be convinced that the assessment grounding his judgment is correct. If John is only pretty sure that Mary is teasing him, he can feel resentful, but he cannot yet resent that she teased him.

In brief, our reactive attitudes normally do *not admit of epistemic qualification*. There are all manner of differences between, say, mild and strong resentment; or between being annoyed, irritated, and offended by someone's actions. But there are no attitudes corresponding to a compromise between a negative reactive attitude toward someone (e.g., disgust, revulsion) and a weak epistemic position (e.g., I am slightly more confident than not that . . .) to judge whether the claims of that attitude are met.

Mild resentment is never resentment caused by what one judges to be a serious offense directed toward oneself tempered by one's degree of uncertainty in that judgment—for example, a student's mildly resenting her teacher's lowering her grade because she refused his persistent personal advances, although she is not sure that the grade wasn't deserved. For similar reasons, there is no actually engaged attitude corresponding to a conditional resentment (anger), whose condition can only later be known to be fulfilled.[5]

One way to reinforce premise (2) is to consider cases where one's fragile predicament is glaring. Imagine that you think that you have been unjustly excluded from a club, group, or organization. Although most of the members opposed you, you cannot be sure how many, and you know that a few supported your case. The corollary of my claim that there is no place for epistemically qualified anger, indignation, or resentment is that you will find no place for straightforward anger, indignation, or resentment directed at any specific individual in this group, moderated by the degree of probability that he or she is one of the blackballers. In such situations one finds oneself in a confused and ambivalent state, and one adopts piecemeal, unsatisfying strategies (e.g., attempting to avoid contact with any members of the group).[6] Thinking of an individual member, one experiences ambivalence or vacillation, but no firm negative judgment-casting attitude with its attendant belief.

This conclusion—that in the envisaged circumstances there is ambivalence, but not firm judgment—appears subject to refutation when a belief is confused with a closely associated action. If, after being blackballed, the anger wells up in you and there is no chance of avoiding some of the potential blackballers, you would prefer to act negatively toward those you judge most likely to have blackballed you. You would rather be curt to these persons than to others in the group; or you are more suspicious of their ostensibly good willed actions toward you. But it does not follow that you actually have formed a negative reactive attitude toward them. The empirical punch is that you will tend to act toward them in ways, like being curt, that allow for "plausible deniability," rather than engage in overt retaliation.

Strong linguistic support for the claim that reactive-attitude beliefs cannot be epistemically qualified follows from the factive nature of the propositional expressions of our attitudes. "John resents Mary's teasing him" is derivative from "John resents the fact that Mary teased him." The latter is true only if Mary did tease John. But if there were an epistemically qualified form of resentment—"probably-resents"—the implication would not hold.[7]

A stronger implication to knowledge follows (Unger 1975: chap.4). If John resents the fact that Mary teased him, then John knows that Mary teased him. It follows then that if John is at all unsure that Mary teased him, he cannot (even mildly) resent the fact that she teased him.

Premise (3) is that there are serious practical obstacles that commonly restrict the evidence available prior to judgment. The most obvious is that the reactor has limited knowledge as to what the actor intended. The restrictions are especially severe when the judgment implies flawed character and the judger has only the single action on which to base his inference. Time, resources, or motivation to investigate further are tightly bound. For ordinary cases, as above, it is often not feasible or worthwhile to learn much more than is immediately apparent as to why, and the circumstances in which, the person acted.

The problem of "moral luck" is promoted by the common examples in which our attribution of blame for the same act is much more severe when actual harm is done (Williams 1981). In a standard example, we blame the truck driver who hits the child, however unavoidably, much more than we blame his colleague, who drives similarly but has the good fortune that no child runs suddenly into the path of his truck. For our ascriptions of blame to be more appropriate to what is within the actor's control, we often need to consider comparisons with how we would judge others who acted similarly, except for the actual harm. Obviously, though, situations come to us one at a time, and we do not store in accessible memory a record of prior judgments in similar situations.[8]

There are, as well, conceptual and social barriers to obtaining further evidence. Conceptually, the attitude toward seeking further evidence, even setting aside the implied full belief, is sometimes in conflict with the spontaneity that is a feature of many of our reactive attitudes.[9] Socially, it is often inappropriate to attempt to settle the open questions that one's judgment implies are foreclosed. The questions needed for judgment are heard as accusatory or presumptuous. Frequently, the policy that the reactor adopts toward the actor is avoidance, at least for the time being, which obviously precludes asking questions at all. If instead one queries others, then that is often to be nosy, or to risk appearing to be so.

These practical limitations apply most obviously to whether a wide variety of excusing conditions hold of the actor in his faulty behavior toward the reactor. Ruling out a wide variety of possible excusing conditions for any reactive-attitude attribution—a bad day at the office, a marital dispute, a close friend or relative taken suddenly ill—is, for practical reasons, normally beyond the reach of reactors.

This premise may strike the reader as especially implausible in light of the conclusion, (5), to which it leads. It implies both that our reactive attitudes are readily adopted and that the conditions under which they are adopted do not permit extensive inquiry. But then reactors' judgments (or beliefs) will frequently be mistaken, and so the actions they guide will fail. Failure would be noticed, and either criticism raised or correction or modification imposed. The lack of a critical stance toward these attitudes itself tells against the conclusion and this premise, in particular.

But the objection is faulty. The objection assumes an intimate connection between the onslaught of a reactive attitude and a correlative action. However, we often have strong reactive attitudes, without doing much about it. Our reactive attitudes typically weaken over time. We do not attempt to erect barriers to forgetting, such as keeping records, and we criticize one another for bearing grudges. It is time alone that is to heal, when there is no expectation that in the interim the actor's character will be altered or compensation (to the reactor) extended.

A number of the values one would ascribe to our reactive attitudes, or emotions, more generally, depend only very loosely on their being firmly established. The reactive attitudes are ways of being engaged with others, of enriching our experience, of caring. The emotions help demarcate "saliences" that direct attention (de Sousa 1987: 196). They are designed for responsiveness or sensitivity to perception, not sustained inquiry (Greenspan 1988: chaps. 1 and 4). At a remove from the evolutionary struggle for survival, the values of our reactive attitudes do not pivot on achieving high levels of certainty.

Finally, the objection falsely equates falling short of a high level of certainty with actual error. The claim I am advancing is that our reactive-attitude judgments are made under conditions of limited inquiry. The objection falsely equates that claim with the much stronger and dubious claim that these judgments are seriously prone to error.

According to premise (4), for social life to continue recognizably as it is, we must form reactive attitudes in a large number of the situations in which they are elicited. The starting point for this fourth premise, as well as for choosing to focus on the reactive attitudes, is, as already noted, Strawson's "Freedom and Resentment." Strawson argued that our reactive attitudes such as resentment, indignation, and gratitude are essential to maintaining anything like our social lives. If our social lives remain remotely as we know them, he concluded, no general thesis, such as determinism, could challenge those attitudes: "The human commitment to participation in ordinary inter-personal relationships is, I think, too thoroughgoing and deeply rooted for us to take seriously the thought that a general theoretical conviction might so change our world that, in it, there were no longer any such things as inter-personal relationships as we normally understand them, and being involved in inter-personal relationships as we normally understand them precisely is being exposed to the range of reactive attitudes and feelings that is in question" (Strawson 1982: 68). Strawson's is an argument for the natural necessity of our reactive attitudes. Given the kind of beings we are, broadly conceived, there is no alternative but to have these attitudes. Limited investigation and spontaneity are the usual conditions under which reactive attitudes are formed. These cases are too integral to our social and personal lives for us to envisage their being lifted out, while everything else remains intact.

The conclusion, (5), is that we must, insofar as we are able, often form full beliefs with limited investigation. (If the illustrations are realistic, we actually do form these beliefs, so we surely have the ability.) How strong is this "must," to recall our earlier question? Although it is nonoptional for us as social creatures to widely refrain from adopting reactive attitudes, and this is a crucial source of the constraints on us, it is less obvious how much room there is either for restructuring them or for at least taking a critical perspective on them, and so on ourselves.

Strawson's response to the question here of whether we can restructure our reactive attitudes is ambiguous. He declares forthrightly that "Inside the general structure or web of human attitudes and feelings of which I have been speaking, there is endless room for modification, redirection, criticism, and justification" (1982: 78). Yet, this criticism must always be internal to the "web of human attitudes." However, when we look at the influence of constraints on us, we can recognize that we are subject to opposed overreactions. As reactors, we are disposed to form reactive attitudes rapidly; and as the target or victim of a (negative) reactive attitude judgment we are disposed to demand of reactors decisive evidence. These overreactions do constitute criticism of the practice as a whole. Although, for reasons already given, there are severe limits on the possibility of restructuring the practice accordingly, it is best to leave open, as an empirical matter, the severity of those limits.

4   Demands on Participants in Assertion, Inquiry, and Argument

In the previous section, I argued for constraints on us both to form reactive-attitude judgments and, as a consequence, to form them as full beliefs. The contrast between full and partial belief will take center stage in the next chapter. Here I want to use this contrast to bring out constraints on more purely epistemic practices than the social practices of forming reactive attitudes.

The advantages of unqualified over (epistemically) qualified assertion explain a related basic role of full belief as the medium of *reasoning and argument*. Reasoning and argument run more smoothly with full, rather than partial, beliefs. With qualifiers one has to assess both the inferences and the weight of the qualification, rather than the inferences alone. Alternatively, one can draw a conclusion that is cumbersome, since stated in conditional form.

If the belief that p is false, then believing that p is incorrect. The falsity of a partial belief, however, does not entail its incorrectness. This is one way in which partial beliefs render critical discussion more difficult. If someone asserts "I am pretty sure that p," it is hard to focus criticism. Criticism may be viewed not as a challenge, but as explaining why one should be only "pretty sure."[10] The focus of discussion is not on the proposition alone, but also on the attitude of the speaker. Only in the case of full belief does the believer disappear from the argument. Recognized differences in partial belief toward the same content do not constitute conflict, a prominent stimulant to argument, unless it is also known that the evidence is shared. Since full belief claims to comprehend all the relevant evidence, recognizing shared evidence is unnecessary.[11]

The constraints on us to offer unqualified assertions for purposes of reasoning and argument extend to complex, controversial subjects. As observed above in section I, participation in informal and social discussion often does not allow us to express our views in their whole complexity.

Our opinions are improved through public argument, and in some ways can only be so improved. But in seeking the benefits derived from participation in the practice of argument, we incur duties and responsibilities. We need to promote forums that improve our beliefs and facilitate reasoning and argument. Full belief accords diverse viewpoints a place in the forum of discussion, resisting the many pulls toward homogenizing of positions. The most prominent pull is due to our respect for the judgments and efforts of others. We recognize the weaknesses of our own abilities as compared to that of many others, particularly when pooled. So we have good reasons to defer to them and to restrain our own contrary views. But if we continually defer to others, the set of views in lively contrast is narrowed.[12] Think of contemporary political positions that you regard as discredited and even denounce. Nevertheless, political debate and argument would be dull without them, and without them your motivation to delve more deeply into your own position would be weakened. Full beliefs protect a plurality of views, since less responsive than degrees of belief to new information. They forcefully motivate pursuit and defense of one's view. Where one holds only a partial belief, one refrains from making a commitment, pending further evidence. Thus the partial believer has less motivation to pursue and defend his view. Consequently, as participants in communities of argument and inquiry, we have a duty to form and express strong opinions (full beliefs) on a large number of subjects, rather than suspend judgment.

These cognitive virtues and demands for full belief apply to science as well, even if more pronounced in our everyday activities with their much greater need for conservation of resources. Consider the comet-impact hypothesis to explain the extinction of the dinosaurs. We, nonexperts, would observe that the hypothesis is strongly supported but far from established. When one looks inside the field itself, however, one finds that many of those who adhere to the comet-impact hypothesis fully believe it.[13] But even if they found the evidence strongly favorable, it seems odd from our outsider's and lay person's perspective that they should take a position so dismissive of their peers who dissent. Wouldn't the more judicious position be one of a high degree of partial belief?

The conjecture is that the adoption of a full belief in the comet-impact hypothesis is a product of constraints on us to believe fully. If so, the constraints are operating on scientists in their role as scientists. Borrowing from Peirce (1957), we can say that partial belief (Peirce's "doubt") is a dissatisfied state that seeks resolution in a definite judgment. Supportive reasons are offered earlier in the discussion of argument and testability. But there are further needs or benefits to inquiry that are operative. Those who represent themselves publicly as fully believing the hypothesis imply a commitment to it, and thereby encourage others to work on a common goal (of elaborating and refining the hypothesis).[14] The most obvious benefit is that once a hypothesis is accepted it becomes the basis for further inquiries. Given that even scientific research needs to economize, keeping inquiry open has opportunity costs—other inquiries are delayed or forsaken. Here, again, is a nonevidential source of our dissatisfaction with the state of doubt and our desire to resolve it through coming to a full belief.

5   Faith

Our standards for evidential adequacy must accommodate to various ways in which we are constrained to form full beliefs. Only in this way can evidentialism be defended against the challenge posed by constraints. How far can such accommodation go? James's argument for the entitlement to "will to believe," which I criticized in chapter 4, looks better in the light of the discussion of constraints. Given the importance of certain beliefs in our lives, we are constrained from regular suspension of judgment on them. However, James's argument seeks to go much further: He is claiming the right to believe in the wholesale absence of evidential support.

Can there be constraints on beliefs severe enough so that we need to form those beliefs even if the evidence in their favor is seriously deficient, rather than merely limited? Arguments for belief on the basis of faith can be construed as answering this question in the affirmative. The most troubling defense of an affirmative answer that I know of is found in Robert M. Adams (1995), "Moral Faith." It is the most troubling because Adams respects evidentialism, though he takes the need for faith to be in opposition to it.

Adams understands faith as "believing something that a rational person might be seriously tempted to doubt, or even not to believe" (1995: 75). The need for faith arises from genuine possibilities of error that "must be recognized, and in a way respected" (84).

Adams starts from a premise very much like the one I have defended concerning constraints—there are activities and practices we must participate in that require full beliefs, yet there is limited opportunity for extensive inquiry. Adams observes that there are fundamental roles in our moral lives that require *commitment,* now understood in a more familiar way than in chapter 3. It is a stance to bind oneself to a position or endeavor. The focus now is on what the person intends to commit himself to in his claims, rather than to what a person's claims commit him. Full belief is necessary for commitment; partial belief is an obstacle to it. A commitment is a stance that one will not readily withdraw, and thus it expresses aspects of our identity and helps secure the trust of others. Partial belief cannot support commitments because its strength is overtly open to alteration.

Although I largely accept the form of argument that Adams advances, I am unsure that the commitment–full belief connection holds for the particular role that Adams assigns to it. Adams is dealing with a special subclass of beliefs—beliefs in morality—that are, on his view, inherently subject to doubt. In that case, commitment may take the precise form of a stance to oneself and others that one will stick by a view—such as that morality is for the good—despite a lack of full belief. The stance is not misleading because, like tactfulness, others are aware of the difficulties of achieving convincing arguments, as we ourselves are when we attend to them.

For the sake of argument, however, I shall concede to Adams that moral commitment requires full belief and proceed to Adams's argument: Many central moral beliefs can be sustained only on faith, as contrasted with evidence or argument.

What are examples of rightful belief for reasons of faith? Adams answers: "The first and most obvious object of moral faith is morality itself, or one's own morality . . ." (76). Other demands for faith are in "moral ends": "it is morally important, in typical cases, to believe that other people's lives are worth living" (78). Related to this moral end and to its role in our concerns with the welfare of others is believing that "the moral life will be good, or is apt to be good, *for other people*" (80). Another example of a moral end is "faith in *the common good*": "believing that the good of different persons is not so irreconcilably competitive as to make it incoherent to have the good of *all* persons as an end" (81). More generally, we need faith that "actual causal circumstances are not so adverse, all things considered, as to preclude realization of the moral ends" (83). Faith sustains one's own morality, particularly in how we treat others and in the virtues of mind that are nourished by beliefs that go beyond mere compliance with moral rules. But it is only faith that can serve, since morality is subject to persistent doubts.

Adams tells us that we need to have faith to "encourage each other to live morally." We couldn't do it if we thought morality would be bad for others. But "while few doubt that it is advantageous to have the rudiments of honesty and neighborliness, it is notoriously easier to doubt that some of the finer fruits of morality are good *for* their possessor" (80). Presumably, the thought is that morality often requires self-sacrifice.

It is unfortunate that Adams is not explicit here. We know from reflections on (repeated) *Prisoner's Dilemmas* that if persons have even a minimal respect for, and trust in, others, then cooperative arrangements can be expected to raise the level of all more than if each tried to maximize his or her own self-interest.[15] When we encourage others toward morality, the basic appeal is to their reasonableness, given the expected gains overall compared to noncooperative alternatives.[16] We can then encourage others to at least cooperate toward the "finer fruits of morality," even knowing that some would be better off not cooperating.

What is remarkable about the solutions drawn from the Prisoner's Dilemma, to which I am alluding, are the weak assumptions about human nature and the conditions for cooperation needed for enlightened self-interest to triumph over pure self-interest. In particular, and as touched on in chapter 5, if one seeks the benefits of cooperation, then it is wise to develop oneself to go well beyond the self-interested calculations that originally motivate one's cooperative acts. Of course, the Prisoner's Dilemma and cooperative responses to it do not alone lead one to the finer fruits of morality such as: charity, kindness, "turning the other cheek," or other forms of ethical self-sacrifice. However, because the success of one's own cooperative acts depends crucially on securing the cooperation of others, one is advised to take steps in advance to head off backsliding and to display one's cooperative intent. A practically and theoretically recommended solution is to develop dispositions toward cooperation that are deep-seated and exceed what is strictly required to garner others' cooperation.

Neither the Prisoner's Dilemma nor the resolutions of it are offered as answers to Adams. The purpose is wholly dialectical. I simply offer it as a way of indicating that Adams's claims are themselves only suggestive and promissory. Reflections on the Prisoner's Dilemma, and far from that alone, show that a great deal of morality can be based on the solid, but minimal, foundations of reasonable self-interest, appreciation of the benefits and vulnerabilities of cooperation, and a normal range of intelligence and sentiments. In concluding that faith is the only alternative to moral nihilism or skepticism, Adams incurs the burden of showing that these foundations are profoundly inadequate.

There is a further methodological worry. The predominant doubts that Adams takes to necessitate faith are from the forefront of abstract moral epistemology. Adams attempts to freely transfer these doubts onto specific moral claims, and, for reasons touched on in chapter 4, I am suspicious of the transfer. Adams tells us that "one cannot live morally without intending to do so," and, he then comments, "one cannot exactly intend to do what one believes is totally impossible" (80–81). But this logical point does not capture the ways that we set aside serious doubts about morality so as to maintain particular moral beliefs. Setting aside these larger questions and doubts is recommended at the crucial moments that Adams cites. When a person is depressed or very ill, Adams reminds us of the importance of believing that a person's life is worth living: "To have faith that a person's life is worth living will sometimes be manifested in clinging stubbornly to that person's life as a project to which one is committed, refusing to give up hope for her" (79). But to accomplish this we must presuppose that life or morality is capable of being worthwhile and a facet of a happy life. The manageable task is then to convince the person that this holds for her. We try to refocus Sally, depressed as she is, on all that is enjoyable and valuable in her life. If Sally can be brought to evaluate fairly the sum of her life, we think she will be persuaded of its value. A friend can be committed to the value of Sally's life, while remaining in some doubt as to whether life in general is truly of value. There are appropriate occasions for abstract inquiry into the meaning of life, but saving a friend from depression is not one of them. (Additionally, if our main purpose is to help save the friend through building up her faith or hope, there is a socially acceptable diminishing of the demand for truthfulness, akin to the workings of tact or politeness noted earlier.)

The bracketing of one's general doubts about whether life or morality is worthwhile is not burying one's head in the sand. On the basis of the arguments in chapter 6, we can see that there is much background evidence supporting the moral ends that Adams posits as objects of faith. We have the evidence of our own lives, as well as the lessons of good literature. We know of communities that thrive in ways we admire, and these are communities with a high degree of moral concern and sensitivity. Diminished decency and fellow feeling tend to have a rapid negative spreading effect.

The background support for morality is more evident when we look at the kind of cases Adams ignores. For example, many would find life without meaning, and without moral value, if they did not believe that we have immortal souls. Still, even if that belief yields hope, and hope crucial for their concern to be moral, Adams's reasoning is unenticing as a justification for belief in immortality. The fact that his reasoning does not extend to this belief is an indication that he is filtering, undeservedly, his selection of cases so as to retain only what is well founded. Yet, his reasoning, insofar as it is opposed to evidentialism, should extend to deeply and personally needed beliefs, even when clearly ill founded.

My overall conclusion is that Adams's argument is of the right form to pose a serious threat to evidentialism. But it is incomplete. Adams ignores background support and groundings for morality that do provide answers to some of the doubts that he raises. He relies too heavily on an unanalyzed notion of "doubt," a claim that will be developed below and in chapter 10. Finally, Adams does not consider the familiar (anti-inflationary) strategy of setting aside fundamental moral (or scientific) quandaries in answering practical, everyday ethical questions.

6   Challenges to Evidentialism (and How to Meet Them)

If constraints are admitted as the normal structures that shape the formation of many of our beliefs, then evidentialism and our conceptual arguments for evidentialism come under challenge. Specifically:

1. How can evidentialism allow for nonevidential limits on our strength of attitude toward the truth of our belief?
2. Do not the limits on inquiry in the formation of beliefs leave reasonable ground for doubts? If so, how is that compatible with full belief in recognition of these limits and as aiming at knowledge?
3. Isn't evidentialism too demanding, since it would deny entitlement to full belief within the vast and ordinary practices in which constraints on us to form full beliefs operate?

Chapters 9 and 10 attempt to answer these implied challenges in a way that is compatible with evidentialism. Part of the answer is that standards for the attribution of adequate reasons or inquiry adjust according to certain *contextual* factors. In the case of directives to action, this adjustment is familiar. If my newspaper is missing, I'll check a few obvious places before I judge that it is lost. But if my wallet is missing, I will search longer, harder, and more frantically, before I judge it lost and take the requisite drastic actions. When Adams raises broad doubts about morality, he overly sensitizes us to possibilities that our moral claims are false. But in the original context of our claims, we still may be entitled to ignore these possibilities.

Of the above challenges, the last two could be raised from the outset of this work. We can all think of beliefs, held honestly and openly, for which reasonable doubts exist and which are so recognized. In attempting to meet these challenges, especially the last, we need to be strict about what will count as reasons or evidence to which proportionality is demanded. In chapter 10, I argue that not all reasonable doubts—including some of those that Adams takes to require faith—are of a kind that constitute evidence against the relevant belief.

The distinctions just alluded to are aspects of a perspective on funda-mental epistemic notions that we accept. The standard perspective is that knowledge, say, is a rare and mighty achievement, requiring great efforts. The alternative perspective is that in the routine cases, which are by far the dominant ones, we can easily come to know and even to have conclusive reasons. If this latter perspective is correct, then beliefs formed under con-straints are not for that reason unjustified. Where matters are not urgent, limited evidence or investigation can still be sufficient. In reading *Pride and Prejudice,* we can both recognize that Elizabeth could have done more to check the ward's story before she accepted it, and also think that her judg-ment was not markedly hasty in the circumstances. There is enormous background support for her proceeding as she does.

I am not entering the benighted claim that we do not have tendencies to hastily form bad or prejudicial judgments. For one among numerous ex-amples, recall the widespread rumor, noted in chapter 5, that a basketball star had memorized the entire Manhattan phone directory. My concern about constraints is not to deny our credulity, but to reject the claim that admitting the role of constraints itself undermines evidentialism and bars knowledge. Worries over credulity arise over the comparatively tiny sub-set of salient beliefs.

The broad constraints on belief that concern us arise at two points: as limits on opting out of a practice, and as limits within the practice either on circumventing its various rules or on shaping them to our circumstances and limits. The practices that we have focused on (assertion, responsibility attributing responses, reasoning, and argument) are too broad and funda-mental for opting out to be at all realistic. The practical necessity reflects the severe limits on opting out of participation—a way we could really live without gross distortion in character or practices. Within these practices, there are structural demands that limit inquiry, and so, unless one has spe-cial reason to object, our disposition to full belief bends to those demands, rather than responding mainly to our individual epistemic positions. Eliza-beth can neither opt out generally from default acceptance of testimony and the formation of reactive attitudes fairly spontaneously nor recon-struct those practices to wait on her hearing and assessing Darcy's side of the story.

9

Interlude—Transparency, Full Belief, Accommodation

The first two sections of this chapter address the distinction between full and partial belief. Important roles in our activities and practices can be played only by full belief, which supports the claim that a demanding notion of full belief is not optional or artificial or peripheral. The distinction is prominent in my arguments throughout, and it is presupposed in the treatment of constraints on belief in the previous chapter.

In section 3, I continue efforts to meet the challenges to evidentialism presented in chapter 8. I need to show, in brief, that evidentialism is not too demanding—we can be entitled to full beliefs across a wide range of our activities and practices when the entitlement still requires adequate reasons or evidence. The appeal in earlier chapters to our forceful, yet effortlessly obtained, background beliefs makes headway in meeting this challenge. In this chapter, drawing overtly on recent investigations in epistemology, I appeal to different standards for attributing adequate reasons dependent on context, particularly in the costs of error and the value of being correct. I do so through an extended dialogue, which continues past presentation of a contextual view and other fruits of recent investigations. The dialogue also foreshadows developments in subsequent chapters that attempt to meet other facets of the challenges.

1 Full and Partial Beliefs
Full belief, though demanding, is ordinary, common belief—the notion that is expressed in assertion. Degrees of belief are most naturally presented with such qualifications as "pretty sure," "very sure," "more sure than not," as well as "think," "suspect," or "inclined to believe"—paradigmatically, "I am pretty sure that p."[1]

Expressions for partial belief are not the same as (objective) probability judgments, for example, "The probability that the coin will land heads is 3/5." Probability judgments attribute properties, dispositions, or propensities to objects. Although they can, of course, be based on evidence, expressions of them are not incomplete without mention of evidence.[2] However, the two are easily confused, since, for brevity, in expressing our partial beliefs, we cut away from reference to the believer or his evidence. Typically, we say "It's probable that Mary will meet us" just as we say "It's possible that Mary will meet us." In either case what is usually meant involves a disguised reference to the asserter (and his evidence)—it's probable or possible, given the asserter's beliefs.

Full (all-or-nothing) belief is issued in by acceptance or judgment of the truth of the proposition. Acceptance is most characteristic as marking the end of successful inquiry. However, by the extensions argued for previously, we can also construe the automatic formation of beliefs from perception or memory or simple reasoning as issued in through acceptance. The acceptance ends inquiry (as to the proposition's truth), rather than continuously altering degrees of belief, thereby conserving resources and time.[3]

In this section, discussion focuses on two basic roles played by full belief that could not be played by partial beliefs or by other qualified or weaker belieflike attitudes (e.g., "inclined to believe"). In the previous chapter three other roles were noted. Full belief is required to dominate argument and reasoning, to back our reactive-attitude judgments, and to support commitments. Because these five roles cover our central practices involving belief, full belief is still ordinary belief, even though its claims are strong and its standards are high.

Full belief, in contrast to partial belief, *facilitates (intentional) action*. Partial belief regularly calls for significantly greater hesitation and calculation.[4] So, full belief will be called on to play a role that partial belief cannot, since we are constantly acting in response to rapid informational changes.

Consider a situation in which you are at a shopping mall and desire a drink of water. You know that there is a fountain at the far end. If you come to believe that there is also a fountain nearby, you go straight to it. But if you are only somewhat sure that the second fountain is nearby, you are burdened with having to assess the value of trying to go to it. You factor in the likelihood of disappointment and then also the additional, longer, walk that you will have to take, instead of going directly to the fountain at the far end. Or, consider suddenly finding yourself approaching an old acquaintance. Memory proves rewarding when you remember her name, but frustrating when you are unsure of it.[5] The advantages of full belief are significantly, not proportionally, greater than virtually any lesser degree of belief. The advantage of definitely recalling—fully believing— that the name of the acquaintance is "Louise" is much greater than being very sure it is, yet to be very sure is only marginally better than to be more sure than not; for in either of the latter cases, you still have to strategize how to discover her name without embarrassment.

Admittedly, not all partial beliefs impede action in these ways. Partial beliefs can become habitual, lending themselves to routine behavior or to planning. But such cases are not sufficiently extensive to undermine the general point. Situational and informational changes are limitless, which restricts the possibilities for advance planning or the fixing of habits.

The advantages claimed for full belief are in comparison with degrees of belief, not to subjective probability. Institutions must constantly work with probabilities. An insurance company that did otherwise would quickly go bankrupt. Similarly, individuals regularly make decisions under uncertainty, relying on expected utilities—subjective values and probability.

Think of a case of uncertainty: should you take the local train that just pulled in to the station, or wait for an express train? Your only objective is to get to your station as fast as possible. You are uncertain because you can only make a good guess as to how long it will take for the express train to arrive. But the uncertainty is constituted by full beliefs; a local train is here; an express is not; both trains stop at your destination; the express trains are spaced about ten minutes apart; the local train makes four more stops. Despite how often we act under uncertainty, we can still be quite certain as to the nature of the uncertainty, as we are not when uncertainty is grounded in partial beliefs.

Full beliefs facilitate intentions or decisions or plans as partial beliefs do not. When, for example, I plan to make gazpacho for dinner, I need to buy tomatoes. But I believe that the store that sells the best tomatoes is closed for vacation, which eliminates this part of the plan as incompatible with my belief. Either I shop elsewhere or I do not make gazpacho. But if I am only pretty sure that the store is closed, the option remains open (Bratman 1987: 36–37).

These demanding and pervasive roles of belief in guiding action also rule out belief-related notions such as "as if" belief,[6] understood as a time- and purpose-restricted attitude. A lawyer who believes that her client is guilty is advised to act and think "as if" he believed in the client's innocence. A scientist continues to work on a refuted theory, "as if" he still believed it, where no substitute theory is in the offing.[7] But, in everyday activities, outside of institutionally defined roles, "as if" belief is not sustainable. Either one is unduly burdened to factor in the pretense involved, since others are put off by it, or one gradually adjusts to it, but only because its "as if" quality is transformed into belief.[8]

The claim that full belief facilitates action is, in one respect, misleading. Full belief expresses a stronger attitude than that expressed by any degrees of belief, and so requires more evidence. Consequently, the demand for full belief rather than partial belief will delay action. But the delay is for the sake of truth. We do not merely want to act; we want our actions to succeed in their purposes, and we expect that to occur only when the beliefs guiding the actions are true.

Of course, we are often called on to act without the benefit of full belief. We frequently act under uncertainty, for example, when we try to determine directions while driving. Richard Swinburne offers a case in which, on a drive to London, he comes to a junction in the road: "clearly if I believe that it is more probable that the road on the right leads to London than that the road on the left does, I shall take the road on the right" (1981: 8). The example is meant to support Swinburne's claim that "to believe that p is to believe that p is probable," which we rejected in chapter 1. The example seems supportive only because we accept an unexpressed premise: He must decide immediately. If not, he would just take out a map. He takes out a map because he wants to turn to the right only if it is the correct road, and, if so, the map will show it. He will then come to (fully) believe it, which will now issue in action. We can assume here, as is typical, that the driver would prefer to continue to drive rather than stop to check the map. Nevertheless, he willingly uses up valuable time to try to achieve full (and ordinary) belief, rather than act merely on a partial belief.

The fifth and last prominent difference in role between full and partial belief that I discuss is one that I have leaned on repeatedly: Only the (full) belief that *p* warrants its simple assertion. If (and only if) I believe that the bread is in the refrigerator am I entitled to assert "The bread is in the refrigerator." In contrast, if I only partially believe it, I am entitled to assert only some qualification of it, for example, "I'm pretty sure that the bread is in the refrigerator." (The whole assertion-belief parallel is outlined in the appendix to chapter 10.)

Unqualified assertion is the normal form, whereas (epistemically) qualified assertion is deviant. As we observed in chapter 1, the former is *unmarked* by virtue of its form or structure—simple, natural, non-attention-grabbing (as a speech act), frequent. But epistemically qualified assertion is *marked*—complex, difficult or slow to process, attention-diverting, infrequent, lexicalized.[9] What is marked burdens the listener, requiring compensating benefits. The epistemic qualifier renders the whole expression more difficult to process, grates on the smooth flow of conversation, and diverts attention (from the propositional content to speaker's attitude, reasons, and self).

Epistemically qualified assertions are not truly assertions. Toulmin captured this crucial point without, however, developing it: "To say 'Probably *p*' is to assert guardedly, and/or with reservations, that *p* (1958: 85).[10] Since the central aim of the exchange is to transmit the information that *p* (all-or-none), the qualified expression (manifestly) falls short. If Harry asks Sally "Whose turn is it to walk the dog?" and Sally responds "I'm pretty sure it's your turn," the task remains unsettled.[11] Sally's guarded assertion is an acknowledgement of unsuccessful communication. In so failing, Sally incurs the burden to present her reasons. Reasons that serve only to back the truth of an assertion are not of focal interest as is the assertion. The default rule relieves the speaker of the demand to present them and so relieves the hearer of the need to comprehend them. But with a guarded assertion the default rule no longer provides this benefit. Thus, Sally might add, without prompting or challenge, "I thought this was your week." Since Sally's reason is backing for her attitude, rather than the assertion, it offers less compensation to the hearer for the additional burden of comprehension.

Since assertion expresses belief but guarded assertion does not, only assertion can be the speech-act whose characteristic function is to present and communicate truths. As noted in chapter 1, reasons are adequate for full belief just in case they are adequate for knowledge. Knowledge can be the goal of full belief because it is *factive* ("*X* knows that *p*" entails "*p*"), and it is knowledge that is the position represented by the speaker in assertion.

2   Truth and Transparency

These differences between full and partial belief in their nature and roles all stem from the fundamental one that only full belief eventuates in a *transparent* attitude toward its content. Transparency is the mental analogue of the semantic relation of factiveness. We look through the belief to the world, but not to our attitude of believing it.[12] The transparency property is modeled on the transparency of truth with respect to any sentence of which it is predicated. Tarski's condition of adequacy for a theory of truth ("Convention T") is:

S is true if and only if *p*

(where "*S*" is replaced by a name of the sentence for "*p*," e.g., "Snow is white" is true if and only if snow is white. Tarski 1983: 187–188). The truth of a sentence does not depend on any intermediary between it and the world—not minds, interpretations, or states of affairs (Davidson 1986). There is no more to understanding a statement's being true than to understanding that statement.

So too, by analogy, belief, from the first-person point of view. I believe that *p* if and only if the world for me is: *p*. From my point of view, I "disquote" *p* from my attitude toward it, and I am left simply with *p*. Belief does not just aim at truth; transparency implies that it aims to be exhausted or constituted by truth. From my point of view in attending to my belief that *p*, there is nothing more to the truth-conditions of my belief than the truth-conditions of *p*. When I regard my believing that *p*, I regard it to be the case that I believe *p* because *p*, just as it can be held that "Snow is white" is true *because* snow is white (Horwich 1990: 111). Aside from secondary matters like attention or interest, my believing *p* is to be explained by its being the case that *p*. Of course, if you ask me why do I believe that *p*, I allude to my reasons or evidence, not to *p* itself. But so too if asked to explain a phenomenon, for example, "Why does ice float on water?"—one offers an explanation in terms of the relation of these properties, not in terms of the presupposed fact that ice does float on water.

Partial belief, however, in this respect is more like desire. It points inward to the believer (his degree of confidence), as desire points inward to how one wants the world to be.[13] (Again, it is essential here that we not confuse "Probably *p*" as an objective judgment with a subjective judgment expressed in the same words.) When one holds a partial belief, one may look to the world for further evidence of its truth. But one cannot look through one's attitude—"disquote" from it, to recall the parallel—to the content as expressing a feature of the world, since one just does not (yet) take the world to be that way. In partially believing that *p*, however strongly, we recognize a gap between our attitude and the way the world is. But with full belief there is no gap—from my first-person point of view there is no difference between my believing *p* and its being the case that *p*.

Since full belief claims truth, there is no reason for one's actual evidence to be retained. From my point of view, what matters is that my belief is established by adequate reasons, not the specifics of those reasons. Compare with assertion: The assertion is of focal interest, and so normally, from the hearer's point of view, what matters is that the speaker has adequate reasons for what she asserts. The specifics of those reasons are not of focal interest. By contrast, since partial belief is an unsatisfactory state, seeking resolution as full belief (or disbelief), it cannot unburden itself of its evidential base. For the specific evidence one has will affect how one treats further evidence—does it extend the force of the evidence one has or contravene it? Consequently, partial belief carries with it a motive to retain its grounds, another facet of nontransparency.

The difference in transparency is more glaring in the large picture than in reference to particular beliefs. You do not understand a domain or process or subject if your grasp of it is suffused with partial beliefs. If you are asked whether you understand how the tenure process works, you would reveal a lack of understanding if you listed various steps under epistemic qualifiers ("I'm very [almost, fairly] sure that a subcommittee sends out for reviewers," for example). If you so hedge your claims you imply some degree of belief in the denial of each step ("But there's a chance that the Provost sends out the request"). Your grasp would also be very limited, not comprehensive. Each new piece of relevant information would have to be evaluated against an extensive background of various degrees of belief. Simple acceptance, by contrast, incorporates new information in previous understandings, and so many new beliefs can be recovered by inference.

Accordingly, we could not expect our grasp of a complex domain to extend to many of its details if our grasp were grounded largely in partial beliefs.

To summarize these last two sections: Only (full) belief will naturally flow toward actions and provide backing for assertion. The simplicity of full belief is crucial if these pervasive activities are to go smoothly and easily. One can surely act if necessary on partial beliefs and assert statements with epistemic qualifications on occasion—but not as a rule. Partial beliefs are cumbersome and their implications too difficult for regular, everyday use. Since full belief is not epistemically qualified, it is much simpler and less burdensome than partial belief. The aim of full belief is realized in transparent functioning, to look through one's attitude outward to the proposition believed, and this transparency underlies these fundamental contrasts in role.

3   Contextualism and Other Forms of Accommodation

In defending significant qualitative differences between full and partial belief—so that the former should not be viewed as merely the endpoint of a continuum of degrees of belief—I sharpen the challenges to evidentialism, particularly that it is too demanding. On one hand, evidentialism enforces high standards. Full belief ought to be backed by evidence or reasons adequate for knowledge. On the other hand, full belief is ordinary belief—much of it easily and routinely acquired and openly expressed. The incongruity, noted in the previous chapter, is that ordinary settings demand that inquiry is quickly resolved to yield full belief. So there are constraints on it, and yet still the resulting claims are to the meeting of high standards.

In this and the following chapters I hope to meet these challenges, resolve the incongruity, and to continue to abide by the principle set out in chapter 1:

(I)   If the belieflike attitude A toward the truth of p is (epistemically) stronger than A' in the same situation, then if the available reasons are insufficient to justify A' then they are insufficient to justify A.

As noted in chapter 6, condition (I) is not formidable. The attitude of full belief can be a stronger one than any degree of partial belief, and so then the adequacy of the reasons demanded for it is the greater. But the greater strength of reasons is what is demanded, not any greater demand for revealing them. Consequently, full belief can be everyday belief, since it does not impose a continuous burden on ordinary practices to show one's reasons or to justify one's belief.

In recent years, various *contextual* analyses in epistemology have gained momentum, and they promise to help us reconcile our incongruous claims.[14] Contextual analyses have shed a new light on the persuasive force of skeptical arguments. The basic idea is this: If you are sitting by a fireplace, then in normal circumstances you can come to know that you are seated by a fireplace. The skeptic then proposes the *counterpossibility* that you may be having a perfectly realistic dream that you are seated by a fireplace. Many are persuaded by the proposal to deny that you can know in the circumstances. The contextualist tries to unpersuade them. When the skeptic proposes this counterpossibility, he subtly *raises the standards* for knowing (or attributing knowledge). In this new context, you do not know that the you are seated by the fireplace. Nevertheless, in the original context, when no such possibility is presented, the standards are appropriately low, and then you can know that you are seated by the fireplace.

The standard-raising that is especially pertinent to constraints is due to differences in potential costs of error. Inquiry is ordinarily very limited because when inquiry is not a professional or institutional activity, as with science, the time and resources we have to devote to it are under severe competition from our other interests, projects, and commitments. An earlier example from chapter 3 (section 2) provides a helpful illustration. The example was of differences in the efforts any of us are willing to invest in determining the number of jelly beans in a large jar as a function of the stakes (a prize of $10 vs. a prize of $1,000,000). We are entering the same judgment, yet we care to increase our certainty and exclude more ways we can err in the one case than the other. The example is, however, obviously imperfect since the judgment we enter is offered as a guess, not as an assertion backed by a corresponding belief.

Here's a more pertinent example that will serve as a reference point for the remainder of discussion: A waiter at an exclusive restaurant published a letter in a local newspaper complaining of customers who asked him whether the coffee he brought was decaffeinated. Isn't it sufficient, he asked, that he brings the cup in response to their request for decaffeinated coffee, which is a very normal request (one well within the competence of waiters)? When customers asked for reassurance they were impugning his competence. However, a later letter-writer, admitting to being one of those second-guessing customers, rejected the waiter's complaint. She is arrhythmatic, so drinking caffeinated coffee is dangerous for her. The cup brought to her is not labeled, there are orders for both kinds of coffee, and there is no way for her to discern by the senses that the coffee is decaffeinated.

The greater cost of error for the arrhythmatic as compared with the regular customer bears on practice. If the waiter learned that his customer suffered arrhythmia, he would feel pressure to check specially that her coffee was decaffeinated. He would, for example, make extra sure that he did not put down the cups at any point en route back to the tables, where they might get mixed up.

Intuitively, we think that the waiter and the arrhythmatic can both be correct: The waiter is correct that the ordinary customer unfairly challenges him. But the arrhythmatic is correct too that, for her, the waiter's assurance that the coffee is decaffeinated is unjustified, even granted that the normal procedures work well. There are further, simple checks that could rule out unlikely, but not wildly unlikely, ways that the cups could be mixed up.

Contextual accounts of justification harmonize these seemingly antagonistic claims. The waiter's implied assertion that the cup he is handing the customer is decaffeinated is justified in the circumstances of the ordinary customer for whom a mix-up will not have dire consequences (at worst, a bad night's sleep). But the arrhythmatic can be right too. Since the threat to her from an error well exceeds that for the ordinary customer, the checks that are forgone as a burden for the ordinary customer cannot be forgone for her. In the context of the arrhythmatic, the waiter is not justified in asserting that the cup is decaffeinated.

With contextualism, we have a good start to answering the problem raised by constraints—the reconcilability of limited inquiry and adequate reasons, and an account of why they seem irreconcilable. Clearly, the waiter's judgment is made under severe constraints. He cannot offer a customer merely a high degree of partial belief that the cup is decaffeinated. But nor can he (practically) devote himself to extensive further checks that no mix-up has taken place. However, the context changes—becomes more demanding—for the arrhythmatic, and then further checks are mandated if the waiter is to be justified in asserting that the coffee he serves her is decaffeinated.

We can understand strategically why there should be this contextual accommodation. If demands for reasons or evidence are too low, then knowledge or justification is weakened as a guide to truth. If demands are too high, then reference to knowledge or justification will be much less useful for distinguishing knowers or those with adequate reasons from those who fail to know or lack adequate reasons, since much fewer now meet the requirements for knowledge or adequate reasons. Unless the standards for reasons find a happy median, the value or critical function of ascriptions of knowledge or justification diminishes.

So a view of constraints on believing as having its greatest impact in ordinary contexts where standards are low allays the worry that full belief will normally arise in a wide variety of practices without adequate reason. But contextual variation alone will not answer all the difficulties raised either by constraints on belief or by the broader objection that evidentialism is too demanding.

Here is one way to present that objection: We grant that at the more stringent standard the waiter would make some further checks that he does not in the original context. The checks are neither idle nor infeasible. They are not idle because by performing some of them he would directly exclude further ways that the coffee cups might get mixed up. They are not infeasible because he would make some of the checks for the arrythmatic. So in not mandating these checks in the original case, evidentialism seems to accord with our ordinary ascriptions of justified believing or asserting only because those ascriptions are sensitive to the practical difficulties in the circumstances. But these practical difficulties are at the expense of the real epistemic requirements. So evidentialism cannot hold on to its high requirements for reasons and broad agreement with our ordinary ascriptions.

In order to assess the force of the complex difficulty just raised, we will consider its import in the case at hand, as a challenge to the waiter. Letting "W" stand for the waiter, and "C" for the ordinary customer, we consider a series of exchanges with commentary:

W: Here is the cup of decaffeinated you ordered.
C: But are you sure it is decaffeinated?

This challenge—or "Do you know that it is decaffeinated?"—suggests that C has a good reason to challenge W, even though he offers none. Speakers, like W, are often inclined to accept challenges—to offer their reasons—even without recognizing or requesting the hearer's backing. But the suggestion and speakers' tendency toward accommodation misleads us to think that W is obliged to present his reasons or to have a reason additional to those C finds evident. But, as noted in chapters 5 and 6, it is C that requires the reason to back his challenge. If, however, C's question is not a challenge but a request for reasons as a matter of interest or curiosity, then presumably W could respond with an account of the restaurant's procedures and the lack of significant complaints from customers.

So if C's response is a challenge, W is entitled to reply something to the effect:

W: What's your reason for thinking I made a mistake?

This is effectively the force of the waiter's complaint in the original letter—the customer offered no reason for thinking the waiter made a mistake, and so his challenge casts aspersion on the waiter's competence. Without entitlement to this response, the default rule lacks force.

What could provide backing to the customer's challenge? He could find the restaurant's procedures inadequate:

C: Look, the cups of coffee are indistinguishable, and there are many places along the route that you could mix them up. You could even have misunderstood the order.

In fact, the owner of the restaurant was sympathetic to this response. The exchange actually ended when he wrote in to apologize for the waiter's rude remarks. The owner had decided to introduce different-colored mugs for caffeinated and decaffeinated coffee.

Alternatively, we could construe the arryhthmatic as offering a backing to her challenge, different from how we presented it above, which we can put in the mouth of the ordinary customer:

C: I admit that your procedures are pretty good, but they have to be good enough for just about all the customers you are likely to serve. Some customers are arryhthmatic, and for them caffeinated coffee is life-threatening. So if you are going to continue to offer both kinds of coffee, you should introduce more stringent standards than you have now, like labeling both cups.

What both of these responses have in common is that they offer *special reasons* to back the challenge of the waiter by the customer—ones that point to the possibility of defects, and that are themselves backed by evidence or argument.[15] If so, and the waiter cannot undermine them, then indeed the waiter's asserting (believing) that the coffee is decaffeinated is unjustified.

The verdict does not raise a difficulty for the evidentialist, since there is neither discrepancy with our ordinary ascriptions nor indication that evidentialism is too demanding. The requirement of a special or specific reason places a limit on what can count as a challenge. For there to be such a reason depends on the facts or details of the case, and then it lacks generative power—crucial to Descartes's dreaming counterpossibility—to undermine any claim to knowledge.[16] The specific or special-reasons requirement is in opposition to the appropriateness in all circumstances of the skeptic's challenge.

The special-reasons requirement satisfies the constraint to economize. It allows a procedure to go ahead unless a reason is offered to challenge it. The special-reasons requirement, as earlier observed, imposes a burden of proof on interferences.[17] The burden in assertion, for example, is on hearers to back a challenge to the speaker. In our extended example, the waiter's implied criticism of the customer is that the regular customer has failed to discharge his burden of proof. The waiter does not need to show (further) that the cup is decaffeinated, but the customer does have a burden to back his challenge with real evidence, even if only for a counterpossibility.

The special-reasons requirement sets a bottom line on accommodation, even though the requirement is addressed to individuals—do *A* (accept the assertion), unless *you* have special reason to object. The requirement demands no effort to obtain such reasons; though there may be some (held by others). The special reasons offered above might be true, but the customer not know them. Nevertheless, we as hearers accept the assertions of various speakers in the absence of any special reason to object. We thereby implicitly endorse the claim that the sacrifice in assurance imposed by the default rule is not a sacrifice in truth. Insofar as we are competent as hearers, we regularly endorse the claim that the vulnerability that the default rule casts on us ends early enough. It ends at the point—the special-reasons requirement—beyond which there is a genuine threat of inducing false belief.

The next response, although initially sounding natural enough, actually represents a radical break. One signal that there is a break is that, as W's reply brings out, the exchange becomes much less natural:

C: Well, I know that there are further checks you would make for customers, like an arrhythmatic, who would be in grave danger from drinking decaffeinated. But if so, I think you ought to make these further checks now. They are obviously feasible, since you could make them. And they would provide greater assurance for your assertion, which you present as true.

W: But you are not arrythmatic. And although it is feasible for the exceptional cases of the arrhythmatic, it would not be feasible for ordinary customers.

C is not offering a special reason. He is not indicating any defect in the restaurant's procedures. So if his proposal is a condition on the waiter's justification for asserting that the coffee is decaffeinated, then it is a proposal to raise the standards and so increase the burdens on the waiter without backing. It is grounded in the aim of greater certainty alone.

C: It seems then that part of your response is that you did not do the further checks suggested because you did not have enough time. But lack of time is mere happenstance. What you are saying is that if you could do the additional checks quickly—if it merely required pushing various buttons, rather than stopping and looking over some procedures—then you would have done so. But these practicalities are not germane to the truth of the belief.

W: You misread the import of the practicalities. The fundamental claim is that the further tests are not worthwhile; so that the contrast you are suggesting between, say, performing tests A, B, C and performing an additional test D is misleading. The real contrast is between performing all necessary or worthwhile checks, which happen to be A, B, C and performing further checks, to be extra cautious, even though not strictly necessary or worthwhile. So practical happenstance is not the decisive grounds in either case for when I stop checking or for my assertion.

C: Well, maybe it isn't worthwhile or feasible to go on. But then you should not simply assert that the coffee is decaffeinated, but only something qualified like "I'm almost certain that the coffee is decaffeinated." For you agree that there are further checks that you could make, and if you made them, there would be greater assurance. So you cannot have adequate or conclusive reasons for the truth of what you assert.

C's reply is illicit, and it embeds an influential conflation, one particularly threatening to evidentialism. The conflation is hinted at in W's prior response: Briefly, it conflates the possibility of greater assurance (or confidence) with lack of adequate reasons. The checks that yield greater assurance do not thereby rule out any further genuine counterpossibilities. If the procedures that the waiter follows for the ordinary customer are adequate then they do exclude all genuine counterpossibilities. The test from the introduction supports this conclusion: Were the cup handed to the customer decaffeinated, would we not say that the waiter did know it was? So the greater assurance or extra checks (for the arrhythmatic) are not necessary for the waiter to know that the coffee is decaffeinated. Consequently, the customer is mistaken in inferring from the possibility of greater assurance to the lack of adequate or conclusive reasons:

W: But I can have adequate reasons for saying the coffee is decaffeinated, given the procedures we follow and their successful workings. You do not find fault with the procedures. The greater assurance I could get from, say, checking that the coffee bags were not mixed up when poured into the different machines does not rule out a way I could go wrong. Either it is so way out that it does not have to be ruled out, or else it is implicitly ruled out by our background reasons as to the good workings of the procedure. I admit that there is greater assurance with the check, so it would not be for nought for the arrhythmatic. But what it yields is greater assurance of the adequacy of my reasons, rather than its being a necessary condition for that adequacy. Were it a necessary condition for that adequacy, then on your view one is never entitled to simply assert anything like "The coffee is decaffeinated" since there will be always the possibility of further checks. The fact that I can successfully perform any one of these now does not mean that I can either perform all of them now or even regularly perform some of them.

C: But even if it is a highly unlikely possibility, it is still a possibility, and hence something that we should rule out if we are to know. Knowledge after all is the highest cognitive achievement. I admit that your background reasons lessen the chances of its occurring. But surely the bags could have been mixed up at that stage, and that is precisely the possibility that the further check would rule out.

In reply, W has to unpack his previous response.

W: However, compare: You are speeding if you go above the applicable speed limit—whether you drive 75 or 85 mph in a 65 mph zone, you are speeding. The fact that at 75 you could be going even faster does not imply that you have not already crossed the threshold for speeding. So too the fact that the extra check would provide more assurance does not imply that I do not already have conclusive reasons.

C: But aren't you then admitting that for all your care, it is possible that the bags get mixed up, whereas if you made the additional check properly you could rule out this possibility?

W: Yes, except that you are neglecting that behind my displayed care there is the background evidence of hardly any previous complaints about, and the rationale for, my procedures. Still, my assertion is *defeasible.* But not every occurrence that could defeat a justification must be specifically ruled out in order to be justified. After all, if I can have inductive knowledge at all, then I can do so without specific evidence that all normal conditions for a particular inductive inference to work hold. I can know that my reliable friend Tim will meet me for lunch tomorrow, even though if he is in a car accident he won't meet me and I cannot specifically rule this out (that is, rule it out over and above my background reasons that such occurrences would be abnormal).[18] If I have to show, as you are in effect demanding, that each normalcy condition is met, then I could never meet the demands, for two reasons: There are too many normalcy conditions; and new normality conditions would have to be checked for each one that I offer to satisfy the original demand. I admit that these restrictions depend on the fact that my time and resources are limited and I need to economize. But this minimal practicality is true of science as well. There are no definite limits on a scientific inquiry; nevertheless, inquiry is shaped to be economical. Hypotheses are accepted after all the relevant tests have been successfully completed, but not after all possible tests (and re-tests).

C: Let me try a different tack. Not only is your assertion defeasible, but since you will admit that you are fallible about such matters, some are actually defeated. Surely the fact that you are fallible should lessen your confidence and motivate further checks to improve that confidence? Your simple assertion does not account for the fallibility that you are willing to admit.

W: While I am inclined to accept your premise as to my fallibility, I do not think the requirements you draw from them are fair. (I am only inclined to accept it because for many beliefs, especially many of our background beliefs, I doubt that there is a serious chance of error.) We should recall what is at stake: my entitlement to assert that this cup contains decaffeinated coffee. My fallibility is not evidence one way or the other about the truth of that proposition. Fallibility is about me as a believer, not my belief. So it can play no role in denying that I have conclusive reasons or even know what I assert. And you agree here too, since you accept unqualified assertions from speakers whom you regard as fallible. It may be advisable, where I am especially fallible, to impose *extra* checks. They are motivated not by any fault in the reasoning backing my assertion (as we agreed), but by an overall aim, or even duty, to better my believing. The aim or duty need not be achieved by extra checks in this case, and even if it were, a failure to perform them would be a failure of mine, still constituting no specific reason for the falsity of my assertion or a failure in the grounds for it.

More on these last responses, and my obvious sympathies with the waiter, in the next chapter.

10

The Compatibility of Full Belief and Doubt

The problem central to this chapter is to explain how there can be, and commonly so, avowed and justified full beliefs maintained in the face of reasonable doubts. Examples that will quickly come to mind are controversial, though strongly held beliefs, such as that abortion is immoral or that capital punishment is a violation of human rights. But in keeping with our methodological injunction to emphasize examples that do not import perplexities, consider the following: You recall (believe) that two acquaintances of yours Dean and John met in a conference in Colorado in the 1970s. You are told, and you come to believe, that John, who is British, rarely left the United Kingdom, and as a result you start to have doubts about your belief. Nevertheless, I claim that you are still entitled to believe it, and that in full awareness, you must.

This claim poses a problem for my fundamental thesis that it is incoherent to recognize oneself as fully believing both that p and that one's reasons do not establish p, on the assumption that reasons to doubt p undermine p or any argument to establish it. The major theme of chapter 8 indicates that there should be many other examples. It was argued there that we are constrained to form full beliefs in circumstances permitting only limited inquiry.

Previous discussion defuses some of these putative counterexamples. In chapter 9, I noted that standards for adequate reasons vary according to certain features of context such as costs of error. Standards in everyday circumstances are accommodating—they can be readily satisfied. But neither this attempt nor others can dispose of the problem. Any one of us could offer numerous variations on the above illustration without any ax to grind against evidentialism.

The problem posed by reasonable doubts with full belief—one of a host of what I will refer to it as *belief-doubt problems*—depends on the *uniformity assumption,* as I'll call it, noted above:

Any epistemic reason to critically reflect on, or doubt, a belief constitutes evidence (reasons) that undermines the truth of the belief or the argument for it.

In responding to belief-doubt problems, I argue against this assumption and urge a distinction between *belief* and *confidence.*[1] One can be entitled to a full belief without having unqualified confidence in that belief, and so it is possible for reasons, such as the rarity of John's visits to the United States, to diminish confidence without undermining one's belief.

My response to belief-doubt problems in this chapter *presupposes* the success of earlier defenses of full belief (chaps. 1 and 9) as qualitatively distinct from degrees of belief in both the former's relation to the claim to truth and in its unique ability to fulfill a range of central (epistemic) roles in our practices. I refuse to avail myself of the neat resolution of belief-doubt problems afforded by withdrawing from full belief to partial belief. The central arguments in this chapter do, however, further the earlier ones: If belief-doubt problems can be handled without invoking an attenuated notion of belief, the motivation for adopting such a notion is dampened.

1   Confidence and the Directionality of Weight Fallacy

There are extremely familiar circumstance in which we distinguish between our belieflike attitude and our confidence. Experimenters in cognitive psychology ask subjects to answer a target question (e.g., "Which city has more inhabitants? (a) Paris or (b) San Francisco"). Subjects are then asked the unremarkable question of how confident they are in that answer (Gigerenzer, Hoffrage, and Kleinbolting 1991; Griffin and Tversky 1992).

What is it subjects so naturally distinguish? A subject's answer to the original question might be put as "Given my evidence, it's more probable that Paris has more inhabitants." The question of confidence is the question of how good one takes one's basis to answer. The question of belief and the question of confidence are different questions.

Variations of confidence depend mainly, but not solely, on judgments of the *weight of evidence,* and judgments of weight answer to how complete one's evidence is. Judgments of degree of belief answer to the *force* of one's evidence. In chapter 4 of his *A Treatise on Probability*, Keynes writes: "One argument has more *weight* than another if it is based upon a greater amount of relevant evidence; . . . It has a greater *probability* than another if the balance in its favour, of what evidence there is, is greater than the balance in favour of the argument with which we compare it . . ." (1962: 77).[2] Keynes's simple presentation makes it clear that the weight and force of evidence cannot be combined—*integrated*—to form a judgment of support or probability. Assume that my evidence renders it more probable than not that the Giants will win the Super Bowl. I realize, however, that this evidence covers a very small fragment of what bears on which team wins a particular game. Still, the probability on the evidence is what it is, regardless of whether it is based on a lot or a little evidence.

The weight of evidence, unlike the evidence itself, has no *direction*, which refers to the function of evidence or reasons to raise or lower the credibility of a proposition. Greater weight of evidence is no greater positive force of the evidence, since further evidence could lessen probability.

When arguments turn on treating judgments of weight as having direction, they commit what I will call the *directionality of weight* fallacy. The distinctive import of the weight of evidence or confidence is missed because it is assimilated to directional judgments on the evidence. Of course, alterations in the weight of evidence or confidence are directional—they go up or down. But they are not directional for the original judgment. If you conclude from a scientific study that there is a two-thirds chance that if you take aspirin, your headache will go away within an hour, and then you read another study with similar findings, your weight of evidence and confidence increase. But there is no directional import for the original judgment.

The directionality of weight fallacy is implicated in the claim and felt sense that full belief and doubt are incompatible. In this section, however, the distinction proposed, in which the claim fails, holds only for partial or degrees of belief. It is only in subsequent sections that we attempt the transfer of the partial belief/confidence distinction to full belief.

An important criticism of the *Paradox of Ideal Evidence* by Richard Jeffrey (1983) exposes one source of persuasive power in the directionality of weight fallacy. The "paradox" is this: Viewing a normal-looking, two-sided coin, you conjecture that the objective probability that the eighth toss will be heads is one-half. But then you are allowed to study it. After subjecting the coin to a thousand trials, where the frequency of heads and tails is close, you conclude that the probability that the eighth toss will be heads is still one-half. Since the conclusion you reached is the same as your original conjecture, what is the value of all the testing?[3] The alleged paradox is that there is none.[4] The balance of the evidence remains constant, and so the judged probability is the same (.5). But the *weight* of the evidence increases with the further trials. Your degree of belief is unchanged, but your confidence in it increases. Without reference to the notion of weight of evidence, Jeffrey points out that divergences between judgments based only on the make-up of coins and judgments based also on the large number of tosses lie elsewhere. Imagine that the coin is now tossed twenty times, eighteen of which are heads. What is the degree of belief that the next toss will be heads? The person whose degree of belief is based only on the observation that the coin is two-sided and looks evenly balanced will set the probability at much higher than one half. His judgment will alter from the original one, since the original one is based on little evidence. But the person whose degree of belief is based on a thousand trials sticks close to his estimate of one-half. The weight of his evidence is much greater, and so too his confidence.[5]

Jeffrey's analysis shows that the air of paradox depends on our attending to only the central judgment that the coin will land heads on the next toss. The result of this misdirection is that the role of differences in weight is hidden.

Judgments of weight simply lack prominence. If one's degree of belief is fixed in accord with the total available evidence, we can understand why Keynes actually disparaged his discovery. Regardless of the weight of the evidence, we can only judge on the basis of the evidence we have, and then it should hardly matter whether the weight is large or small.[6]

The weakness in Keynes's reasoning is the one noted in chapter 2. The weakness is to view the endpoint of theoretical reasoning, reasoning toward belief, as the same as practical reasoning—the best judgment on the available evidence. Rather, the goal of theoretical reasoning is an all-out affirmation of truth or falsity, and that demands a judgment of high weight.

In typical arguments toward belief, particularly when in the service of practical ends, judgments of weight not only lack prominence but take on the appearance of directionality, giving rise to the directionality of weight fallacy. The three main, and related, ways this can occur are through first, the unrecognized intervention of factual assumptions, second, the practical demand for a single judgment, and third, the belieflike role that variations in weight or confidence play in facilitating or impeding action.

Here is an example illustrating the first and second difficulties: A witness, called by the prosecution, testifies that he is very sure he saw the defendant at the time and scene of the crime. You, as a juror, take his strength of conviction to be high—say, around 85 percent. But you also notice that his eyes are shifty and he becomes visibly agitated on cross-examination, especially when his relation toward the defendant is raised. What degree of belief in whether the defendant was present at the crime scene do you now assign?[7] The natural response is that it will be lower. So discovering that the witness is not very trustworthy leads you to alter your judgment downward. Thus the diminished weight of evidence is absorbed into the directional judgment of how likely it is that the defendant was at the scene, since the juror's deliberation must issue in a single verdict.

But the hidden component is actually a matter of weight, lacking directionality: A lack of truthfulness itself need not issue in testimony that unfairly favors or unfairly disfavors the defendant. The unnoticed factual assumption effecting the illusion is that the untrustworthy witness, since called by the prosecution, will lean toward error on the side of harming the defendant.

The third way for judgments of weight to be obscured and assimilated to evidential matters arises because alterations in confidence in a belief affect one's willingness to act on it, as does an alteration in subjective probability. So if we infer from action to degree of belief, a nondirectional alteration in weight will be bypassed (and, again, by assimilation to an evidential influence).

Viewing belief in its action-guiding role is not a narrow or specialized one. Traditionally, belief is understood as a disposition to act (Braithwaite 1932–33). Although I do not share this understanding, I accept that the prime function of belief is to guide action, and one's actions are the best evidence of one's beliefs, given one's desires.

Consider an example: In response to an query, Paul affirms that it is very probable that Bridget is devoted to the environment. As a result he is strongly disposed to invite her to join him in protesting the granting of a logging permit to a lumbering company. However, the inquirer then asks

Paul how sure he is about Bridget's commitment. Realizing that he does not know Bridget well, Paul responds that he is not real sure. The lack of surety does not, retrospectively, diminish the probability that Bridget is devoted to the environment. Further evidence could go either way. Nevertheless, given Paul's awareness of his weak confidence, he is more reluctant to invite Bridget to join his crusade. The greater reluctance is indistinguishable behaviorally from Paul's reaching further evidence in which, say, Bridget displays a lack of concern with the environment (e.g., he observes her one day driving an SUV). Because these behavioral consequences are the same, the alteration in the judgment of weight is not recognized as distinct from a directional, evidential one.[8]

2 The Task Ahead: The Difficult Transfer to Full Belief

Were my account to rest here, I would be home free on my main task. For belief-doubt problems would dissolve. Low confidence would not only be compatible with a belieflike attitude, but it would explain one's doubts. "I have doubts about my judgment that Paris is more populous than San Francisco because my evidence is pretty thin."

But the application to full belief is hardly automatic. The claim to full belief requires that one's evidential support is *maximal,* by which it is meant that we have reached the *threshold* of adequate reasons. For the partial belief/confidence distinction, the lack of confidence can overtly be due to weak evidence. But if the evidence is weak, full belief is unwarranted. I need to transfer the partial belief/confidence distinction to full belief, but I cannot do it over variations in evidence.

The broad claim is that full belief is compatible with variations in confidence (with diminished confidence corresponding to doubt). Looking back to chapters 6, we realize that there are a slew of examples. Linda may fully believe both that Plato admired Socrates and that there are dogs, but the latter is much more certain. Indeed, our discussion of tacit confirmation begs for something like the belief/confidence distinction. For the background beliefs that are subject to ongoing tacit confirmation, confidence in them is overwhelming and much greater than for our run-of-the-mill full beliefs (like that Plato admired Socrates).

Normally, belief and confidence go together. Our beliefs could not function well in easily guiding actions against the tension and self-consciousness induced by a diminution in confidence. Since our confidence normally depends on our evidence, to have evidence adequate for full belief is to have correspondingly strong confidence. The distinction is rooted in an analytical one—between the facet of full belief as an epistemic condition (adequate reasons) and as an attitude (strength of believing).[9]

What the opening example already shows, and which the examples below will bring home more forcefully, is that the distinction occasionally surfaces in our attitudes as well. Unfortunately, it generates a locus for the directionality of weight fallacy. The objects of assessments of confidence are judgments, whereas the objects of directional judgments are statements or propositions or types of events. The question asked in the psychological studies is which city has a larger population. The subsequent question is how sure (confident) are you about that judgment (e.g., that Paris has a larger population). In answering, one is assessing how well founded one's judgment is, not reforming that judgment, given further information.

However, before I can present the directionality of weight fallacy for full belief I have to show that the clean distinction between partial belief and confidence transfers to a full belief/confidence distinction. One's confidence can vary while one's full belief is stable, and it can do so because there is a component of confidence, that is separable from the force of evidence. I will then undertake to show that the analogue of the directionality of weight fallacy applies to full belief. The application would explain why the distinction is missed and explain away the felt incompatibility of belief and doubt.

3   Fallibility, Controversy, and Mill's Pragmatist Reasoning

Let me begin with an example of the directionality of weight fallacy that concerns full belief, which I analyze as if I have already made good on the transfer from partial to full belief. If the analysis is plausible, it will promote the transfer. The example is from a famed argument of Mill's, whose central epistemological reasoning is important to the ethics of belief generally. Mill argues: "Those who desire to suppress it [a disfavored opinion or doctrine], of course, deny its truth; but they are not infallible. They have no authority to decide the question for all mankind and exclude every other person from the means of judging. To refuse a hearing to an opinion because they are sure that it is false is to assume that *their* certainty is the same thing as *absolute* certainty. All silencing of discussion is an assumption of infallibility" (1978: 16–17). Without claiming textual authority, it is natural to reconstruct the pivotal subargument as follows: Since you are fallible, you are only entitled to a degree of certainty less than absolute certainty—you can only be morally certain that p is false. The argument reflects the pragmatist insistence that a criterion of knowledge or certainty or conclusive reasons is too demanding for us finite and fallible mortals.[10]

Recognition of one's fallibility in regard to a belief may lessen one's confidence in it without constituting any negative evidence. The analogue of the direction of weight fallacy is to construe recognition of one's fallibility as evidential. It is clear enough that fallibility alone is nondirectional: You can be fallible in underestimating, as well as overestimating. The would-be censor could have underappreciated his evidence that the opinion he wants to suppress is mistaken, just as he might err by thinking it too decisive. So the admission of one's fallibility cannot be integrated with one's evidence to yield a new assignment of support—specifically, of diminished certainty.

Were the integration to be allowed, the Millian reasoning lands in a self-defeating regress. For at whatever new, lesser level of assurance is proper, reaching that level will still involve a fallible inference, subject to a possibility of error. But, however tiny, this possibility must be factored into determining whether we have reached that level,[11] in accord with the reasoning itself. But to this latter determination a further, if tinier, possibility of error must be factored in. The result is a regressive erosion of any degree of assurance. The argument just sketched is borrowed from Hume, though, notoriously, he did not view it as a reductio (Hume 1975: 181–182)[12] The question is why Mill's implied integration appears to go so smoothly, and the answer calls on the direction of weight fallacy for full belief.

Mill's reasoning seems to work because the attitude that we start with is a strong, threshold one (certainty), which might as well be full belief.[13] This starting point is the analogue of the background, factual assumptions that we earlier found to hide the weight/force distinction. Given that the position to which Mill is objecting is a threshold one, the only "direction" to go is down, and to go down below the threshold is vastly more important than where one lands. As a consequence, the matter of confidence is not recognized as a (non-integratable) judgment of weight. Instead, it is itself taken as having direction (downward) and so is construed as a kind of evidence.

Treating Mill's reasoning as involving the directionality of weight fallacy undermines the rationale for taking full belief and doubt as incompatible. That rationale, at its broadest, is precisely that we are fallible. This same line of criticism applies to related fallibilist inferences: from the falsity of past scientific theories to the conclusion that our current theory is not true or not well supported or that the terms in it fail to refer (Putnam's "meta-induction," 1978: 24–25); from the claim that since an argument is defeasible or corrigible it cannot be conclusive or yield knowledge; from the discovery of controversy surrounding a belief to the conclusion of diminished support. The fault in this last inference is particularly well suited to illustrate my main claim.

At one time, in the early-nineteenth-century United States, say, it was controversial that slavery was wrong. We can plausibly conjecture that those who opposed slavery offered an argument roughly like the following: Slaves are persons; persons are entitled to liberty and respect; slaves are denied, in the extreme, liberty and respect; hence slavery is terribly wrong. Presumably, if the attention of those who endorse this argument is directed to the serious controversy about the topic, doubts will be generated among some of them as to the force of the above antislavery argument. Nevertheless, the controversial nature of the antislavery position, which is the source of these doubts, does not undermine that argument.

Currently, there is no serious debate about whether slavery is wrong. Its wrongness is uncontroversial. But if asked what argument shows that slavery is wrong, something akin to the informal argument just presented is the argument that many of us would offer today. On the assumption that a core of similar grounds for the truth of the premises were available then, as today, if the argument is strong or conclusive now, it was so then. It's the same argument. The intense disagreement over the slavery question does not challenge the belief, since the fact of dissent itself exposes no failing in either the content of the belief or the (above) argument for it.

Neither controversy nor fallibility in regard to a full belief can undermine it (or any argument for it). A judgment of the probability of a proposition on the evidence, although a subjective or epistemic judgment of someone, purports to capture an objective fact (how genuinely probable is the proposition). When the appeal to fallibility or controversy are germane at all, they answer not to the question of the support for a belief, but to our confidence in that support.

4   The Uniformity and Focal Assumptions: Counterexamples

Fallibility and controversy vividly lack direction and so help to make the case that their relevance to belief is distinct from support or justification of a belief. I now want to pursue the transfer to full belief with examples that involve overtly negative reasons, and yet which I will argue still do not amount to undermining reasons or evidence.

The four examples to follow I interpret as illustrating the compatibility, if uneasy, of full belief and doubt. I will provide a theoretical underpinning for this interpretation of them in due course. The underpinning will relieve any burden of argument on them, beyond that of illustrations. But, as a prelude to doing that, in the next section (5), I attempt to corroborate through assertion this interpretation of these examples, and in the section following it (6) I try to show how the interpretation casts light on some familiar psychological studies that I have touched on elsewhere.

Example (1): You are a pretty good student in logic, and you have just worked out a complex proof from the rules of logic alone. You fully believe that the last line is a theorem, based on the proof. If your proof is correct, you know that the last line is a theorem. However, there is an advanced student, Kate, who you know is very good at logic. Kate, in passing, remarks that there is an error in your proof. Your confidence is shaken. You are less sure that your last line is a theorem (or that the proof of it is correct), although Kate's testimony is no refutation of the soundness or validity of your proof.

Example (2): Jones has reasons adequate for knowledge to justify his belief that

(A)   Picasso is a greater artist than Duchamp.

Hearing Jones's argument, a friend remarks that

(D)   Smith believes that Duchamp is the greater artist.

Jones accepts (D), and that Smith, though not a connoisseur, is considerably more knowledgeable than he is about art, and that broadly they have shared tastes. (D) is not counterevidence to Jones' belief that (A), yet it can be, like Kate's dissent in the previous example, a reason for Jones to be less sure of (A).

The discrepancy between Picasso and Duchamp as artists is meant to be wide, so that it is a fairly easy judgment to justify in ordinary circumstances. (Compare: Kant was a greater philosopher than Plotinus; Lincoln was a greater U.S. President than Coolidge.) For this reason and for the sake of argument, I ask you to grant that Jones could know (A). Otherwise substitute your own example.

Neither this example nor the previous one implies any skepticism about knowledge transmission through testimony. Normally, a speaker transmits his knowledge that p to the hearer by asserting it and the hearer accepting his assertion. (For a more careful formulation, see Adler 1996.) But the default rule for testimony does not apply in these cases. I allow, of course, that one can have evidence that one's argument or reasoning is mistaken without knowing wherein lies the mistake. But that would apply to this case only if either Jones knew Smith's reasons (presuming they were related to Jones's argument for (A)) or Smith knows that (A) is false. It takes no realism away from the case to assume that neither of these disjuncts holds. In example 1, Kate's testimony is not related to the theorem in the internal way that a proof is—it is the very condition for the last line to be a theorem that there be such a proof, not that anyone testify to it. Testimony in this setting, as with opinions, cannot override proof or argument.

Example (3): This example is a neighbor of the opening one, and it is of independent interest. Variants of the example play a prominent role in the debate over the interpretation of the experiments on probabilistic reasoning (the "base rate" studies) that we turn to in section 6.[14]

You are assigning final grades in a large class, which are mainly based on a term paper. One senior received an A- on it, which you fully believe is deserved. But you learn that this student's average is around C/C–. (For the sake of the example, put aside professional duties associated with grading.)

The student's average is not counterevidence to your belief. It is an instance of a statistical truism that grades on some papers or tests may well exceed a student's long-standing average. But your confidence is reasonably lowered.

Example (3), unlike examples (1) and (2), assumes that you do not retain knowledge of the student's paper. It represents typical beliefs where we do not retain the specific grounds for accepting them.

Example (4). This is just an earlier example extended to full belief. Paul judges that his neighbor Bridget is morally devoted to protecting the environment. However, he observes her throwing away, rather than recycling, today's newspaper. Even as Paul understands his observation, it is not incompatible with his judgment. One can be morally devoted to a cause without being a stickler in regard to the actions that comply with it. Still, if he sets aside—brackets—his belief, Bridget's current action is more in keeping with someone who is not too concerned about the environment. So his confidence in his judgment of Bridget diminishes.

The defense of these examples so far is mostly intuitive—they ring true. In each case, you empathize with the believer whose confidence is diminished. But in no case does the source of the diminished confidence constitute counterevidence or undermining reasons of the belief. If our intuitive judgment is correct, and the bulk of the defense comes later, then these would constitute counterexamples to the uniformity assumption. Recall:

Any epistemic reason to critically reflect on, or doubt, a belief constitutes evidence (reasons) that undermines the truth of the belief or the argument for it.

In the opening section I observed that this assumption inspires our belief-doubt problems. The examples all offer epistemic reasons that, though they diminish confidence, do not undermine the belief.

The above examples show that one can have reasons to doubt or to critically reflect on a (maintained) belief. My twofold conclusion goes, in fact, further: There are actual cases, and lots of them, where we have reasons to be self-critical of particular beliefs. These reasons derive from the possibility, also illustrated by these cases, of reasonable doubts or diminished confidence in a belief that do not require abandoning it.

Behind the uniformity assumption is an influential, though vague and unstated, assumption that I will call the *focal assumption*:

Any reason relevant to accepting or maintaining a belief has its reason-conferring or doubt-conferring force only in its impact on the justification of that belief.

In the Paradox of Ideal Evidence, the focal assumption licenses the mistaken inference from the sameness of the probability assigned to the worthlessness of the further trials.

The focal assumption has going for it that our attention in inquiry, argument, or criticism ought to be on the truth of our beliefs or candidate beliefs. But it wrongly licenses the conclusion that nothing else counts.[15] An obvious line of reasoning moves from the focal assumption to the uniformity assumption, since if, according to the focal assumption, a negative reason can have impact only by diminishing one's justification, then it is undermining evidence of the belief. Reasons to doubt will then either be counterevidence (and so incompatible with belief) or irrelevant (not really epistemic reasons). To reject the focal assumption and with it the uniformity assumption is to reject this disjunction as a false alternative.

If we surrender the focal assumption, it is evident that examples (1)–(4) are just the tip of the iceberg.[16] For an example suggestive of many others, consider a student Jill, who takes an exam consisting of fill-ins of great precision (e.g., Kant's year of birth is ___). If each of Jill's answers is correct, then her grade will be 100 percent and not at all accidentally. Jill knows each answer.

Nevertheless, we can easily imagine that during the test or afterward various kinds of information will upset Jill's confidence. Jill notices that most of her fellow students are still working and sweating away, including those whom she expected to do much better. Or, she recalls that her average in the class so far is not stellar. Or, afterward she compares answers with the better students, and a number of their answers diverge from hers. And so on. The upsetting information constitutes reasons for Jill to lesson her confidence, and the first and second provide reasons for Jill to check over her answers. But however racking Jill with doubt, none of this information amounts to undermining reasons—ones that show that Jill's answers are mistaken or that her grounds for them are defective.

This model assumes, of course, that it is genuinely possible for Jill to have earned the perfect score and for her to know these various facts as negative. But it would be desperation to deny this assumption. Such reasonable nervousness and rechecking is the everyday stuff of the modest, capable student's life. Underlying this compatibility is the difference between satisfying a condition and showing or knowing that one has satisfied it. Whatever condition is necessary for a belief p to be justified, call it "C" (most prominently, that the evidence for p rules out various possibilities that p is false), will be satisfiable without comprehending all facts correlated with whether one has satisfied C. So there can be information that renders it less probable that one has satisfied C, and yet, one has satisfied it.

Examples (1)–(4), as well as these latter ones, further my extension of the partial belief/confidence distinction to full belief. The reasons that diminish one's confidence do not thereby undermine one's full belief. Once we cease to view the myriad cases in which confidence in belief is reasonably disrupted, through the focal and uniformity assumptions, it is apparent that such reasons readily arise for many beliefs, especially the salient or forefront ones. The compatibility of belief and doubt now appears as evident as it is banal that persons in love occasionally, and reasonably, feel anger, dislike, or even hate for each other.

5   Assertional Corroboration

In this section, I try to corroborate our interpretation of these examples by reverting to the parallel with assertion. The examples accord with our assertional practices. According to the default rule for testimony, to challenge an assertion is to incur a burden. So one's challenge must itself constitute a specific reason to doubt an assertion or its backing or the speaker's position to know it. A parallel claim applies to legitimate withdrawals of an assertion:

(W)   If S asserts that *p*, then S is entitled to *withdraw* the assertion if and only if S offers a specific reason for the withdrawal.[17]

(W) implies that to withdraw an assertion incurs a burden. The speaker must present as his reason what amounts to a challenge, were it to be presented by the hearer. Only then is S bound to withdraw his assertion, since he can no longer affirm (all-out) that *p*.

Let us slightly vary example 3 so that the term paper is not the main basis for grading:

(C)   The student's grades on exams are well below the grade given on his paper.

We want to contrast the evidential import of (C) with (E):

(E)   The student's overall average after three years is C/C–.

The assertion we are considering is yours that

(A)   The student's paper deserves a grade of A–.

Since you assert (A), you imply that you know it. To challenge your assertion is to deny the implication to knowledge. Now (C), but not (E), constitutes a challenge. Compatible with the evidence from your evaluation, only (C) implies that it's possible that (A) is false (e.g., the student plagiarized). (C) is a *defeater*—incompatible with successful justification or knowledge—but not (E).[18] (Recall that our talk of evidence here, as elsewhere, is a convenience. The claims made are not peculiar to empirical statements, as the examples above indicate, and so the broader notion of epistemic reason can always be substituted for evidence, readability aside.)

In example (2), the denial that (D) is counterevidence implies that Jones is not entitled to withdraw the argument he presents for his acceptance of (A). It does not constitute a basis to challenge Jones's assertion of that argument or conclusion. It would be something of a Moore's Paradox for Jones to justify his withdrawal by saying: "(A) follows from p1 and p2. But I no longer endorse it because of (D), although (D) shows nothing wrong with my argument." Jones's endorsement of (A) resides in p1 and p2 and the validity of the argument from them, and these remain intact. So were Jones to withdraw his assertion he would fail to compensate us for considering his argument in the first place. More pertinently, he undermines his entitlement to assertion, whose point is to present relevant truths, for he retains his basis for taking (A), his conclusion, as true.

In examples (1) and (2), the speaker may very well wish he had not offered the assertion in the first place, given the dissent. However, that is an expression of his loss of confidence only. To offer an assertion is to enter claims, which the speaker is responsible to make good on. So, once a claim is entered, the speaker is not free to simply withdraw it. The speaker incurs the burden to justify a withdrawal. Of course, in real discourse, we can hope to slink away from many assertions through the expected forgetfulness of our listeners. But that is not to withdraw an assertion, any more than forgetting a belief is to withdraw it.

The cost of withdrawal would be loss of the information transmitted. The question to ask is this: In examples (1)–(4), if you imagine yourself the hearer to whom the believer asserts his belief, would you want the speaker to withdraw his assertion, given the negative reason that he learns? Would you criticize Jones as irresponsible for not withdrawing his argument and conclusion when he learns of Smith's dissent? The answer seems to be "no." That is an answer we offer not primarily to be sociable or to further democratic ends (of encouraging persons to give voice to their opinions). We offer it primarily for our epistemic interest in receiving good information.

The extent to which we would lose good information becomes apparent if we attend to the natural generalization of these examples. The natural generalization of the first two cases would be that if you assert *p*, and someone whom you take to be more knowledgeable about the subject of *p* dissents, then you should withdraw that assertion (or not assert it at all if you know of the dissent earlier). For the opening and the third and fourth examples, the generalization would be that you should not offer an assertion if the property it ascribes to an object occurs very infrequently among members of the kind to which the object belongs. Undoubtedly both of these generalizations could be tightened up to bring in relevant qualifications of the example. However, no uncontrived tightening will undercut the point. We would lose a great deal of good information if these negative reasons are construed as sufficient to challenge an assertion.

In claiming that despite reasons to lower confidence, the corresponding assertions would still be warranted, I really enter a much stronger claim. In the full awareness that is presumed in assertion, the speaker *cannot* offer in, say, example (3) the student's overall average as a basis to withdraw his grade of the paper (as opposed to offering it as a reason to reexamine the paper). The "can" is the conceptual "can" that has dominated this work from the outset.

6   Competence, Constraints, and Base Rates

These claims about assertion correspond with prior arguments, particularly in chapters 8 and 9, of the qualitative distinctness of full belief. We are constrained not to continuously modify our assertions according to the reasonable ebb and flow of our confidence. What pressures us toward the integration that allows continuous modification is the focal assumption—that a reason is either evidential or irrelevant. The pressure has been succumbed to by commentators on the important *base rate* studies in psychology (Kahneman, Slovic, and Tversky 1982). In a standard study, subjects are told that a sample of biographical sketches is of seventy lawyers and thirty engineers. Subjects randomly select one of, say, Jack, whose sketch sounds like an engineer. Most subjects judge it highly probable that Jack is an engineer, seeming to ignore the base rates altogether.

The psychologist Thomas Gilovich in application of these findings observes that individuals judge the prospects for success of their own marriages almost wholly on the basis of the perceived quality of their personal relationships with their future spouses, moderated hardly at all by the divorce rates, as base rates. Gilovich comments: "To be sure, we should not discount our current feelings and self-knowledge altogether; we just need to temper them a bit more with our knowledge of what happens to people in general. This is the consensus opinion of all scholars in the field" (1991: 106). The consensus that Gilovich reports bears the scars of the focal assumption and a failure to appreciate the constraints on us to full belief. To temper our judgments implies that no one is justified in fully believing that their marriage will succeed or that their marital prospects are excellent (or whatever the prominent belief is that is falsified by divorce). If these beliefs maintain their close association with actions, then the practical import is that prospective spouses should hedge their commitments in marriage, as with prenuptial agreements, out of deference to the high rate of divorce.

But it is difficult for commitment of one partner to be lowered without stimulating a downward spiral, when the other partner follows suit. The full belief is constrained, but it is not thereby unwarranted or illusory—we form such full beliefs without obliviousness to the divorce rates.[19] I claim that we can find a place for Gilovich's concern as a tempering of confidence, not belief.

The marriage-divorce case is problematic in some obvious ways—it is emotionally charged, and we all come to it with the baggage of personal knowledge or experience. The downward spiral cited as a danger of integration or "tempering" seems specialized to the demand for strong commitment and to an abstract view of marriage as having features of a two-person competitive game. Nevertheless, the critical point holds in general. Consider Gilovich's "consensus" recommendation as applied to our favorite practice of conversation or assertion. Imagine that we acceded to the recommendation to temper our acceptance of testimony by an estimate of the degree of reliable and honest truth-telling in the relevant community, however rough. The result would be that much more of what we standardly accept as true, we could now accept only as bearing some high degree of probability. Tempering issues in tempered acceptance. The layers of complexity would be unmanageable. We would undermine the trust and normal flow of information between speakers and hearers. No conversational practice corresponds to it, assuming, as before, that the relevant beliefs serve in their usual function as guides to action.

The cases that concern us are ones where the relevant base rates do not point to any specific fault in the current judgment. The specificity that the base rates require to undermine a judgment reflects the Jamesian trade-off between seeking truth and avoiding error. As we loosen up on that specificity, more believers (and their corresponding beliefs in conflict with those base rates) are excluded, just as more speakers (and their assertions) would be. In example (3), if the student's average is posited as a challenge to the grader, the challenge cannot be restricted to this particular case, since the appropriate description is not "sharp discrepancy between the grade on this paper and the student's overall, longstanding average," but "sharp discrepancy between grades on any paper and the student's . . . average." So, if in the case of grading, and similarly one's marital prospects, discrepancy with the respective base rates do undermine judgments, then they will do so in virtue of a very strong consequence: In these areas, none of us can claim competence to make similar judgments.

However, in taking the impact of the base rates on full belief to be located in confidence, I restrict their epistemic role, not eliminate it. The data that constitute the divorce rates or the student's average are more objective and reliable than those that constitute either your own self-knowledge or self-assessment. In neighboring areas, the relevant base rates can penetrate to require the withdrawal of full belief. Consider those base rates studies that show personal interviews to be much less reliable as a basis for evaluating clients or applicants than bland data from dossiers and standard testing (Nisbett and Ross 1980: chap 5). Here the findings may very well reach to specific judgments, when they turn on the personal interviews. If so, you cannot know that judgment. We now have evidence of a likely deficiency in forming that judgment. But you can know that your grade of the student is accurate, even if it is discrepant with the student's average.

The direction of weight fallacy is involved when it is argued that because the base rates are relevant to your judgment, and they run counter to it, you should cease to hold the corresponding full belief. In example (3), if your assessment is correct, then the student's overall average does not have a negative impact either on the judgment or the basis for it. But the discrepancy is a reason to lessen your confidence and recheck your grading. Since the judgment is all-out that the student deserves an A–, there is a pull to withdraw the all-out judgment. But if it would be wrong to lower the student's grade because of her average (and wrong epistemically, not just ethically), it is because the student's average does not play an evidential role in evaluating the student's paper. The direction of weight fallacy is to ignore that to become less confident of one's judgment is itself nondirectional.

7   Negative Clues as Tolerable Doubts: Summary of Argument

We have defended our examples and the full belief/confidence distinction along a number of lines: intuitively (the examples ring true), theoretically or epistemically (the distinction is backed up by the distinction between the weight and the force of evidence), psychologically (the distinction is readily obscured in practice) and practically (the distinction explains alterations in dispositions to act.) In effect, our attempt to respond to belief-doubt problems has been complex, yet a single, extended argument.

In this closing section, I will try to present and clarify the argument explicitly, using for illustrative purposes examples (1)–(4). For ease of reference, I summarize those examples:

(1)   You are a pretty good student in logic, and you have just worked out a complex proof from the rules of logic alone. However, there is an advanced student, Kate, who remarks that your proof contains an error.

(2)   Jones has reasons adequate for knowledge to justify his belief that

(A) Picasso is a greater artist than Duchamp.

Hearing Jones' argument, a friend remarks that

(D) Smith believes that Duchamp is the greater artist.

Jones accepts (D), and that Smith, though not a connoisseur, is considerably more knowledgeable than he is about art, and that broadly they have shared tastes.

(3)   You are assigning final grades in a large class, which is mainly based on a term paper. One senior received an A– on it, which you fully believe is deserved. But you learn that this student's average is around C/C–.

(4)   Paul judges that his neighbor Bridget is morally devoted to protecting the environment. However, he observes her throwing away, rather than recycling, today's newspaper.

Each of the examples is supposed to be a case in which there are reasons to doubt, and so lessen confidence, but these reasons do not undermine full belief. Let us refer to the negative information in these cases as "negative *clues*," or "clues" for short. (If one suitably adjusts the examples, it becomes evident that there can be positive clues as well. But since my concern is to show the compatibility of belief and doubt, I ignore positive clues.)

The argument involves five interrelated claims: First, there is a conceptual and psychological distinction between full belief and confidence. Second, the possibility of variations in confidence, while belief is stable, is of sufficient epistemic value that the distinction must have a prominent place in our practices. Third, the negative clues are nonevidential for a person in relation to a specific belief (or judgment). Fourth, it can be reasonable for a person to become less confident of his belief at a time in learning of a negative clue, and in this way, to have doubts about it. "Reasonable" will cover psychological and epistemological territory. The diminished confidence is psychologically reasonable given our limits, a theme picked up under the fifth claim; and the agent has an epistemic reason to lessen his confidence. Our second, third, and fourth claims are effectively premises for our first claim, as conclusion. Fifth, there is a tendency to fallaciously misconstrue the grounds to lessen confidence as evidential. Ascription of a fallacy helps explain why the compatibility of belief and doubt is so readily denied.

First, in each of the examples, a plausible telling of the story is that the main character's confidence in his full belief (or the argument for it) diminishes, and yet he is entitled to maintain the full belief. The conceptual basis for this duality (between belief and confidence) is the central burden of the argument. One way to account for the duality is by reference to the threshold nature of full belief. Just as we can ask how confident one is in the subjective probability one assigns to a proposition, so we can ask, though more awkwardly, how confident one is of a judgment issuing in a full belief. You can be much more confident if you take your evidence or reasons to place you well above the threshold for establishing the proposition. (Suppose that I believe that Joe's wealth is around two million dollars and Jane's is around five million. Then, in awareness of this difference, I will be more confident in claiming that Jane is a millionaire than that Joe is, though I fully believe that both are.)

Second, the diminished confidence acts as a check or restraint on one's belief; and gives salience to it as vulnerable to alteration. Kate's dissent, in example (1), provides you with a reason to recheck your proof. In example (4), Paul will become hesitant about asking Bridget to join his environmental crusade, upon observing her tossing out the newspaper. He is made sensitive to whether his current observation is of a mere lapse, or whether it instead is part of a pattern of deviation, which would undermine belief. Although each of the examples assumes full belief as a starting point, a primary value of negative clues is at the stage of determining that inquiry should close, as a precursor to acceptance and full belief. In example (2), if Jones just started to look closely at the paintings of Picasso and Duchamp, and he is near to forming his judgment that Picasso is the greater artist, he will not yet end inquiry if he learns of Smith's dissent.

Third, the negative clues, though epistemic, are not evidence against the belief. In examples (1) and (2), a certain amount of dissent on one's judgments is unexceptionable; in example (3), from a broader perspective, we simply and unproblematically have a case of a datum that is discrepant from a long-standing, overall average; and in example (4), one can be environmentally concerned without being a stickler about recycling. More specifically, Paul can know that Bridget is morally devoted to protecting the environment, and he can know this without investigating each time she throws away her newspaper, rather than recycling it. In example (1), Kate's dissent signals no falsity in any inference. The proof is what it is, regardless of Kate's dissent, and it is that proof alone which constitutes the justification for your belief (that the conclusion is a theorem).

From the first-person point of view on one's full belief or the argument for it, these clues lose their negative import for the proposition believed. Given a clear grasp of the careful evaluation by which you assigned the student a grade of A–, in example (3), the discrepancy with her average loses its force. (To borrow from a different vocabulary: Your evaluation *screens-off* the import of the student's average.)

Nevertheless, the loss of confidence in each case seems intuitively reasonable—in each case the person can offer a reason, in the form of the negative clue, for diminishing his (default) confidence. Even though, strictly, the belief and your reasons for it undermine the negative force of the clues on the judgment, *were* your evaluation in, say, example (3) to be defective, the discrepancy would be a good indicator of it. But the catch for this truth-indicating feature, the key feature of epistemic reasons, is the "were." You yet have no reason to believe that your evaluation is defective; otherwise, of course, you could not come to, or maintain, the full belief. The subjunctive "were" acquires force, to render the discrepancy a negative clue, only if the discrepancy is conceived at a higher-order level as a member of a set of related judgments, for example, gradings, among which there are likely to be some that are erroneous. Since negative clues, like the discrepancy with the student's average, are good indicators of where you are likely to be mistaken, were you mistaken, you have reason to treat some of them as epistemic reasons, whose impact is realized in its bearing on confidence.

On this analysis, the negative clues for a particular judgment are not relative, like evidence, only to the proposition believed and one's background evidence. They are relative, as well, to one's higher-order policy in regard to the possibilities for error among certain beliefs. We cannot *generalize* to claim that whenever one has a negative clue c for a judgment p, then one's confidence should be reduced by amount s. What is generalizable is only that sometimes one has to be sensitive to such clues, through alterations in confidence, not any particular ones. Unlike genuine counterevidence, other believers, in similar situations, may reasonably dismiss the new information as irrelevant. In example (3), you do not feel any epistemic obligation to check your final grade for each student against his or her overall average, even if this is easy to do (by computer).

At this point our central argument is complete. Full belief and doubt, construed as diminished confidence, are compatible, since there can be reasons that justify the diminution, which do not constitute undermining reasons or counterevidence. (Of course, this does not show that belief is compatible with any reasonable doubts. Specifically, there is no compatibility with evidentially grounded doubts.) As a further consequence, we can reject the uniformity assumption, which assimilates all epistemic reasons to evidential ones.

However, although the argument is complete, it will not be highly persuasive without an account of why it seems just obvious to many people that belief and doubt are incompatible. The claim of incompatibility is not the imposition of theorists alone, since many people in everyday judgments often affirm the claim as well. Specifically, I expect that many people are disposed to treat negative clues as either irrelevant or evidential. The seeming support of the incompatibility within our practices is worrisome. In this chapter, as elsewhere throughout this book, I am concerned to corroborate the evidentialist ethics of belief through our ordinary judgments and practices. So now we must proceed to our fifth claim above that there is a tendency to fallaciously misconstrue the grounds to lessen confidence as evidential.

The most obvious problem is just that terms such as "believe," "sure," "certain," "confident," and their cognates are often used interchangeably, which obscures distinctions between them. It is odd to speak of yourself as fully believing something, and yet to lack confidence in that belief. The oddity of the talk is not readily noticed because a disparity between belief and confidence must be transitory lest there be a serious interference with the smooth flow from belief to action. These ways in which the belief/confidence distinction is obscured are clearly not grounds for denying the distinction. In this regard, our favorable reaction to the responses of the characters in the examples is more telling.

Still, the very presentation of these examples introduces a bias toward a fallacious denial of the belief/confidence distinction. For each of the examples, I am trying to elicit from you confirmation that the ambivalence I project—the loss of confidence and the hold of full belief—rings true. However, you would be much less inclined to find the loss of confidence genuine across a large number of similar cases. You would start to think that I have selected an especially anxious or insecure group of characters to focus on. My analysis above embraces this change in sympathy: epistemic responses to the negative clues are not directly generalizable. But, as actors, of course, we are embedded in particular situations to which we must respond accordingly. Alterations in confidence are emotion-like in their spontaneity. Thus our perspective is constricted to the particular situation, and that encourages us to misconstrue the negative clues that affect us as of greater evidential significance than is really warranted.

This constricted perspective is psychologically reasonable given our limits. Earlier, we emphasized limits on our on-line grasp of our reasons or epistemic position. In examples (2)–(4), much of the actors' reasons for their beliefs can be understood as not explicit. As we observed in chapter 3 and elsewhere, keeping our reasons implicit, or even losing them, is a practical and epistemic necessity.

Even when explicit, comprehension may be limited. In example (1), we can imagine that your proof is set out—it is explicit. Nevertheless, you may not fully understand it. Were you to fully understand it, the confidence-threatening force of Kate's denial is surrendered. Consider, for example, the simple proof that John is taller than Jim on the grounds that

John is taller than Tim and Tim is taller than Jim. With a proof so simple, where we perfectly well comprehend the inference, it is of no consequence for our epistemic position to learn of someone who questions the reasoning and even that simple proofs do sometimes turn out to contain subtle fallacies.

In examples like (1), we assume your proof is very complex. When you are shaken by Kate's dissent, it seems to reflect recognition of a flaw in your proof. But what is really going on is that you do not perfectly well grasp your proof, even if it is, as we are assuming, impeccable, not that additional support is necessary to justify your belief. Given the centrality of the full belief/partial belief distinction, we cannot avail ourselves of the proposal for you to slightly weaken your strength of belief, given Kate's dissent. Withdrawal from full belief marks a sharp—qualitative—difference in one's position in regard to a belief, not merely a minor difference in degree, and so incurs a burden to justify the withdrawal. To withdraw from full belief, given that you have the best of reasons—in particular, a manifestly correct proof—for it, would be to effectively imply a lack of competence to offer proofs in this domain. Rather, you find yourself in one of those uncomfortable, but familiar, situations, in which you stand by your reasons, and thus imply that your more competent, but not infallible, peer Kate has erred.

The direction of weight fallacy applied here consists in inferring from the relevance of the negative clues to lessen confidence in a judgment that they constitute undermining evidence of it. Since the import of the negative clues always depends on assessments of the judger, their primary import is nondirectional. Their primary import is by way of the error-proneness of the judger, and error in judgment can always go either of two ways. That is why fallibility of various kinds is primarily nondirectional. Of course, secondarily, there can be an indication of the direction that the error is more likely to fall. But once the primary nondirectionality is recognized, the information ought no longer to be viewed as evidential for the judgment. In examples (1)–(4), the negative clues are avowedly negative, unlike the appeal to fallibility and controversy. Nevertheless, if the force of these clues depends on what they signal to the believer about his own judging, then to that extent there is a nondirectional step.

However, since the believer's starting point is one of full belief, which standardly goes with high confidence, the only direction to go is downward. If the role of this fact is not recognized, the path is greased for the direction of weight fallacy.

A related source of the fallacy, as noted earlier, can be in the very advantages of alterations in confidence to yield alterations in dispositions to act. In example (1), Kate's dissent will have a greater impact in restraining you, if you are about to exhibit your proof publicly than if it remains merely private. Similarly, in example (4), Paul will become hesitant about asking Bridget to join his environmental crusade on observing her tossing out the newspaper, as he would if his belief had gone from full to partial owing to receiving undermining evidence. Consequently, viewed from the perspective of how one acts, reasons to lessen confidence are readily confused with genuinely undermining evidence.

The main argument and claims of this chapter, just reviewed, are easy enough to grasp intuitively. But they required development because they are meant to overcome the deeply felt incongruity of maintaining both that full belief is ordinary belief, yet that it aspires to knowledge, and that this aspiration can be regularly realized, despite certain doubts.

The argument is also lengthy because it implies a complex view of reasons and of knowers. By contrast, the uniformity assumption excludes epistemic reasons that have a higher-order rationale and do not function as straightforward evidence. The argument is also opposed to a simple view of the epistemic agent as in complete grasp of his reasons. On both counts, I sought to verify our claims by their accord with our epistemic practices and judgments, suitably sanitized. The possibility that one's confidence can vary while full belief is stable corresponds to our attitudes, judgments, and practices. But it does not correspond perfectly. Belief can erode when confidence sinks. Even though I deny that one can in full awareness withdraw one's full belief invoking a negative clue as the ground of one's withdrawal, the condition of full awareness is one that we know from discussion in chapter 3 to be difficult or unusual to meet. Aside from clarifying a distinction that is essential for the ethics of belief defended here, the account just presented avoids a dilemma: We treat these negative clues either as counterevidence or as irrelevant. If the former, we embrace a sweeping skepticism about the justification of many of our humdrum beliefs. If the latter, we dismiss these clues as at most anxiety producers of no further epistemic significance for the maintenance of one's belief. By finding a role for these negative clues as altering confidence, we find a way out of this dilemma.

APPENDIX: OUTLINE OF ASSERTION/BELIEF PARALLEL

Below I outline the parallel between assertion and belief that has been invoked to support the conceptual argument for evidentialism. The parallel, however, operates under abstractions to clarify focus on the core parallel that both aim at truth. If we follow out the parallel, we will conceive belief as assertion to oneself. That conception undoes prominent disanalogies. You can insincerely assert that p (not believe or disbelieve it, while asserting it), but you neither insincerely believe that p nor insincerely assert that p to yourself.

1. Assertion-Belief Connection
Assertion expresses full belief.
Shared ambiguity:

a. "Assertion" refers to the act (asserting) or to the content.

b. "Belief" refers to an attitude (believing) or to the content.

2. Transparency

a. Assertions are put forward as true. The content alone is put forward, detached from the speaker's attitude. The normal form of assertion is not "I believe that p," but p.

b. The normal way to activate one's belief that p, as in guiding action, is to take it to be the case that p, detached from one's attitude of believing. So the normal role of the belief that p is as directing the believer to p (the world) itself, not one's attitude toward p.

3. Truthfulness/reasons

a. Assertions are accepted only if they are backed by adequate reasons. The presumption that the speaker believes what he asserts is important to assertion only as indicating that backing.

b. Beliefs are justified only if they are backed by adequate reasons. If one can recognize p as true, then it is not essential to belief's aim of truth that there is the actual psychological attitude of believing.

4. Epistemic normativity

a. Inherent in the nature of assertion itself (not just warranted assertion).

b. Inherent when one attends to a belief (not restricted to justified/rational/warranted belief).

5. Claim, Responsibility, and higher-order recognition

a. In asserting that p, one enters a claim (to the hearer) that p is true. Speakers are responsible to satisfy that claim, and they do so only if the speaker has evidence of the assertion's truth. The hearer's acceptance of the assertion, depends upon higher-order, but routine, presumptions: The hearer takes the act as one of assertion, whose content is a judgment that is believed by the speaker.

b. In attending to one's believing that p, one regards oneself as entering a claim that p is true. The claim (to oneself as hearer) is fulfilled only if one has adequate reasons of p's truth.

Reason-responsiveness as a responsibility of speakers in regard to challenges to assertions is matched by a corresponding responsibility for reason-responsiveness in belief.

6. Knowledge

a. Assertions are proper only if the speaker knows what he asserts. (The standard form of challenge to the assertion that p is "How do you know that p?")

b. We treat our beliefs effectively as knowledge. ("Effectively" because one need not, and usually does not, take oneself as knowing, under that description.) From the first-person point of view, one treats one's belief as factive, which is the central property of knowledge.

7. Adequacy of reasons

So, adequacy of reasons for belief and assertion is adequacy for knowledge.

8. Context-sensitivity

Standards for adequate reasons for (justified) belief or assertion can be raised owing to shifts upwards in contexts—if the costs of error or the value of being correct increases. The default rule for the acceptance of an assertion or the maintenance of a belief can be overruled when the context shifts.

9. First-person awareness

a. The speaker is inherently aware of the contents of what he asserts and as expressing his beliefs. The speaker is committed to the collection of his unwithdrawn assertions, as if he remains fully aware of them.

b. First-person awareness of one's belief is not the normal condition of believing, but it is the proper condition for grasping the demands of belief. It is in first-person awareness that one grasps the demand inherent in one's believing.

10. Moore's Paradox

a. It is a contradiction to assert "p, but I do not believe that p" or "p, but I lack adequate reasons or evidence that p is true", though both conjuncts may be true.

b. One cannot think (judge) that p is true, but that one does not believe it. Nor can one think that p is true, but that one lacks (adequate) evidence or reasons of its truth, though both conjuncts can be true.

11. Default rule and conditions for withdrawal

a. Accept an assertion unless you have a specific reason to doubt it (or the veracity/reliability of speaker). The default rule imposes an asymmetry that places the burden of justifying on the challenger (hearer), rather than the speaker. You can withdraw an assertion only if you can discharge the burden of providing a specific reason (that the assertion or the grounds for it are incorrect).

b. Maintain your belief that p, unless you have specific reasons to doubt it. Withdraw a belief only if you have specific reasons to question it or your grounds to believe it. (For qualification, see 8 above.)

Some reasons bear only on one's attitude in asserting or believing. They can lessen confidence in what is asserted (believed), but since they do not cast doubt on one's position to know, they do not count as specific reasons to withdraw the assertion (suspend belief).

12. Full/partial belief; qualified/unqualified assertion: markedness

a. Epistemically qualified assertions are marked, but not unqualified ones.

b. Partial belief is marked to oneself. We do not see through it to the content, as with full belief.

13. Full/partial belief; qualified/unqualified assertion: success

a. Assertion of an epistemically qualified statement is not fully successful (the content of what is asserted is not transmitted to the hearer). If Sally asserts to Harry "I am pretty sure that p," Harry will still transmit this as "Sally says that she is pretty sure that p" not "I am pretty sure that p." Not so for (unqualified) assertion.

b. Partial belief (suspension of judgment) is unsatisfying, for propositions that interests the believer. He undertakes inquiry to seek resolution in full belief.

14. Full/partial belief; qualified/unqualified assertion: dangling

a. Epistemically qualified assertions dangle, and so reasons need to be produced. The default rule is overruled or suspended.

b. Partial belief is unsatisfactory, and, in particular, require the retaining of evidence.

15. Full/partial belief; qualified/unqualified assertion: transparency

a. Epistemically qualified assertion is not transparent. It communicates speaker's attitude not just the main propositional content, unlike simple assertion.

b. Full belief is transparent to its content; partial belief is not transparent—the content is attended to only with one's attitude toward it.

16. Implicit qualification

a. Simple assertion of overt chance or controversial statements generate mutually expected audience qualification—e.g., Sally: "The Yankees will win next year's pennant." Harry understands Sally's assertion as something like "I [Sally] am pretty sure [willing to bet] that. . . ."

b. Simple storing of propositions as (unqualified) beliefs whose content is that of overt chance or controversial propositions is recognized as qualified—really, as a partial belief—e.g., Sally stores her belief that the Yankees will win next year's pennant as such. But when she attends to it, she treats it as only a partial belief.

17. Cognitive economy

a. Assertion is under constraints to economize. The preference for unqualified over qualified assertions, as well as the related default conditions, are devices to economize.

b. Belief and its associated mechanisms and procedures are under constraints to economize. The preference for acceptance or full, over partial, belief, as well as the related default conditions, are devices to economize.

18. Everyday practice

a. Assertion (unqualified) is common, pervasive, and ordinary, despite high standards of backing.

b. Full belief is common, pervasive, and ordinary, despite high standards of backing.

19. Abstraction/idealization and overt disanalogies

a. Assertion is subject to demands on the social activity of conversation. To focus on just the epistemics of assertion, there is need to abstract from its natural embedding in conversation. So, for example, an assertion must be construed as a lasting claim, unless withdrawn for a specific reason (see 11 above). Even if a speaker forgets an assertion, to which he no longer wants to be committed, a hearer to whom he asserted it is still entitled to demand that other assertions be consistent with it.

b. Belief is constantly subject to multiple interests, influences, and mental and social demands. In order to focus on just the epistemics of belief, there is need to abstract from its natural embedding in our psychology. The focus is achieved by considering belief in full awareness and as assertion to oneself.

20. Background

a. We do not assert to hearers what we believe to be uninformative to them, though what we do assert presupposes a massive set of shared background beliefs. So what is assertible under normal conversational conditions is only a tiny subset of what we believe.

b. Beliefs that are obvious and long-standing become background beliefs that are not salient, and so less available in on-line justification and reasoning. Still, these background beliefs constitute the bulk of our beliefs and reasons.

Prospects for Self-Control: Reasonableness, Self-Correction, and the Fallibility Structure

1 Self-Correction: Means and Motives

Science is taken as a model of knowledge and inquiry because of the rudiments of its methods. First, a hypothesis is proposed to explain a range of data and observations. The hypothesis is accepted only if a varied and significant range of its implications pass rigorous tests, and none fails. Second, scientific method is *self-correcting*—continued use of it, under the usual conditions, will correct prior mistakes.

In this chapter, I reflect on the prospects for self-correction of our beliefs. Strictly, a procedure is self-corrective only if continued operation of that very procedure can correct its own prior, erroneous judgments. I will, however, apply the label "self-correction" to systematic corrections of one's own prior judgments, even if not through the same procedures by which they were acquired. Both self-correction strictly construed and that which falls under the looser labeling are forms of *self-control*. Self-control is the ability to resist inclinations contrary to one's best judgment.[1] What concerns us is our ability to resist our own beliefs for the sake of furthering their aim of truth, so I will sometimes refer to it as "epistemic self-control."[2] The central problem I address in regard to personal self-correction or epistemic self-control is this: How can one have reasons to impose controls on beliefs that one regards as correct, and what forms can those controls take?

The methods of science largely avoid this problem because to abide by scientific method is thereby to be subject to its self-corrective restraints. However, in this contrast and in others, the picture of scientific method that I invoke is extremely simplified. What concerns us, though, is the illumination cast not on science but on our prospects for our own self-correction as individuals. Those prospects stand out clearest against a simplified model of scientific method.

What is self-corrected in science are full beliefs, which is a link to chapter 10's argument for the compatibility of full belief and doubt. Indeed, without chapter 10's belief/confidence distinction, simple reasoning implies that self-criticism of a belief is not possible. Isaac Levi writes, "Contraction [removal of a belief from one's corpus] occurs when X concludes that some item in his corpus ought to be subjected to critical scrutiny and test and should, *therefore,* cease being an assumption or evidence and should become, instead, a hypothesis" (1980: 25–26; similarly, see Katzoff 2000). I emphasize the "therefore," which is natural to unpack as resting on the conditional: If we have reason to subject an item to critical scrutiny, then we have reason to doubt that item and must suspend judgment on it. If a reason to be self-critical of a particular belief thereby undermines it, then, of course, justified self-criticism of it, as a belief, is precluded. The framework I offer to interpret the examples rejects the presupposition that any reason to critically reflect on a belief is thereby a reason that undermines it.

In keeping with our orientation, the examples in chapter 10 focused mainly on everyday belief, but the same points apply in science, which is Levi's chief concern. The discovery of an *anomaly* to an accepted theory is the discovery of a prima facie falsification. Research is then directed to decide whether the falsification is genuine. The theory is not surrendered with the doubt cast, however, but only with establishing that the anomaly cannot be explained away.

In chapter 6, we observed a number of routine ways that our ordinary methods of believing are self-corrective. Use of our beliefs can generate opportunities for detecting failures through conflict with the findings of basic reliable processes like perception, testimony, or simple reasoning. To take a trite example: you fully believe that your friend Bill is in Alaska. But you see someone who looks just like Bill drive by, wave to you, and call your name. You immediately surrender your belief.

What is requisite for routine self-correction is that the processes on which it depends, like perception or testimony, work in good part *independently* of the beliefs that they correct. In the previous example, the results of your use of perception is the judgment that Bill is driving. You do not decide that your perception should not be relied on because its output is in conflict with your belief. You are compelled, rather, to accept the findings of perception. The independence has limitations, and there are, of course, cases in which belief corrects perception (e.g., we judge the stick that looks bent in water is really straight), as well as memory and testimony (e.g., your belief that used-car salesmen are untrustworthy). But these complicated cases should not obscure the manifest ways that the output of our perceptual mechanisms or the reports of our informants are not subject to evaluation by the beliefs that they may challenge.

We display our endorsement of this independence in deliberative settings. When we argue with someone else we *bracket* the beliefs of ours under dispute. To bracket a belief is not to invoke it as a basis to judge further claims. Bracketing, unlike suspension of judgment, is a genuine action or activity, something we can do willfully.[3] If I believe that the library is open this Monday, and my wife disagrees, she may point out that the library is open only when the school is and that the school is closed this Monday for a holiday. I cannot reject her argument by claiming that if she is correct, then the library is not open this Monday, and that is incompatible with the fact that the library is open on Monday. Without bracketing, we could not hope to learn—to open ourselves to self-correction—through critical discussion and argument.

For these routine self-corrective processes to confer their enormous advantages, they need to operate, as in science, not only independently, but without the burden of systematic and purposeful checks on our beliefs. Routine self-correction takes place as a mere by-product of the use of our beliefs to guide actions. In the routine cases, we easily detect failures, both that the action failed and that the culprit is a particular belief. But no deliberate and ongoing system of self-checks is feasible, as will become vividly clear below, especially in section 2. We cannot divide our consciousness (and bodies) to both act on our beliefs in rapidly changing environments, and to check up on them.

However, as already indicated, we can rely on effortless and routine devices of self-correction to a much more limited extent than in science. Most obviously, many of the beliefs that we care to correct do not have sharp or clear falsification conditions.

As individuals, and even as members of social communities, we cannot nearly match the capabilities of scientific communities, whose shared goals are to discover, establish, and unify important truths about the world.

Social communities are not formed based on a concentrated interest, let alone a professional interest, in explaining phenomena and testing proposed explanations.

Inquiries are threatened with distortion due to the biases of investigators. Science succeeds fairly well at neutralizing biases in efficient, indirect ways: by welcoming a diversity of investigators, by its insistence on exact and publicly reported methods of testing, and by competition in discovery. This indirect neutralization obviates the need for investigators to purify their motives. They are permitted to care and invest more in their favored hypotheses and to pursue research with an eye toward rewards for discoveries. In fact, purification of motives would actually impede scientific progress, since it would diminish competition.[4]

Outside science and other institutional settings, however, we cannot expect to easily neutralize our own biases, some of the most forceful of which are likely to be common in our social communities (Janis 1972). An effort to set aside our biases, so that we display no preferences for our own views, would undermine motivation to inquire. As noted earlier, we will be less likely to keep our opinions open for modification if we cannot allow them to guide our everyday studies. If a political conservative is obliged to increase his exposure to the "liberal press," which he detests, for the sake of immersion in an alternative point of view, there is a good chance that he will just cut down on his political reading. We cannot aspire to science's effortless means of neutralizing biases without dampening the motive to inquire.

Actually, I have so far understated the efficiency of science's ability to neutralize biases. Given that the neutralization is a by-product of the workings of scientific method, there is no need to even recognize or identify biases. However, as we discuss starting in section 4 below, one of the great barriers to our weakening the influence of biases on ourselves is just to recognize them. They work best only when they are not perceived either as operative or as biases.

These reasons for why we can less avail ourselves of routine self-corrective methods than science are the more urgent because we acquire our beliefs according to standards and tests far less exacting than science. Given the constraints on us to form full beliefs, as discussed in chapter 8, many of our forefront, rather than background, beliefs are formed without anything like the rigorous testing of science. From brief observation and interactions with someone at casual social gatherings, we will often form far-reaching judgments of character or personality.[5] These ordinary and rapidly formed judgments, and many others like them, are fraught with high risk of error. Yet, we cannot hope to check on them merely as a by-product of our regular activities.

The urgency arises, however, not primarily from this greater liability of error, but from its costs. To a large extent, science can afford to be Popperian in freely seeking to falsify hypotheses and so detect errors as a goal in itself. But when we falsify our beliefs through everyday activities, we fail to achieve the goals of these activities. It is rare that the aim of our activities is just to test our beliefs. We go to the beach to enjoy the ocean, not to test out the accuracy of the weather reports. Consequently, those failures are, to varying degrees, serious or costly.

2   Artificial Self-Correction

These motives for self-correction beyond that of scientific method apply to manufacturing as well. We can look to the latter for another model of self-correction. In order to exploit this comparison, however, we will assume that the manufacturer's operation is overall good, though it still produces too many defective "widgets." Like us as individuals, manufacturers cannot just wait on the use of their products to ferret out the defective ones. The costs of learning from experience are high. The manufacturer does not want to learn of defects by way of the complaints of his customers.

As a safeguard, the manufacturer might impose an explicit quality-control rule or policy to be applied subsequent to the completion of the manufacturing process:

Every sixth widget is to be checked.

The proposed policy is triggered by an overtly arbitrary but determinate sign. The selection of a widget to be examined does not require the detection of any defect in it. We seek the same for the vulnerable beliefs to which our natural forms of self-control are inadequate: We want to pick them out by a property that is readily detected, yet which does not require us to determine that the belief is defective and so warrants rechecking.

That said, there really can only be a very limited role for an analogous explicit policy to check on our beliefs. Even for manufacturing, the proposed policy is crude. It is introduced mainly for expository purposes—to serve as a contrast. One problem for it as a model is that whereas the manufacturer produces only a single or a few kinds of widgets, the beliefs we want controlled are much more numerous, even when categorized. So we would need to impose a substantial number of rules or policies to achieve an equivalent level of safeguarding, and thus we would need a means, to select which rule to apply. This problem is the more severe if the rule worked like the quality-control policy—the worker complies with it explicitly. For us, however, and aside from the burden on memory, regular checks as to whether a rule applied to a belief would impede the flow from belief to action.

But there is a further obstacle. When a worker applies the widget policy, he checks for defects in that particular widget, regardless of his own judgment of its quality. He is externally compelled to check by the demands of his job. But how does and why should one turn over a belief to uncover defects, when one does believe it? There is little difficulty with the how or why if there is an available, independent source for checking, as when I check on a subway route by consulting the handy maps. But in the absence of a readily available checking mechanism, what is to sustain the effort to examine a belief, or set of beliefs, that one continues to accept?

3   The "Each, But Some Not" or "Fallibility" Structure

The obstacles just discussed ultimately derive from the underlying structure that motivates imposing mechanisms of self-control or self-correction, and to which we now turn. The structure I will refer to as an *each, but some not* or *fallibility* structure. Each object has a certain property, but at least one does not, though not all do not and typically, as in the cases that concern us, only a tiny fraction do not. More carefully, to remove the obvious inconsistency, we have *reason* to believe that each object has a certain property, but we are convinced that some (few) do not. Applied to our beliefs, the structure is realized as follows:

For *each* belief, we fully believe it and take ourselves to have adequate reasons of its truth. But *some* of our beliefs or the argument for them are wrong, though *not all*.[6]

The structure explains why we seek self-correction, instead of just improvement on the basic methods or procedures of belief formation, which work well. The defects and errors are comparatively few, and since these basic methods and procedures have themselves been subject to long-standing opportunities to uncover weaknesses, we can presume that there are no real, nearly as efficient alternatives. So the more accurate but cumbersome way to express our fallibility structure is this: "each . . . are, but some . . . are not, though actually very few are not, though still too many."

Whether in its abbreviated or its cumbersome form, the structure embeds a tension. There is the old tension of maintaining that we have knowledge, and yet we are fallible—since the former appears to exclude the possibility of error that the latter endorses. This tension has been handled by others and we addressed it, in part, earlier (chapter 10). We will address it further here only indirectly through addressing the more pertinent tension, which concerns how we represent constraints on our judgments from the "each" side as a result of reflection from the "but some not" side.

This tension has been on the tip of our tongues in chapters 7, 8 and 10. The tension is sharpest in the Preface Paradox (it's probable that some statements in a complex book are mistaken, but not all; yet, for each one the author is justified in asserting it). But the structure applies in other domains. If you are a devoted political partisan (e.g., a liberal) with a healthy sense of humility, you may reject each of the opposition's (e.g., conservatives) legislative proposals, and yet hope that some few of them succeed. The hope expresses your commitment to the democratic value of a plurality of contending positions. But, more relevantly to us, the hope also reveals an interest in maintaining a self-corrective check on your own position. You know that while your position is informing your political judgments you will regard its implications as correct, even when they are not and detectably so.

A neighbor of the fallibility structure figured prominently in chapter 8's account of how certain central belief practices like assertion constrain us to form full beliefs, yet without recognition. We can have great flexibility in particular instances of a practice to violate its implicit rules, yet hardly any flexibility to violate it regularly. As hearers, we often do not follow the default rule that dictates acceptance of a speaker's assertion unless we have special reason to object. We can, privately, just ignore the speaker's assertion or accept it only tentatively. But even if this withdrawal from the rule and the practice is available in any particular case ("each"), it does not follow, and it is not true, that we can opt out in any general way ("but some not").

The fallibility structure helped explain the category of negative clues from chapter 10. In example (1) of that chapter, Kate's denial that your proof works counts against your belief that it does. Now you can dismiss Kate's denial as simply mistaken, given your proof. But you know that you could do this for *each* of your proofs, yet *some* of them will be erroneous. Since you care to know which, and since you can only reconsider a select few, you become sensitive to clues as to which ones are more suspect. The mere fact that you learn of Kate's dissent is not alone significant, even granted that she is considerably better in logic; for a certain range of dissent is always expected on these matters, and you have no evidence that Kate's dissent falls outside this range. Perhaps most other good students in logic would agree that your proof works. Instead of the burdensome effort to determine if her dissent is specially significant, you adopt the cautious, self-corrective policy of allowing certain dissents, like Kate's, to stimulate you to doubt your belief. So long as you do not take these doubts to constitute undermining evidence, you do not violate the concept of belief (specifically, to withdraw a belief only if you have specific reason of its failure or the argument for it).

The reasoning just presented reflects the tension inherent in the fallibility structure. Since full belief enters strong claims and constitutes our understanding of what those beliefs are about, we need to impose mechanisms for checking on them. But these mechanisms need to operate outside of the attentional space occupied by those beliefs in their normal workings. The uncomfortable resolution is to have a system of checks shadowing our beliefs, which is, in effect, to hedge our bets.

4 Meno's Paradox–like Problems

What is particularly troubling in the tension generated by the fallibility structure is that it arises within only one side. The normal workings of belief is to "blind" us to what might be described from the outside as clues to the contrary. The absence of any tension is the real bite of the "each" side of the problem. In an earlier example, when the car drives by we would normally not even notice the driver as Bill, unless, as in that example, it is thrust in our face. The "blindness" problem is deep because to solve it, we cannot just attempt to remove the blinders, since they are a facet of the good workings of belief (i.e., transparently).

The problem is a variant of the "Paradox of Inquiry" from Plato's *Meno* (80d–e): How can we see (detect, recognize) what we do not see, since, trivially, we do not know that we are not seeing it? How can I recognize that I have, for example, misspelled "Wilfrid" as "Wilfred"? If I suspected my spelling of being incorrect, I wouldn't have offered it; and if I do not suspect it, I can hardly recognize that it needs examination, let alone correction.

Here's a more developed, but still everyday, example that extends an earlier suggestion: On the New York City subways, I believed that the Grand Army Plaza stop was an express stop. Sensing that I had been riding too long, I checked the map only to discover that I had passed Grand Army Plaza, which was not an express, but a local, station. You might say to me, as I said to myself, "Dummy! Why didn't you look at the stations as you passed them or check the map earlier, rather than waiting for the announcement?" This way of posing the objection presumes that I neglected to check and so knew that I ought to check. But the problem is not neglect, but "blindness"—I did not know that I needed to check on my belief, by attending to the stations passed or to the map, by virtue of my believing itself. Since I had no clue to question that Grand Army Plaza was an express stop on my line, I had no reason to even attend to that belief, let alone check on it.[7]

We have already brushed up against Meno's Paradox–like problems, although without acknowledgement. In chapter 3, I recommended deductive reasoning as a way to force presuppositions to become explicit. Charles II's question "Why does a fish dead weigh more than that fish if alive?" presupposes that the dead fish does weigh more. The recommendation is to bring this presupposition out explicitly by deduction and, thereby, redirect focus to the presupposed "fact." However, if the recommendation is to make the deduction only when needed, since one can not just generate deductions, the Meno's Paradox objection surfaces: Either I have reason to perform the deduction or not. If not, then merely performing endless deductions does not help except by accident. With no clues to work with, I will not identify that consequence to which I should attend. But if I do have reason to perform a specific deduction, it will be because I recognize a suspect presupposition. In that case, the very recognition eliminates the need for the simple deduction or the rule to perform it.[8]

The psychological studies that I've alluded to a number of times provide interesting illustrations of the paradox in question. In the *conjunction studies,* subjects are given the following biographical sketch: "Linda is 31 years old, single, outspoken and very bright. She majored in philosophy.

As a student, she was deeply concerned with issues of discrimination and social justice, and also participated in anti-nuclear demonstrations" (Tversky and Kahneman 1983). They are then asked to rate the probability of various alternatives among which are "Linda is a bank-teller" and "Linda is a bank-teller and a feminist." The finding is that most subjects answer that "Linda is a bank-teller and a feminist" is more probable. The finding is striking because to be both a bank-teller and a feminist one must be a bank-teller, and thus the choice "Linda is a bank-teller" cannot be less probable than that "Linda is a bank-teller and a feminist." And this principle extends from one we all learn as young children—if A is a (proper) subset of B, then there cannot be more of A than of B.

Subjects judge Linda as a feminist and bank-teller more probable because her biographical sketch fits the stereotype of a feminist more than a bank-teller. But the subjects do not select this answer over the formal solution (Margolis 1987: chap. 8). They just do not see these alternatives in the pattern of "A" to "A and B," that is, under the relation of "is a deductive consequence of" or "is a proper subset of."

These and related psychological studies are sometimes misrepresented because subjects are viewed as favoring one analysis over another (the experimenter's). But the real problem is that subjects do not even attend to the latter analysis. However, since the failings are in subject matter domains, especially probability and statistics, we are entitled to cautious optimism of educational improvement through teaching. With practice, deductive relations become salient, and so subjects are cued to break from their dominant assumptions and modes of reasoning. But in related studies the "not seeing" problem does not lend itself to reduction through teaching since the fallacious reasoning is not restricted to some formal method (probability, logic, statistics).

The *belief-perseverance* studies show that persons will hold on to a belief, even if the reasons that generate it are discredited. So, for example, you might be informed by experimenters that you scored high in detecting genuine versus fraudulent suicide notes. You come to believe it. But then the experimenters inform you, backed by a variety of evidence, that the scores you received were, in fact, randomly assigned. You actually showed no marked talent for suicide-note detection. Subsequently, however, you continue to form judgments that imply that you still regard yourself as a good suicide-note detector (Ross, Lepper, and Hubbard 1975; Ross and Anderson 1982; Goldman, 1986: section 10.4).

The "not seeing" problem here is crucial: subjects experience no conflict in dismissing the experimenters' "debriefing" because they do not recognize that their judgment depended on the source discredited. Unsurprisingly, the immediate presumption that belief-perseverance is a flaw in our reasoning has been disputed, though the objection is distinctive to this particular kind of perseverance. The objection does not apply across the board to the wide range of studies, which allege to expose flaws in our reasoning.

Gilbert Harman (1986) claims that subjects lose track of the reasons for why they formed their beliefs (the scores reported to them), and that they should. When the experimenters provide evidence that the scores were phony, subjects dismiss it as irrelevant. Characteristically, they will report something to the effect that they have always known that they were good at detecting genuine expressions of extreme depression from "mere" cries for help. Consequently, the claimed fraudulence of the test scores is dismissed as irrelevant.

No analogue of the belief-perseverance problem arises for our widget manufacturer. Any defect in a widget is traceable back to a defect in the process by which it is created, and the workings of that process are manifest. But there are a number of potential sources for why we might hold a belief, and within each source a huge number of potential routes.

Although Harman's account of why we should lose track of our beliefs is persuasive, it does not follow that belief-perseverance should be endorsed. We rightly resist it further than the point at which we accept positive evidence that our reasons are mistaken. The belief-perseverance phenomena may be initiated by the loss of one's reasons, but that loss alone is not sufficient for it. Subjects reject the discrediting information because they take their belief not to be dependent on the information discredited, even if by confabulation. Given that confabulated account, they just do not "see" the discrediting information as relevant. This observation is supported by the main body of experimental studies that characteristically concern judgments about oneself. These are judgments for which subjects are bound to have extensive, further beliefs and so strong motivation to preserve coherence and self-understanding.

To take the belief-perseverance studies as having no critical import is to attend to only the "each" side of the fallibility structure. We are ignoring efforts toward self-correction that can be motivated from the "but some not" side. Think of the ordinary devices that serve self-corrective ends, even if unintended: wide reading and listening to a variety of media, discussion with peers without prior certification of their views, and just sensitivity to failed expectations. By these ordinary means, we increase the chances of coming across discreditation of our reasons. We weaken the import of our tendency to belief-perseverance without strain on our need to economize (by losing track of our reasons). These self-corrective mechanisms work, and can be given more prominence, without flouting Harman's strictures. Their operation does not require a prior identification of the belief that is to be corrected. They thereby circumvent the Meno's Paradox "not seeing" problem. These mechanisms induce opportunities to expose evidence of flaws in reasoning leading to a belief without a prior selection of the belief as likely defective. Consequently, these devices of self-control need not interfere with the smooth workings of belief to blind us to many potential discreditations.

5   Everyday Self-Corrective Impositions

To develop the whiff of optimism that concluded the previous section, I'll use as reference point a domain in which we readily impose self-corrective checks—buying a car. I assume that we are willing to make firm judgments here, and so to hold full beliefs, for example, that the Camry is the better buy than the Subaru. Nevertheless, we check on our judgments, particularly by consulting authorities or experts. How are we to understand this form of self-correction within the fallibility structure?

We do not consult the assessment of expensive products in trustworthy publications like *Consumer Reports* merely as an informational source or for its entertainment value. In domains where the cost of error is significantly lower, for example, purchasing socks or cans of tuna fish, we leave freer rein to whimsy, bias, arbitrariness, habit, and indulgence.

In reasoning from the "but some not" side to the imposition of self-corrective controls, we first need to recognize a certain set of beliefs as in need of controls. These beliefs are too important and prone to error to be tolerated. This first step is important theoretically, not just practically. It shows the workings of *detachment* from our own beliefs. Detachment provides the opportunity for a critical perspective on our beliefs from within any one of which ("each") no such criticism seems appropriate.

Detachment, however, also gives rise to a tension between different levels or perspectives on our beliefs that is an instance of a general philosophical tension.[9] The "each" perspective is a distributive one that is about the objects of belief, and it expresses our internal or participant understanding. The "but some not" side is a collective perspective, understanding our beliefs as a class. When we claim "but some not," we are not claiming this of any specific belief. If we were to do so, we would simply have a qualification, and withdrawal, on the "each" side. What collects these disparate contents is just their being one's belief or one's beliefs of a certain kind (e.g., beliefs about the quality of cars). This perspective or level is a *second-order* one. We view our beliefs as what we believe, and not simply the propositions believed. We view them externally, bracketing our reasons for them.

Clearly, to take the external or detached view does not require any special reflective abilities or dispositions. It is part of our everyday practices, however varied the role accorded to detachment by different individuals. Think of confronting arguments, such as those of Peter Singer, for vegetarianism or extreme obligations to assist those suffering from poverty. What is in the forefront of the confrontation is whether the arguments work. But what is going on simultaneously, though well out of focus, will last, even if you come to reject the arguments. Beliefs that you took for granted are challenged in forceful and simple ways. The confrontation reinforces the value of engaging with disparate views as a form of self-control.

6   A Conundrum of Self-Criticism

In taking the next step to improve on a suspect category of beliefs through self-corrective means, we are assuming that routine forms of self-correction will be inadequate. These beliefs lack clear falsification conditions or it is of special importance that we be correct. But the Meno's Paradox–like "not seeing" problem remains. When biases operate well they not only distort one's evaluations; they obscure their workings on one.

It is not enough, then, to impose independently operating mechanisms of self-correction, as with turning to expert self-help books or to *Consumer Reports*. I must also grant independence in the admission of the findings of these mechanisms. They will not provide self-corrections to my own judgment, or not as effectively, if I retain command of whether to believe those findings. In fact, there is little difficulty in this case with *ceding control*. Anyone who turns to *Consumer Reports* is hardly going to position himself to censor its findings. But, in other cases, where expertise is not so clear-cut or available, there is a serious difficulty, and even a *conundrum*.

We glimpse the conundrum in the remark of a researcher subsequent to presenting studies that show that personal interviews are distorting as a basis for evaluating clients or applicants. The researcher commented (ironically, I suppose) that we can, nevertheless, rely on his interviewing skills because it just so happens that he is very good at it.[10] The conundrum is sharper in conflicts of interest reflections, as when a mother coaches her son's baseball team and worries that she is favoring him (or disfavoring him, as an overreaction to the former worry). In more detail:

> My son ought to bat third because he is the team's best hitter. But batting third is the favored position, and since he's my son maybe I was biased in determining that he is best. After all, it required lots of judgments of my own. But if I was favoring him, it will show up as an error in my detailed evaluation, which I can recheck. However, since I know in advance the import of alterations in the evaluations for my son's batting position, how do I know that in looking over that evaluation the same favoritism will not be operative? But I cannot just refrain from judging or handing this over to someone else, since making these judgments is the competence I claim in serving as coach. So I will just have to check very carefully on my evaluation. But what if. . . .

Of course, we end such thoughts not with resolution, but with confidence or trust in our own fairness, moderated by the humility of an extra check or two and a tolerance for uncertainty. To check on one's judgment is normally to strengthen it. The error, treated in chapter 10, is to confuse strengthening confidence that one made the right judgment with adding a new reason on behalf of that judgment. If honest reassessment does not find flaws, then it approaches mere skeptical neurosis to continue to ask whether one might have erred. But this is not a resolution of the line of thought, which has a characteristic self-referential pattern that precludes perfect resolution. One's reason to incorporate assessment of oneself as judger into the judgment is itself a ground to doubt oneself as a judger (of that very judgment).

The conundrum retains bite even as a practical matter because it is often infeasible or imprudent to impose a self-corrective rechecking mechanism. That is why realistic rules against conflicts of interest recommend that, if feasible, one remove oneself from the position of authority altogether, even when there is only the appearance of conflicts of interest. Usually, the purpose of this overreaction is taken as a social or public one—to keep up appearances. One should remove oneself from a position of authority that will cast suspicions on the fairness of the institution, even if those suspicions are unfounded. But we now realize that the extreme advice to exclude even the appearance of conflicts of interest is directed not, or not solely, to others, as usually suggested, but to oneself. The advice is to remove oneself as a judge of whether one is caught up in a conflict of interest. (A similar rationale can then be offered for the business ethics motto, "If you have to ask, it's unethical," or better, "If you have to ask, don't do it.")

7 Ceding Control and Meta-Fallibility Conundrums

In recognition of a version of the problem at the center of the conundrum Aristotle recommends overreaction, as well as ceding control:

> We must also examine what we ourselves drift into easily. For different people have different natural tendencies toward different goals, and we shall come to know our own tendencies from the pleasure or pain that arises in us. We must drag ourselves off in the contrary direction; for if we pull far away from error, as they do in straightening bent wood, we shall reach the intermediate condition.
>
> And in everything we must beware above all of pleasure and its sources; for we are already biased in its favour when we come to judge it. Hence we must react to it as the elders reacted to Helen, and on each occasion repeat what they said; for if we do this, and send it off, we shall be less in error. (Aristotle 1985: 1109b2–11).[11]

The insight in Aristotle's recommendation is to reject the seemingly sensible advice that you should ignore a consideration only if you know that there is nothing to be said for it. The insight is that typically to know that there is nothing to be said for a consideration requires examining it. But given our own foibles or weaknesses that very examination may distort our judgments. As a consequence, it may be a wiser policy to ignore considerations in advance, even though that sometimes means ignoring relevant considerations. Nevertheless, when it comes to our beliefs, we cannot comply with Aristotle's recommendation. We cannot just send away our own beliefs without specific evidence of a failure.

Perhaps, though, we can adopt something like Ulysses' clever strategy when faced with a problem akin to the one that worries Aristotle, yet without the radical solution that Aristotle proposes. When his ship approaches the island of the dangerous Sirens, Ulysses has his men bind him to the mast and stuff their ears, so that they cannot hear his commands. By ceding control, he manages to hear the beautiful song of the Sirens, but evade the danger.

Ulysses nullifies in advance his future judgments (Elster 1984: chap. II). But he does so not through a mechanism by which his future judgments are evaluated and dispreferred, but one through which they cannot be heard. The option is only narrowly open to us, since the beliefs that we would need to cede control of are already our own. Ulysses can not play the roles of both commander and sailor. If I recognize that I detest Albert, and then I am asked about how good a tennis player he is, where I have a quite definite low opinion, I cannot wholly defer to the fair-minded Oscar. For although his word can lead me try to reexamine my evidence, his word alone, even given my greater faith in it than my own, cannot simply make it the case that I do see my evidence differently.

Even if we could comply with Aristotle's final recommendation as applied to belief, it would be unwise to do so. Unless many of us on occasion refuse to defer to authorities, say about purchasing cars, there will be few constraints on their judgment, lessening the pressure on them to be accurate. Also, we would undermine our own autonomy and the development of our critical faculties. Except in isolated areas, we should not impose self-corrective devices where we wholly cede control of both the operation of these devices and the acceptance of their findings. Better to live with the conundrum, and attempt only to diminish its force, than to try to fully resolve it. Indeed, to claim to fully resolve the conundrum, as a response to it, would require a confidence in one's judgment that the conundrum itself casts under suspicion.

We now, in fact, have a kind of meta-fallibilist argument about ceding control as a way out of the conundrum. The fallibilist structure leads to the imposition of control by way of, for example, deferring to authorities. The meta-version concludes that I ought not always or completely so defer, since then I would lose autonomy.

To review: At an initial stage of reflection on the "but some not" part of the structure, I recognize the inferiority of my judgments to various experts. So I find adequate reason to defer. This control is applied to "each" of a range of judgments from the "but some not" perspective. But then this control now itself provides an "each" side to a new structure, which is itself subject to correction from the "but some not" side. I am directed to institute a control on my corrective to overcome my own judgment that someone else, the local "guru" or authority, is more competent.

The meta-fallibilist reasoning nicely applies to the example of buying the car. If I attempt to impose the control of following the dictates of *Con-*

sumer Reports, I am binding my own whims, fancies, and inclinations. In each case of buying an expensive product, there is good reason to impose the control. But should it happen that the verdict of *Consumer Reports* is usually contrary to my tastes, I ought to impose a further control on my prior one ("but some not") that allows for the occasional carefree indulgence. Our lives would be monotonous if we followed Aristotle's advice to always "send off" the Helens that enter them. A self-control on our beliefs that called on us to always defer to *Consumer Reports* would turn off our critical faculties across a wide range of judgments.

There is no limit to the level to which the meta-fallibilist reasoning applies. At each level to which an argument for a controlling device applies we impose a further device to realize a higher-level call for corrections, which will take the form of exceptions that themselves will require exceptions, if we ascend to another level. However, although further iterated meta-fallibilist arguments are possible, they are not compelled. There is no regress, since there is no mandate that the completion of an argument at any one level requires that one impose a further control from the "but some not" side at a higher level.

Even without a regress, though, the possibility, and frequent actuality, of fallibilist and meta-fallibilist conundrums capture the perplexity of first-person arguments for epistemic self-control. I participate in a practice in which I must form judgments, while also needing to judge whether those judgments are well formed, and when, if they are not, it reflects back on my abilities to judge.

My response is to defend what we can refer to as "uneven" policies of self-control. These are themselves susceptible to further controls. In accord with the fallibility structure, these uneven policies do not enforce a visible consistency of response. So acting on these policies runs the risk of misconstrual. For buying a car, a refrigerator, a canoe, or a TV, I swear by *Consumer Reports.* But then I ignore it when purchasing the Infinity stereo system, and so give the appearance of practical inconsistency.[12]

A greater danger is the oft-noted one that rules or policies with latitude for exceptions risk defeating themselves. Familiar examples, though outside of the domain of the ethics of belief, are diet plans. You decide not to eat sweets after lunch, but only dinner, and then you allow yourself to do it just this once, since it will hardly make any difference.[13] Pretty soon, for many dieters, the exceptions ruin the diet altogether. The "but some not" appeal to pleasure that applies to "each" lunch is itself not subject to any higher control.

If the uneven policies that I have suggested as appropriate to epistemic self-controls escape the danger of erosion, however, they promise two major benefits or strengths. First, they reduce the "strains of commitment" (Rawls 1971, sections 25 and 29). It is easier to stick to self-controls that allow for the spontaneous indulgence. Second, these complex policies— ones that incorporate deviations or exceptions—are more resilient than simpler ones in confrontation with the occasional failure. If the authoritative self-help manuals that I consult give me bad advice, which I so recognize, then an uneven policy of deference to those manuals will lead to a more balanced response than a policy that completely defers and wholly cedes controls. With the uneven policies, the occasional failure is anticipated, and so it can be accepted with equanimity, since the advice is generally sound.

8   Fanaticism, Self-Control, and the Emotions

We impose, and listen to, epistemic self-controls because of anticipated weaknesses in belief or reasoning. Earlier, especially in chapter 6, we observed that our on-line reason will often have a skewed or limited grasp of its own resources. The weakness is one source of the everyday dilemma that is recalled by Dennett: "Surely the following has happened to you . . . : somebody corners me and proceeds to present me with an argument of great persuasiveness, of *irresistible* logic, step by step by step. I can think of nothing to say against any of the steps. I get to the conclusion, *but I don't believe it!* This can be a social problem. It is worse than unsatisfying to say: 'Sorry, I don't believe it, but I can't tell you why. I don't know' (Dennett 1978: 308). We sympathize with Dennett, not only in his discomfort at belief's refusal to be moved by argument,[14] but in the implied judgment that his refusal is well taken.

We can capture something of these dissonant sympathies within the fallibilist structure. Presuming we are competent to assess arguments we confront, we ought to endorse any conclusion whose premises we accept, if we also accept the cogency of the reasoning. But sometimes we will be wrongly persuaded, and where the matter is not trivial, we will need to resist both our own judgment that the argument is cogent and our commitment, as rational agents, to argument as a basis for belief. How can the resistance be discriminating, blocking only the arguments that should be blocked, and not impede our disposition to align our beliefs with the arguments we accept?

The resistance that we feel in Dennett-like situations presumably resides in our emotions and our background beliefs. It is not, as I am treating the case, one in which the person, whose argument Dennett is resisting, does not refuse to allow him more time to reflect. Dennett judges the argument cogent. Yet, there remains something fishy either about the reasoning or the conclusion. Our inability to articulate an objection explains our discomfort, since we know that we ought to be responsive to the force of argument. Yet, the resistance finds a rationale in our knowing that sometimes ("but not each") we will be wrongly persuaded by bad arguments. We want to impose, or accept the dictates of, a handy and discriminating overruling power. Our emotions and our background corpus of beliefs lend themselves to the task since they are stubborn when in conflict with on-line reason.

Our intelligent resistance to moving in lock-step with the course of arguments promotes as well a healthy social environment for learning. Arguments that we now regard in a broader perspective as specious were once taken as persuasive. During the "Lockner" era in the American judicial system, the libertarian argument that persons should be able to contract their own services free of any regulation was dominant. The argument went: If an adult wants to work an eighty-hour week that's his private business and that of his prospective employer only. The gut revulsion many felt at persons laboring extraordinarily long hours encouraged mounting political opposition that eventually won overwhelmingly in the forum of argument.

The danger of a dominant argument resides not only in the chances that it is fallacious, yet many believe and act on it. But, by virtue of its popularity, pressure is exerted toward extending its dominance. We all have reason to defer to it as representing a greater collective intelligence than our own. The resistance we are now applauding represents a meta-fallibilist argument against uniform deference—a self-control on the self-control of deference.

Without the meta-fallibilist resistance, the way is open to *fanaticism* for all but those with perfect reason. The fanatic's thought, I argue, is characterized by resistance to detachment, and the consequent demands to impose independent controls. I offer this account as a way of unpacking the comment we want to make to the fanatic that he should take seriously that he might be mistaken. The comment makes sense as implying that the fanatic has not imposed the required critical controls on his beliefs.

The account to be developed is meant to explain what puzzles us about fanaticism. Theoretically, the puzzle is how anyone sane can maintain those beliefs. Practically, we are puzzled, and frustrated, by the veneer of reason that the fanatic can sustain.

I will understand fanaticism as involving the long-term maintanence and pursuit of a view, and of actions in accord with it, that are well outside the wide bounds of accepted positions and values. The view is dismissed by many respected and diverse sources, which otherwise have no relevant shared ideology or interest. This characterization is intended only to fix us on a range of examples, and I am otherwise not invested in its accuracy.

Noticeably absent from the features just picked out is the claim that the fanatic's views are false. This is in keeping with the fallibility structure. We no doubt have good reason to reject each fanatical position and we will mostly be right to do so. But sometimes the fanatic will be correct, and accepted views wrong (perhaps, the Abolitionists provide an example).

In "The Conscience of Huckleberry Finn," Jonathan Bennett (1974) contrasts different perspectives on how conscience should be restrained by feeling, emotion, or sympathy. One perspective is that of the Nazi military leader Heinrich Himmler, who commanded his soldiers that when they were sickened and revolted at the killing of Jews, they should not hide from themselves their victims' anguish. Confrontation with their own hesitancy and ambivalence would help steel their conscience. Acting on that troubled conscience would keep them "decent" and make them "hard."

In using Himmler's advice to better understand fanaticism, I treat it as embedded in the context of his abhorrent, genocidal views. In other contexts, as an example below illustrates, the advice need not be revolting or even bad.

The feelings of revulsion and emotional distress are viewed by Himmler as sentimental obstacles. They are to be overcome without concession or mollification. Their value is exhausted by their role as an exercise in military character-building. So Himmler's recommendation is a rejection of an undemanding form of self-correction. Feelings of revulsion, guilt, or sympathy engage independently of conscience, and so can serve as a check on its judgments.

It would be a mistake, however, to report the benefits of the retarding force of our sympathies as emotion opposing reason. For whether the resistance will be accepted, or itself resisted on the ground that it is "merely" emotional or inarticulate, is itself a judgment of reason.[15] After all, control is not completely ceded, and we can confront situations where a meta-fallibilist argument overrules deference to emotion. Most feel revolted by the thought of harvesting dead human bodies for their parts. But, arguably, we ought to overcome, or steel ourselves to, such revulsion, if its source is superstition and if the harvesting will do enormously greater good (for transplants and research).

Himmler locates feelings and emotions as merely other sources of reasons, in conflict with conscience, and so to be overruled. He refuses to view them from a detached point of view as constituting a higher-order reason, that overrules his direct reasons to kill Jews without being weighed on the same scale with them. Of course, you might respond that he is not motivated to take the detached point of view, and so to impose independent controls. But, of course, this is to ignore a control we are all bound to impose. We should rethink a belief when it occasions a "gut" negative reaction and there is extensive dissent on it from numerous persons of otherwise respected and diverse views.

Why should the fanatic be open-minded to this dissent? Our response joins the emphasis here on everyday detachment and imposition of controls with our discussion of explicitness and commitment in chapter 3. When these are brought together the obvious critical judgment immediately surfaces: The fanatic is involved in incoherence since he is violating commitments he must make through his everyday activities. He can avoid exposing the incoherence, and so destabilizing his beliefs, only because of a lack of explicitness about those commitments. Himmler's claims display the high costs of error and likely intrusion of bias and prejudice by which, in other areas of his life, he would have to view his judgment in a detached way and impose self-corrective controls.

Of course, if pressed by this objection, the fanatic will respond that the case at hand is distinctive. But the response is inadequate unless it can overcome the controls we impose on ourselves to avoid the "special pleading" of judging one's favored case distinctive; for we know in advance that, like forceful biases, we will not recognize it as special pleading. (Of course, we also learn from the above meta-fallibilist conundrums that, on pain of quashing any opportunity to upset a "herd" mentality, we had better on occasion resist these controls, even though it will appear to us, if we are intellectually honest, as special pleading.)

The prima facie inconsistency in the accusation of special pleading is really an accusation of incoherence in the case at hand, since the conflicting beliefs and commitments are near the surface and from many directions. The costs of error are severe and the self-corrective controls easy to impose. Motivation to impose those controls is compelling in the varied range of potential counterevidence that must be ruled out. Relevant prior commitments are salient or manifest. These commitments in turn justify taking a detached perspective on one's beliefs from which the need for controls follows. The fanatic resists evident forms of control that he endorses, especially that of the dissent of others and often, as in the case of Himmler's soldiers, his own emotional reactions.

The second-order account I am developing is meant to address the above puzzles. Its practical value is limited to diagnosis. As emphasized in chapter 3, there is a wide gap between a diagnosis of incoherence and the person's taking it to heart or psyche. There is an even wider gap between the wrong of incoherence and the possible wrongs one can do in acting on it. More important, the second-order account does not imply, what is surely false, that Himmler otherwise had good evidence for his judgments, even by his own standards, let alone objectively.

But a purely first-order account will still not answer our puzzles, because they arise over the fanatic's stance under practical constraints, not within the relatively unconstrained space of pure research and scholarship. Even under practical constraints, the fanatic's position, being outrageous, should be easy to refute and hard to maintain, mental derangement aside. But neither holds.

However, my account may be questioned on a different matter of practicality. In relying on the example of Himmler, or, similarly, if I had focused on examples of terrorism, I may be thought to have shifted domains from belief to action. Although the belief/action distinction is of course real and methodologically fundamental, to adhere to it here would be deeply misleading. For the fanatic's willingness to act itself expresses the fanaticism of his beliefs.

The truism that needs to come under scrutiny is that you act on your beliefs, given your aims and desires. You want an egg-cream, and you come to learn that there is an ice cream parlor at the local shopping center, and straightaway you drive to it. But this case and the vast number of cases like it mask a further, implicit belief effecting action. Roughly, it is the belief that if opportunity arises, you should act on your first-order belief, or that it should be your will. Obviously, this meta-belief is a constant for our actions, so it normally does not appear to thought.

However, consider a case in which you are convinced that your child's friend, when he was in your home, pocketed the $10 that you left on the microwave. You did not catch him "redhanded," but the evidence is still compelling. Had you caught him red-handed you would have admonished him and spoken to his parents. However, now you do not. In either case, you have the full belief. What's the difference?

The answer recalls our discussion in chapter 10: The difference is one of diminished confidence, given the serious costs of error were one to act on the belief. In this case, the meta-belief gains salience, and you do not endorse it. You hesitate to act.

The belief-action truism holds, then, only generally. It is overridden when the costs of error are high or where the relevant beliefs are suspect. When an issue is of political or social urgency, integrity often calls on us to act on our beliefs. The appeal to integrity, however, acknowledges that the truism is overridable.

Because the fanatic attempts to operate under the belief-action truism, his actions express or exhibit his relevant fanatical views, since it is in just such circumstances that the truism is overruled. Our self-controls kick in to upset the smooth flow from belief to action, since on these occasions one's first-order judgments are noticeably likely to be ill based.

The self-controls that are especially germane to the case of fanaticism are those that are familiar and natural to us—the emotions, the views of authorities and diverse, respected peers, traditions of civility and mutual respect, and our background beliefs. Although I have spoken of the everyday controls as impositions or policies we adopt, they really serve naturally so long as we do not intervene on their independent operation and voice.

The fanatic does not merely refuse to impose controls on his judgment; he *withdraws* various natural forms of control. These are just the ways we are compelled to operate in forming and modifying our beliefs. You can rarely rely just on your own judgment about whether, for example, a house you want to purchase is free of carpenter-ants, and you will go badly wrong if you do so. Consequently, subjecting one's views to these controls is a common committment and a mutual expectation of discussion and argument.

Understanding fanaticism as a failure of epistemic self-control accords with the extremes of the fanatic's position. The fanatic is dismissive of a varied range of undermining evidence without suspicions about himself in that dismissal. This understanding of fanaticism as a failure of second-order belief-control also contributes toward explaining the practical puzzle stated earlier, as well as the theoretical puzzle, on which we have so far concentrated.

The second-order diagnosis involves the dual claims that the higher-order reasoning is ours and that it is easily overlooked. The only way to understand the phenomena of how our belief-practices work is to ascribe to ourselves a competence or grasp with such second-order reasoning. The examples above, such as the conflict of interest reasoning of the baseball coach, display reasoning with which we are familiar. But the reasoning is not itself typically a direct object of our thought or reflection. So we need not have the awareness of it as an abstract object of thought to be brought into the forefront of attention.

Reverting to the second-order level in critical discussion is a distraction from the focus of first-order inquiry on disputing the issues. Consider the fanatic's position in on-line argument, which brings us to the practical puzzle. On the "each" side of straightforward disagreement, the fanatic is difficult to argue with simply because his views and presuppositions are extreme. We lose footholds of shared agreement to test claims and theses. But because first-order argument—disagreeing about the issues—is the natural form of argument, a critic of the fanatic incurs the burden to justify greatly shifting the discussion to the personal and to the meta-levels. The Holocaust denier, for example, must reject the numerous historical documents by respected and diverse scholars. Outside scholarly journals the rejection cannot seriously be disputed. The nonexpert critic is not in a position to certify the validity of these documents. But he also does not want to leave it as an open question, as if to concede the fanatic's entitlement to withdraw these sources as somehow tainted just by virtue of his dissent. Rather, the critic's claim should be that in rejecting these sources the fanatic is violating meta-criteria as to what sources are legitimate, as well as meta-controls on one's dismissal of such sources.

In violating these meta-criteria and withdrawing the meta-controls, the fanatic effectively relieves us of the duty to assess the cogency of his arguments; just as when someone commits a fallacy, it preempts the arduous task of evaluating the truth of his premises. But, of course, since the fault occurs at the meta-level, the critic places himself in a difficult position to actually expose the faults. Aside from the critic's burden of shifting discussion away from the main issue, the critic has to articulate a meta-level of reasoning for critical controls. Even if the reasoning is articulated, the further task remains of explicitly representing the fanatic's incoherence. The latter requires that the critic also bring forth related commitments and claims of the fanatic, which will not be readily available on-line, as they are usually presented outside the current context of discussion.

My diagnosis of the stance of the fanatic and my response to the puzzles have been guided by the fallibility structure. It is a virtue of reliance on that structure that it provides a way to explain the difficulties of criticizing the fanatic without the least concession to his position. The sense that the fanatic's position is way off, and is yet the facade of reason by which he is able to maintain his position, makes sense of the frustration we feel. But the credibility that the position achieves merely by virtue of its sustainability is just a reflection of limits on our on-line efforts to articulate the fanatic's underlying reasoning and commitments.

9   Reasonableness

We contrast the fanatic with the reasonable person (in a domain) to bring out the extremes of unreason of the former. In imposing or tolerating self-controls, the reasonable person exhibits unremarkable humility, where *reasonableness* fits the very ordinary, if easily obscured, conception set out by Brand Blanshard: "What do we mean when we call a man reasonable? We mean at least this, that in his thinking and acting he shows objectivity of mind. And what is that? It means being realistic, impartial, just; seeing things as they are rather than as fear or desire or prejudice would tempt one to see them. The reasonable person will suit what he thinks and claims to the facts. He will be ready to give up an opinion in the face of inner and outer pressure if the facts require it" (1973: 130).

Blanshard goes on to list two conditions for reasonableness: "In the first place, there must be a set of independent facts to be grasped. . . . The second condition is that this common rule should at times control the course of our thought" (1973: 130). Similarly, Peirce finds the scientific method of inquiry an advance over the methods of authority, tenacity, or a priori reasoning, for its attunement to the world: "To satisfy our doubts, therefore, it is necessary that a method should be found by which our beliefs may be determined by nothing human, but by some external permanency . . ." (1957: 24).

In expressing reasonableness as responsiveness to the world and to evidence, Blanshard captures its unavoidability as an ideal and its *minimal* demands, so that not to be reasonable is to be unreasonable. By contrast, not to be rational, at least by cooperating in Prisoner's Dilemma situations, is not to be irrational. The minimal demands explain away two seemingly opposed ascriptions to it. On controversial matters, we often remark that it is a subject on which reasonable persons may disagree, thus embracing a pluralism. (In chapter 10, I so described the plurality of potential responses to a negative clue as reasonable.) Yet, in other attributions of reasonableness, we imply that only one judgment can be reasonable. Thus, when reasonableness is used in the law, as when we speak of what precautions a "reasonable man" would take in cases of alleged negligence, we imply that to not even recognize certain dangers is to be unreasonable.

The minimal demand of reasonableness reconciles these seemingly opposed outcomes. The reasonable person is one who responds to evidence and reasons without serious sacrifice in other parts of his life. Neither reason nor evidentialism demands that we drop everything to gain ever more certainty, and reasonableness in this regard is the analogue of basic decency or civility as minimal social and ethical demands. On controversial matters, the reasonable person will devote a certain amount of effort to discussion and argument to reach consensus, but he is not going to devote himself singularly to that effort. One is reasonable to stick by a judgment on a controversial issue, despite a plurality of conflicting views. However, in the law case, it requires little effort to recognize certain dangers (e.g., if one does not clear the ice from the pathway to one's house, it will be a danger to pedestrians), and so here the reasonable judgment, and probably also the correlative action, has no real alternative.[16]

Even given its minimal demands, deviations from reasonableness are unsurprising. Our reasons for a judgment both support it and deny the need to impose controls (the "each" side). Since the dictates of these self-controls are opposed to the judgment of on-line reason, to comply with them is to accept a diminished, and so discomforting, loss in self-understanding. Were a soldier of Himmler's to acquiesce to his emotional suffering, rather than openly defy it as Himmler recommends, he would puzzle himself and regard his inaction as weakness of will; for, at the time, he shares Himmler's principles and conscience. Correlative with the reasonable person's humility is his tolerance of diminished self-understanding.

Earlier, I noted an area in which we impose self-corrective controls—buying a car. Of course, the "we" here is many of us, and the real claim pivotal to the discussion of fanaticism is that all of us impose these controls in some related areas. As throughout this work, I emphasize the ordinariness of such examples not to appeal to popularity. Rather, the ordinariness provides evidence that the ethics of belief I have been defending is ours and that at its rudiments it issues in necessities. Given that belief requires responsivity to the facts, we are compelled to impose these controls, which restrain judgment influenced by our biases. Since, though, we are not compelled to impose any particular controls, we do not perceive them as necessities, as discussed in chapter 8.

The natural forms of control can keep us responsive to the facts because they are not highly susceptible to our intrusions. In chapter 2 I observed that we would not want any overall control of our beliefs, however much we would want it in particular cases. The control would render our beliefs sensitive to us, rather than to what those beliefs claim. Were epistemic self-controls as freely imposed as the manufacturer's widget policy, we could gain control of our beliefs through a back-door. Fortunately, however, we have comparatively little to say not only about the workings of these natural forms of self-control, but also about their operation . You cannot tell the expert what judgment he should reach within his area of expertise. Or, when you take stationery from the office for personal use you feel guilt, unless you have already intervened to weaken your moral character, and so it is not up to you to impose this control. These natural forms of self-control recommend themselves to us, then, not only for the wisdom they inherit, but because they are not freely subject to our manipulation.

The self-controls are justified to reason via our interest in the truth of our beliefs. The self-controls address anticipated weaknesses in reason, especially on-line. These weaknesses extend to the selection of self-controls themselves, and that is why we noted the meta-fallibilist arguments to restrain prior controls and that the policies to cede control ought to be uneven.

The controls are in a delicate balance. They must be independent of the judgments that they are to check on. Yet those checks appear to make claims in opposition to our judgments. So we have reason to reject them. This tension, I argued, is endemic to the fallibility structure. Correspondingly, there is typically no neat resolution of the tension, and there should not be. In the case of the fanatic, and in our discussion overall, I have emphasized, and criticized, resolutions that diminish the role of controls. However, the reasonable person is in danger of the opposed resolution. The danger is that he so subjects himself to controls that he bars himself from trusting his judgments, or putting forth, or acting on, his own views. He is under the glare of the fallibility structure without appreciating the meta-fallibilist check on it that generates the conundrum.

Despite the delicacy of judgment in determining where to cut off controls at a higher-level, reliance on mechanisms of self-correction is not supererogatory—a concern for greater certainty through a system of double checking. The goal is simply self-correction. The objective of imposing or tolerating the self-controls remains responsivity to what our judgments or beliefs claim. It is because the objective is so common and what it seeks so fundamental that I attribute the underlying reasoning widely, even though when stated abstractly, via levels and meta-levels, it sounds esoteric and of specialized interest. In restraining or controlling ourselves, we try to ensure that belief is determined by what is being judged, and the best way to ensure it is through following the evidence. Evidentialism offers, then, a very ordinary, but compelling, standard for our aspiration to be reasonable.

Notes

Introduction

1. It may be a common error to think of all practical or prudential reasons as nonepistemic. See Harman (1997).

2. For a related discussion, see Evans (1982): 224–235.

3. Some exceptions are to be found in chapters 6, 9, and 10. Also, sometimes I stretch ordinary usage. Since, for our purposes, what is central in the notions of evidence or epistemic reasons is that they indicate the truth of a proposition, I allow direct observation to count as evidence: e.g., its appearing to you visually that the light is on, I count as evidence that the light is on.

4. For forceful defense, see Stalnaker (1987).

5. Because I rely on conceptual implications, it may be thought that the framework is at variance with Quine's (1980) challenge to the analytic-synthetic distinction. I do not think that maintaining that a concept has a certain structure commits me to the view that some statements are true purely by virtue of meaning, but the issue is too complex for treatment here. However, I do try to show (in chaps. 1 and 8) that one can defend the understanding of belief presented here on grounds of function or role, and so centrality to our corpus of beliefs, which is a rationale palatable to Quineans.

6. Adler (1981). But I am also moved by recent challenges to the force of skeptical intuitions in Williams (1991), and in the contextualism of Cohen (1988), DeRose (1995), Lewis (1996), and Unger (1984), among others.

7. But not because skepticism does not cut deep. Intense discussion of skepticism in recent years has made it clear that any healthy skepticism must be radical, casting doubt on satisfaction of the most rudimentary epistemic notions like reasons. For critical overviews, from respectfully opposed perspectives, see Williams (1991) and Stroud (1984).

8. For forceful criticisms of the notion of conceptual scheme, see Davidson (1984): 183–198.

9. Among the problems in moving from this rough formulation to an exact one is the following: Lots of sentences are said but not asserted, as when embedded, e.g.,

"John believes that the number of stars is even." I assume that the basic point will go through, when the needed qualifications are entered.

10. This is the primary function to which Grice (1989) applied his account of conversational reasoning in regard to the confusion of pragmatics and semantics (or logic).

11. The importance of background beliefs in contemporary debates about knowledge is shown by Vogel (1990), and for its bearing on broader epistemological issues see Rorty (1979): chap. 6. For approaches to roughly this understanding, though deriving from considerations of language and intentionality, see Dennett (1987): essays 2–4; Davidson (1984); and Searle (1983): chap. 5.

12. Wolterstorff (1983): 142. See also his (1986), which begins with a persuasive definition of "evidentialism" via rationality (38–39).

Chapter 1

1. Clifford's ringing motto is often quoted: "it is wrong always, everywhere, and for anyone to believe anything upon insufficient evidence" (1999: 77). See also Blanshard (1974: 401).

2. Of patients suffering "Capgras delusion," who "claim that one or more of one's close relatives has been replaced by an exact replica or impostor" (Stone and Young 1997: 327), Stone and Young write: "the patients can be aware of the normative aspects of their belief claim; they realize that the belief is hard to understand and needs defending" (335). Surprisingly, in trying to explain away why those suffering from Capras delusion do not report the impostor to the police, Stone and Young deny the force of their observation: "We do not have to attribute to the patient any exotic projects to make this kind of action appropriate. For example, the deluded patient who acts in accordance with the delusion . . . will cause distress and may experience recriminations or the unwanted attentions of the medical profession. It is surely a perfectly understandable project for the deluded person to try to avoid these consequences" (353).

   Really? Put yourself in the place of deluded person. You are convinced that your spouse is an impostor. Do you allow your concern that people will think you loony to stop you from running to various authorities? Not at all. In not going to the police those suffering from Capras delusion ought not to be construed as surrounding their delusional belief with many ordinary ones that allow them to avoid the exposure, as Stone and Young contend. Rather, the inaction is part of the delusion; it is related evidence of the disturbance. See further chapter 3, section 7 below.

3. Nisbett and Wilson (1977).

4. As discussed later, in chap. 8, attending to and maintaining one's belief amounts to a commitment. Compare to van Fraassen's (1984) reading of "I believe that p."

5. For comprehensive discussion and references, see Sorensen (1988): chap. 1.

6. For defense (of the iteration and conjunction principles) with some qualifications, see Shoemaker (1996). In chap. 7 a related argument is offered, although without the iteration condition.

7. On a related point, see Marcus (1990).

8. There may be need for an explicit assumption that the "one" is a believer. See Velleman (2000): chap. 8.

9. It is telling that rarely does one find anyone who claims that his upbringing compelled him to hold a belief, which he rejects as false.

10. See Unger (1975): 260–265. For broader defense of the assertion-knowledge connection see Brandom (1994): part one, chap. 4, sections I–II; Austin (1970); and, especially, Williamson (1996).

11. A slight variation on Grice's (1989: 27) maxim of Quality.

12. See Dretske (1971) and Fogelin (1994): chaps. 1, 4, and 5. Cohen (1977) analyzes inductive support as a gradation of necessity.

13. On truth as the aim of belief, and much else of value, see Williams (1973). Two recent works developing this theme are Railton (1994) and Velleman (2000): chap. 11.

14. Peter Strawson's writes that "being reasonable" *means* that one proportion the degree of one's convictions to the strength of the evidence (1952: 257).

15. On the implied dual-view of probability, see Hacking (1975): chaps. 1–2 and Carnap (1962): chap. 2.

16. Compare with similar principles in Feldman and Conee (1985) and Williamson (1996).

17. More exactly, parenthetical uses of these qualifiers. See Urmson (1966).

18. Reid (1969), the anti-evidentialist hero, affirms that "In every case, the assent [to a conjecture] ought to be proportioned to the evidence; for to believe firmly, what has but a small degree of probability, is a manifest abuse of our understanding" (43). See too p. 290, though some of the passages are equivocal for our purposes.

19. See also p. 119. Alston identifies this view, which he favors, with James and Reid. A Reidian view is endorsed in a number of Plantinga's writings; most recently it is a main theme of his (1993). In other writings, Alston is more sympathetic to evidentialism. See the essays in parts II and III of his (1989); and especially his (1993): 129. Alston's default view should be contrasted with that of Harman (1986): chap. 5.

20. Contrast with Locke (1975): book IV, ch. 17, section 20.

21. A crucial claim of Plantinga (1983). Plantinga, although arguing that foundationalism is "self-refuting," endorses a kind of externalist foundationalism—some beliefs are "properly basic." The endorsement distances him from the view that there are "groundless" beliefs and brings him actually close to evidentialism. In later works, Plantinga (1986) considers the possibility of evidentialism resting on foundationalism's competitor coherentism. He even considers the evidentialist criticism to be of a "noetic defect" (111–112). But the incoherence he looks to, and does not find, depends on accepting a view (a further belief) incompatible with a non evidentialist one (127–128).

22. See Alston (1983) and (1989): "The Deontological Conception," and Plantinga (1983).

23. Compare with a major theme in Williams (1991), that the alleged intuitiveness of radical skepticism depends on imposing substantive assumptions on very innocent doctrines, such as the possibility of error in any knowledge claim, without noticing the imposition.

24. See the continuation of the opening quotation from Plantinga (1983), p.30.

25. Zemach (1997) argues that the attempt to evaluate believing for its practical utility leads to a (vicious) infinite regress.

26. In a critical work (already cited) to which I am indebted, Feldman and Conee (1985) are moved by such a practical "ought" and our finitary predicament to offer an emasculated version of evidentialism that lacks prescriptive force. See pp. 17–18; but see also p. 19.

27. Contrast the response of Pojman (1993) with that of both Code (1987) and Govier (1976).

28. But see Foley (1987).

29. Priest (1998, and elsewhere) defends the thesis that some contradictions are true, and so he would claim that he can believe them. I am addressing neither this position nor Priest's overall defense of paraconsistent logic. Even if correct, the central cases that he calls on in support are well-known paradoxes (the sorites, the semantic paradoxes) that are problematic in the extreme, independent of issues in the ethics of belief.

30. Unsurprisingly, I take the complementary view of other so-called epistemic virtues like *conservatism:* "The less rejection of prior beliefs required, the more plausible the hypotheses—other things being equal" (Quine and Ullian 1978: 67). Conservatism so understood is nonoptional. To favor a less conservative hypothesis is simply to deny the force of evidence, and so to undermine the individual's understanding of the world and his (evidential) basis for it. It is one thing to realize I made a mistake; it is another to hold that hypotheses are to be preferred in inquiry on grounds other than truth-indicating ones.

31. For other reasons to reject the dichotomy, see Harman (1986): chap. 1; Kim (1993); and De Sousa (1971).

32. Compare to Frege's judgment-stroke:

A judgment will always be expressed by means of the sign

⊢ ,

which stands to the left of the sign . . . indicating the content of the judgment. If we *omit* the small vertical stroke at the left end of the horizontal one, the judgment will be transformed in a *mere combination of ideas,* of which the writer does not state whether he acknowledges it to be true or not. (Frege 1967: 11)

33. There is dispute as to whether Meletus's admission before the court is a Platonic contrivance, particularly because the twin claims (of atheism and belief in new gods) are so manifestly contradictory. (It should, however, be recalled that Socrates does lead Meletus from his actual claim that Socrates believes in divine ac-

tivities to his believing in gods.) But it is enough for my purpose that something akin to the assertions and beliefs represented in this scenario are realistic, not whether they were real. Nevertheless, a lucid defense of a fairly literal reading of Socrates' arguments is mounted by Reeve (1989): section 2.2.

Chapter 2

1. On indirect control of belief formation, see Alston (1989), "The Deontological."

2. See the discussion of Nozick's "experience machine" in chap. 3 of this volume. See also Wiggins (1970).

3. What of the desirability of partial control? But if we control just some beliefs, how are we to select just the proper ones without reinserting the problem of responsivity to us, not the world? The difficulty here is an instance of the problem of (epistemic) self-control, treated in chap. 11.

4. For analysis, see the early pages of Bennett (1990).

5. Williams offers a second, related argument, but for our purposes it introduces nothing new. See Winters (1979) for an extended reconstruction of the argument. In her critique, she makes much of Williams's term "acquire." But it is used by him only to exclude other bases for the belief. The belief is acquired and sustained only by the act of will.

6. In reply to a descendant of Williams's argument (Scott-Kakures 1994), Radcliffe (1997) rightly distinguishes between my not believing myself justified and my believing myself not justified (as well as my being not justified). But, contrary to Radcliffe's assumptions, the former, weaker of these is adequate for the argument. A positive epistemic evaluation is requisite to acquiring a belief, not merely the absence of a negative one.

7. See Bennett (1990); Winters (1979); and Cook (1987). See also Velleman (1989): 128–129. However, Velleman (1989: chap. 4; 2000: chap. 11) recognizes that his self-fulfilling examples, although strictly counterexamples, do not dissent from the spirit of Williams's argument. See also Millgram 1997: chap. 2.

8. Ginet observes that it is not "in my power now to acquire, just by deciding, the *intention* to run over pedestrians with my car" (2001: 74). But the lack of "power" in the case of intention is psychological or empirical—an inability. It can be in someone else's power to run over pedestrians. But the corresponding lack of power for belief will be conceptual—an impossibility. It will not be in anyone's power to decide to believe (with the evidence available to us) that Abraham Lincoln's existence is myth.

9. Consider Spinoza's response to the Cartesian assumption that we can suspend judgment rather than assent to a belief, when we lack a clear and distinct perception (Descartes 1996: Meditation IV). For Spinoza, "suspension of judgment is really a perception, not free will" (Spinoza 1982: IIp49 Scholium; p. 99). For helpful commentary see Curley (1975); and Williams's (1978: 175–183) circumspect defense of Descartes.

10. See Dennett (1978): "How to Change Your Mind."

11. For general discussion, see Alston (1989): "The Deontological Conception . . ."

12. However, although we do *try* to be happy, less sense can be attached to trying to believe, for reasons prominent in section 1 above. Aside from this disanalogy, I agree with the substance of Stocker (1982).

13. For some qualification, see Adams (1985): 27.

14. Adams slightly overstates his case. He assumes that responsibility for a state (or attitude) implies blameworthiness for any defects in that state. However, although a person born in ancient times is responsible for his false belief that the sun revolves around the earth, he is not blameworthy. He could not believe otherwise, given the limits of his understanding and that available to him.

15. See Fischer (1994): 164. He takes this to be a condition of "guidance control" (roughly, freedom to act that does not require that one could do otherwise).

16. For expansion on this theme, see Petit and Smith (1996).

17. A related disanalogy is that we cannot insincerely believe as we can insincerely assert. Again, however, this difference requires qualification. The speaker's goal is to have the hearer discern the speaker's intention, and if one's intention is open to others, the possibility of insincerity is lost. Also, to assert insincerely is to misrepresent oneself, so that an insincere assertion is a failure to meet the conditions for proper assertion.

18. For the (self-referential) causal efficacy of intentions, see Searle (1983): chaps. 3 and 4.

19. The problem of not losing a grip is clear in Aristotle's discussion. He begins reasonably by denying the Socratic Paradox (no one knowingly does wrongly) for contradicting "things that appear manifestly." But then part of Aristotle's own "solution" is that the akratic's thought at the moment he acts is like that of the drunk. Aristotle (1985): book vii, chaps. 2–11.

20. Following Hempel (1965), essays 1, 2, and 12.

21. Some of these are suggested by Heil (1984).

22. For a relevant distinction between avowed and central beliefs, see Rey (1988).

23. The position is not "overly optimistic about human rationality" as claimed by Mele (1987: 114). If the connection is conceptual, rationality is not yet involved.

24. Mele (1987) argues that these kinds of cases are improperly excluded by Heil's account.

Chapter 3

1. For a detailed analysis, see McLaughlin (1988).

2. Along these lines, Descartes's standard of absolute certainty can be motivated. See Williams (1978): chap. 2.

3. Reason detached from emotion appears as well to be ineffectual at reaching decision. See Damasio (1994).

4. For evolutionary speculations on this connection, see the discussion and references in Pinker (1997): 201–205.

5. Recently, Stich (1990) has attempted to deflate the importance of truth: chap. 5, especially 123–124. For a defense of the value of truth against Stich's arguments, see Loewer (1993). For further criticisms, see Peacocke (1992): 25–27, as well as Haack (1993): 195–202.

6. See Whyte (1990). Whyte credits the rudimentary idea to Ramsey (1978a: 46).

7. A number of the studies depend on very restricted options. In the case of selecting among pairs of stockings, most subjects opt for the rightmost pair, while denying that as their reason. Yet, the setup is one in which all the pairs are, in fact, identical. The normal setup in stores is that there are some identical pairs, but not all pairs are alike. Many pairs vary in look, quality, or price. Standardly, there is a rational (and so acknowledgeable) basis for choice.

Where time is limited and products are indistinguishable, we helpfully develop tie-breaking mechanisms. "Buridan's ass" problems explain why. The "ass," facing two equally inviting bales of hay, starved because he could not find a reason to prefer one bale to the other. He didn't appreciate that the failure to find a discriminating ground, given his need to eat, engaged his higher-order reason to just pick one bale. In contemporary society, we regularly face Buridan's ass situations. When we go shopping, we look through rows of identical products such as indistinguishable jars of tomato sauce. The subtle bias toward the rightmost is presumably one of many instant tie-breakers allowing us to "just pick" (Ullmann-Margalit and Morgenbesser 1977). These tie-breakers determine choice without reflection. Otherwise they would return us to a deliberative understanding of our dilemma from which we need to escape.

Further, a requirement for exact sorting into ties and nonties before application would be self-defeating. So our use of tiebreakers ought to be carefree and un-self-conscious, and we ought to develop them independently of the cases to which they will be applied. In fact, the empirical studies overall—not just ones offering near ties—show our sensitivity to differences or ways of generating differences that are external to judgments of merit, and so cannot ground those judgments. Standard examples involve using a semantic cue ("ocean-moon") that influences a classification judgment (selecting "Tide" as a response to the category "detergent"), though it is not so acknowledged. See Nisbett and Ross (1980): 207.

8. Related claims are made by Williams (1973) and Burge (1993).

9. On related issues, see Kornblith (1983).

10. Darmstadter (1971). On cognitive limits and consistency, see Cherniak (1986): chaps. 1 and 2; and Goldman (1986): chaps. 6 and 10.

11. Psychological studies attest that this is a regular consequence of categorization, which is a practical necessity. For a review, see Smith (1995).

12. Following the analysis of Reeve (1989): sections 2.1–2.2.

13. But see Elgin (1997): 169–170.

14. See, for example, Cherniak (1986): 50–51.

15. These specialized cases, including the Descartes/student ones, pose a difficulty—exceptions—to my assumption that sincere assertion expresses belief. However, in these cases, the speaker (Jones) does "on-line," sincerely, though mistakenly, take himself to cease to hold the belief.

16. A subtle illustration is presented by Wood (1988): 211. On these mechanisms in self-deception, see Bach (1981).

17. For recognition of the importance of this condition, as well as arguments against it, see Dretske (1970), and Nozick (1981): chap. 3, sections I and II.

18. For a critical analysis, see Thomas (1997).

19. For defense of this complaint, see Hogarth (1986) and Margolis (1987): chap. 9. But the complaint holds only "typically." See, for example, Janis (1972). To secure my criticism below along the lines of this complaint I would need to test it out against naturalistic studies of cognitive dissonance as in Festinger, Riecken, and Schacter (1956).

20. See Hare's (1981: 169–187) discussion of the pure and the impure fanatic.

Chapter 4

1. I am borrowing in these two paragraphs and in some of the next section from Adler (1998).

2. Sidney Hook writes: "'It is not impossible' is a preface to an irrelevant statement about human affairs. The question is always one of the balance of probabilities. And the evidence for probabilities must include more than abstract possibilities" (1980: 122).

3. Contrast (1)–(7) with the traditional structure: It is not disproved that p; So, p. See Woods and Walton (1978), and Sorensen (1988): 129–159.

4. Some arguments from ignorance resemble inferences to the best explanation. The latter inferences require the substantive empirical claim that there are no better or alternative hypotheses. When this substantive claim is undefended or defended only very weakly, it is likely that the failing is due to the influence of arguments from ignorance, even if not clearly of that structure. See further Adler (1994; 1997a).

5. Referring to the traditional structure, Robinson (1971: 102) observes that arguments from ignorance license conflicting conclusions.

6. The second premise also ordinarily has a stronger consequence. As a working hypothesis: "a state of affairs is possible if it is not known not to obtain, and no practicable investigations would establish that it does not obtain" (Hacking 1967: 149; and for proposed emendations DeRose 1991). Lack of proof (or knowledge) of falsity yields the first conjunct only. This second conjunct holds only if the original hypothesis has been subject to our best efforts to falsify it. But for the really far-out hypotheses, neither heavy resources nor time will be invested.

7. The criterion goes back at least to Hume (1977), discussed in chap. 5.

8. For related discussion, see Levin (1998): 27–29.

9. Even if the first premise of the argument sketch above were the stronger "It is not disprov*able* (refutable) that *p*," rather than merely "No one has disproved (refuted) that *p*," the premise still would not establish a real possibility. There are propositions such that they and their negations are (logically) unprovable, yet either those propositions or their negations are necessarily true. For example, consider a sequence like "77777." Either it occurs or it does not occur in the expansion of pi, and whichever is the case will be necessary. But we may never know which. It is conceivable that 77777 is in the expansion of pi, even if it turns out not to be logically possible.

10. There are neighboring scope of negation problems in argument from ignorance reasoning: If no one has disproved *p*, then it is seems reasonable to hold that one should not believe that *p* is false (or disbelieve *p*). But if the latter is (mis)construed as a "double-negative," it yields that one believes that *p* is true. Woods and Walton (1978) observe that the fallacy in one form can be "exhibited as confusion between the pair"

$\sim Ka \sim p/p$ with $Ka \sim p/p$. (92)

("Kxq" = "*x* knows that *q*"; "a" is a denoting expression.)
A related confusion expressed in ordinary English would be: "*x* doesn't know that *p* is false. So *x* knows that he hasn't shown that *p* is false. So it's possible (for *x*) that *p* is true."

11. A correlative of this misleading focus is that we accord forefront evidence too great a role in explaining decisions or actions. "Monday morning quarterbacking" involves assuming that the coach on Sunday had the same evidence that you have on Monday.

12. The relevance of pragmatics is most simply exhibited in the misleading effects of emphasis. If in an accusatory tone, the second juror is pressed "Do you *really* know that the building's falling down is not possible?" he will tend to back off, just as he would from "But do you *really* know that the building won't fall down?" One way to realize that something fishy is going on here is that the manipulative question would work for any inductive knowledge. See further chap. 9.

13. Findings that children maintain starkly contradictory ideas are easier to swallow when it is observed that the children are able to keep these ideas apart. See, for example, Carey (1990). Consistent with the main themes of this work, my doubts about Piagetian conservation apply only to where the contradictory ideas are brought together.

14. For one of numerous examples of James-like reasoning in everyday settings, consider the following excerpt from a thoughtful essay by George Johnson, "Science and Religion: Bridging the Great Divide" (*New York Times*, June 30, 1998, p. F4): "If certain physical constants had slightly different values, stars would not have formed to cook up the atoms that made the biological molecules. Since early in the century, some truth seekers have taken this sort of argument as a reason to believe that the universe was created with people in mind.

But one is also free to choose the opposite belief: that the coincidences simply show that life is indeed an incredible fluke."

15. See Popper (1959): 42, 82–83. An application of this meta-criterion is my response to the reply to the proposed variant cognitive dissonance study (chap. 3, section VII above). Larry Laudan (1983) underestimates the value of falsifiability as a critical tool because he disassociates it from the "meta-criteria" that must govern its workings, especially the avoidance of ad hoc maneuvering, specification of falsification conditions in advance, and burdens of proof.

16. Bryan Appleyard, "In Science We Trust," *New York Times,* op-ed, April 8, 1993.

17. But see Alston (1983): 128–130.

18. For a plausible account of these not as full beliefs, see Sperber (1985).

19. But see also Gutting's (1982: 83–92) criticisms of both Wittgenstein's "groundlessness" view and Plantinga's external foundationalism.

Chapter 5

1. On the distinction between generating and sustaining, see Dretske (1981): 88–89; and Sellars (1963): 132.

2. Where the testimony is used and passed along without opportunity for checks, the "telephone game" problem arises whereby the continued transmission of testimony degrades its informational value.

3. Coady (1992: 47) is also not a fan of the opposition between "the attitudes of critical appraisal and of trust."

4. Coady (1992): 82–83. Coady is here objecting to only one interpretation of Hume's view.

5. See Davidson (1982): "Mental Events." The absence of laws governing intentional human actions (so described) is an obstacle to any purely externalist—reliabilist—account of testimony. For the internal-external issue in regard to testimony, see Fricker (1987).

6. Recall the recommendation for off-setting this form of skeptical question in section 1 of the introduction.

7. That there is a difference between trust and reliance is defended by Baier (1986): 234; and Garver (1994): chaps. 5 and 6.

8. See Fricker (1994) for a forceful defense of a neutral position. But it is so nuanced that the contrast with the default position becomes hard to maintain. Fricker allows for default entitlement of sincerity, but not reliability, and she rejects only a default view that is not engaged if the speaker's critical faculties are active or which is indifferent to subject matter. See especially pp. 144–145 and 150. Notice that her characterization of reductionism and anti-reductionism (e.g., p. 154) does not neatly classify our view.

Jones (1999) also opposes the default view. Her account, however, ignores the demands of the practice (for a tacit cooperative arrangement maintained despite regular threat of defection and which is under severe time constraints).

9. Fricker (1994: 154) requires that "the hearer must always be monitoring the speaker critically . . . if there were any signs of untrustworthiness, she would pick them up."

10. Coady (1992): chap 9. Although shared values are also included, the objection to be offered stands. Additionally, Coady offers an argument from coherence as best explained by the truth delivery of various sources to which my objection does not apply.

11. As Bradley Armour-Garb suggested to me, an argument like Coady's might be recast to rely directly on assertion as governed by the maxim of truthfulness. If there is an a priori rationale to accept this rule, then the rationale would extend to any application of it. But the recast argument is subject to the same limits as noted for Burge's argument. It would be too easy to override in most ordinary empirical circumstances.

12. For helpful discussion of Foley, Coady, and related issues of testimony, see Schmitt (1994): esp. 13–15.

13. This is broadly the position taken by Blais (1987).

14. Hardwig (1991: 703, 705–706) appeals to lack of funding and motivation in challenging the power of replication. Hardwig also neglects relatively cost-effective checks on the validity of reports through statistical analysis. For one of a number of recent such studies, see the discussion of Cyril Burt's IQ research in Kamin (1974).

A recent investigation of the most well-known accusation of fraud in the 1980s turned on subtle differences in interpretation of a small portion of a large amount of data. The report indicates extensive government checks on fraud, internal checks from coworkers, as well as, although much less prominently, replication. The report favors the view that no fraud or serious error went on, and among the author's conclusions is this: "No reliable data exist on the incidence of scientific misconduct, but it is likely that the serious form of it—fabrication and falsification of data—is rare" (Kevles 1996: 109).

15. Knowing of this general reliability does not require any credibility ratio for the reliability of informants, a notion that Coady (1992: 210–211) ridicules, given how context-sensitive such judgments would be.

16. It is the lack of recognition of background evidence that undermines much of the criticism of traditional empiricist views, as, for example, in Schmitt (1987): esp. his criticism of Hume on pp. 48, 54.

17. See Faulkner's (2000) distinction between the justification for acceptance of testimony and the justification (or warrant) for the proposition accepted.

18. For an incisive treatment of this topic, broader than my focus on testimony, see Kitcher (1990).

19. Broadly, this is the perspective one finds in Brandom (1994), Burge (1993), and Ross (1986). The significance of the ethical dimensions of testimony were brought to my attention by Timothy Williamson, in comments, and by Richard Moran, in a paper he delivered at New York University and in subsequent correspondence.

20. However, as noted earlier, the hearer has leeway not to accept the speaker's assertion in the privacy of his mind, whereas with social norms, noncompliance would usually be visible.

21. See Axelrod (1984) on the virtues of "tit-for-tat."

22. In this paragraph, which derives from Adler (1994), I am grateful to discussion with Catherine Elgin.

23. Correspondingly, the overhearer would pass other tests for knowledge (such as the subjunctive test):

If the directions are not correct, the overhearer would not believe they were (since the competent speaker would have reported otherwise).

24. The thought that if one claims that there are background reasons supportive of testimonial acceptance that one is reducing or explaining away testimony as a fertile source of our beliefs is due to an unwarranted assumption of a kind of transitivity:

If our background reasons support adopting the default rule, and the default rule is the ground for accepting a particular piece of testimony, then those background reasons are sufficient to accept that testimony by themselves. So we can cut through testimony's distinctive default rule.

But this is not a plausible principle because the imposition of the default rule creates a different justificatory structure. See Rawls (1968). In Adler (1996a), Rawls's account of justification in a practice is taken as opposed to this kind of transitivity.

25. See Coady (1992), and also Audi (1997), who observes that testimony can give rise to beliefs that are basic among our beliefs, even if not a basic source of beliefs.

26. This pseudo-challenge is to be distinguished from a genuine one like "How do you know, I thought you're just visiting New York City?"

Chapter 6

1. For background, see Sosa (1999), Williams (1977): chap. 3 and Elgin (1996): chap. 2.

2. For the last example, see Wittgenstein (1969): 153, 163. Some of these cases raise the question of "implicit beliefs"—how should we understand propositions that follow closely from explicit beliefs but which one has never thought of before? See Audi (1982), and Crimmins (1992): section 2.3.

3. This need for auxiliary assumptions is central to the "Quine-Duhem thesis." See Duhem (1954): chaps. 6–7, and Quine (1980).

4. See Quine (1980): 41. Duhem's (1954) doctrine is nonisolationism, not holism.

5. It is this thesis that is enough for Quine to challenge his main target—that some statements are not falsifiable because they are analytic or confirmable in isolation. With the falsification/revision distinction, I would try to answer criticisms of Quine (1980) due to Katz (1998): 73 and Field (1998).

6. Mimicking Goodman's (1983) famous "grue" hypothesis. On the unrealistic nature of the problem of underdetermination see Kitcher (1993): chap. 7, section 6.

7. Specifically, I avoid the vexed issue of the "converse consequence condition" (if e confirms h and h' implies h then e confirms h'), and of whether the project of qual-

itative confirmation should be surrendered for a quantitative or at least comparative inductive logic. The classic work on qualitative confirmation, which rejects the converse consequence condition, is Hempel (1965): esp. 31–33.

8. Field (unpublished) argues that not only logic or certain basic logical laws are exempt from empirical falsification, but so too inductive rules, though for different reasons.

9. We may also be mistaken in what hypotheses actually receive tacit confirmation. If, as some have argued, there really are no colors, then the success of our color-ascription practices do not tacitly confirm that there are colors, but something more like that we have regular and reliable color-experiences owing to certain (noncolored) properties of objects.

10. This string of objections is found in a number of places. It is a central theme of Plantinga's Reidian views in (1993). See also Alston (1989): 70–72.

11. For an example of such an objection in the context of testimony, see Plantinga (1993): 187. Plantinga makes similar claims about memory and perception as part of his Reidian view.

12. On early developmental pragmatics, see Ochs and Schiefflein (1979). For a more recent and broader survey of the surprising degree of intelligent responses and activities of even infants, see Rogoff (1990).

13. Millar (1991), esp. 61–63, account of competence (with reasons) as "pattern-governance" does not require conceptualization or reflective thoughts.

14. In accepting some sort of belief requirement for reasons, I place on myself a burden that may be unnecessary. For others who reject it, see Haack (1993) and Pollock and Cruz (1999).

15. Grice (1989), Davidson (1984), Dennett (1987), and Burge (1993) offer versions.

16. For discussion of skills, see Ryle (1949): chap. 2. Although Ryle is insistent that intelligent practices or know-how do not presuppose reflective operations, he does not deny that these practices and know-how are the workings of reasons.

17. The example is borrowed from Kirkham (1992): 252–253.

18. Pollock and Cruz (1999) argue that epistemic norms are matters of know-how. My views in these paragraphs are closest to that of Pollock and Cruz.

19. Thus I reject the allegedly internalist "constraint that all justification determiners must be *accessible to,* or *knowable by,* the epistemic agent" (Goldman 1999: 272).

20. The essays in Jerome Kagan and Sharon Lamb (1987) take as a starting point that rudiments of moral thinking or judgment emerge at around age two.

21. In taking this view, I offer one line of argument toward Sellars's (1963) claim of the epistemic and conceptual dependence of particular judgments like that this screen is blue and general judgments like that perception is reliable. The view is also, I think, at one with Wittgenstein's remark (1969: at 141) that "When we first begin to *believe* anything, what we believe is not a single proposition, it is a whole system of propositions. (Light dawns gradually over the whole.)"

22. Contrast my discussion of this principle with an analogous one treated by Wolterstorff (1996): 67–69. Notice, specifically, his endorsement, here and elsewhere, of association of this principle with the regress problem.

23. Although Plantinga (1983) is well known as a refutation of evidentialism, it is overwhelmingly about foundationalism. The entire argument that evidentialism entails foundationalism is that the evidentialist "does not mean to suggest that *no* propositions can be believed or accepted without evidence, for if you have evidence for *every* proposition you believe, then you will believe infinitely many propositions; and no one has time, these busy days, for that. So presumably *some* propositions can properly be believed and accepted without evidence" (39). I do not find the appeal to psychological storage pertinent. First, the evidentialist claims backing by adequate reasons or evidence. He does not claim that one has to know the specific reasons or evidence for which one came to believe. Second, and related, Plantinga assumes that all the reasons or evidence have to take the form of explicitly represented beliefs, excluding our believing that we can generate the further reasons (beliefs) as we can be held to believe that the number of stars is greater than 1, 2, . . . 3489, . . . n, without explicitly representing each.

24. The alleged connection is also judged starkly implausible by Kretzmann (1992).

25. The discussion bypasses a difficult issue as to whether perceptual experiences have a nonconceptual content. For defenses, see Dretske (1990) and Peacocke (2001).

26. Further backing derives from the knowledge I acquire second-hand by deferring to scientists who study visual perception.

27. Millar (1991: 176–178) moves from a denial that we retain specifics to the "groundlessness" of our believing, though his understanding of groundlessness is sensitive to evidentialist concerns.

28. On the self-corrective nature of science, see Sellars (1963): 170.

29. It is along these lines—of diminishing epistemic dependence due to ongoing testing—that I would try to answer the problems raised by Post (1980) that an infinite chain, since it would be merely a chain of conditional justification, is too easily satisfied.

30. Although Wittgenstein's groundlessness view is well motivated as a response to the infinite regress problem, I do not claim textual authority for ascribing that motivation to his argument. However, for a defense of Wittgenstein as a kind of foundationalist, see Stroll (1994): chap. 9.

31. Fogelin (1994): 216–217 does not overlook our actual response. But he too sides with Wittgenstein in just dismissing its significance.

32. The confusion is reified in common ways to represent confirmation—e.g., $\text{Conf}(h,e)$ if and only if $\text{prob}(h,e\&b) > \text{prob}(h,b)$—in which the probabilities are subjective.

33. Only "can," because other conditions are involved in confirmation, as we observed earlier.

34. In a number of publications, John Post has argued that the circularity objection depends on the assumption that the justification relation is *transitive,* and he has vigorously challenged this assumption. See especially Post and Turner (2000). Post is on to something important. In the case of a prominent neighbor of justification—probability—various probabilistic relations are not transitive e.g. p can be positively relevant to q and q positively relevant to r, where not only is p not positively relevant to r, it is negatively relevant.

35. See Alston's "Epistemic Circularity" in his (1989), especially 347–348. The fullest development is in Alston (1993). At the end of both "Epistemic Circularity" and his (1993), Alston explicitly tries to mitigate the skeptical import of this circularity problem.

36. The argument just sketched could also be stated in terms of the reliability of perception for given individuals (so that the one whose reliability is in question is not one of those checking on that reliability); and then an inference from each of these reliable perceivers can be made to the reliability of perception for creatures like us generally. As an answer to epistemic circularity, however, Alston (1993: 115–116) holds that inductive inference or the success of science cannot be invoked.

The conclusion could also be argued for by appeal to the *converse consequence condition.* In his development of the "epistemic circularity," Alston does not consider the possibility of transmission of confirmation from instances of the success of a process of belief-formation like perception to confirmation of the reliability of that process. (The transmission holds only under assumptions that restrict alternative hypotheses that would also entail the successful instances.) At one point, Alston suggests sympathy for arguments that effectively deny the special consequence condition (Alston 1993: 133, n. 14). But it is the special consequence condition itself that is the chief argument against accepting the converse consequence condition (see Hempel 1965).

37. For a detailed defense of coherentism with important criticisms of foundationalism see Bonjour (1985).

38. Fogelin (1994), part II, esp. chap. 10, also rejects these responses. Regrettably, he then concludes that the infinite regress problem is unanswerable.

39. As on any external foundationalist view, e.g., Plantinga (1983; 1993). For a general statement of reliabilism, see Goldman (1986): part I.

40. The criticism is influenced by Bonjour's (1985) extended critique.

41. Goldman writes: "Practically speaking. it is difficult to see how a cognitive agent could know that relevant justifiers exist without knowing which particular ones exist" (1999: 275). If the account I offer is correct, this is the opposite of the practical and the theoretical truth.

42. The response I am developing is an "internal" or "everyday," as opposed to an "external" or "philosophical," response. See Stroud (1984): chap. 3. But I take reliance on an internal response not to be itself a philosophical stance, as it is with G. E. Moore. My response is Moorean "everyday" without Moorean ambition ("philosophical").

43. Compare with Austin (1970): 113, n. 1.

44. Walton (1978) makes it plausible that the experience of powerful emotions is compatible with a make-believe view of the object to which one is responding. However, there are various degrees of pretense, and the kind I posit is mild and diffuse. Specifically, I do not claim that the subjects in Milgram's study are involved in the kind of pretense that is paradigmatic for Walton, as when children play act that, e.g., the broomstick is a horse.

Walton's article supports a number of my earlier claims, including that distraction is easily accomplished (so that in make-believe we distract ourselves from the belief that what is going on is not real, and then experience a full gamut of emotions). Walton also removes a prominent role for partial belief (in explaining our response to fiction), and he denies, as well, that our response to fiction should be described as a willing suspension of disbelief. At no point while we watch a horror film that terrifies us do we seriously suspend our disbelief. We know all along that it is real, and so, I would add, we cannot just suspend disbelief.

45. This expresses a thought of us as detached commentators. In fact, subjects who are asked to observe the Milgram study judge that obedience was much more a product of personality than situation. See Nisbett and Ross (1980): 120–122.

46. See further note 44 of this chapter.

Chapter 7

1. What of Moore's Paradox for partial belief? The following is no Moore's Paradox:

I am almost sure (certain) that p, though I have some doubts about it.

For example, "I am almost sure that the fox is hiding in the garage, though I have some doubts that he is." This is not heard as contradictory; indeed, the second conjunct explains the qualifier on the first. But it may be suggested that the closer analogue is:

It's highly probable that p, but I am not at all inclined to believe it.

For example, "It's highly probable that the Yankees will be pennant contenders next year, but I am not inclined to believe it." The coherence of this assertion is supported by claims that subjective probability and partial belief are distinct (Bach 1984: 49). I'm not convinced that the alleged coherence goes beyond psychological interferences—the actual state of partial believing does not ensue, though it would under full awareness. The latter result is in accord with the conceptual connection claim—that to believe p to degree n is to take it as supported to degree n by all one's evidence.

2. See references in chap. 1, especially to Williamson (1996).

3. Hawthorne and Bovens (1999: 242, n. 3, 244–245) allow that we can reduce the "curious doxastic situation" of the Preface and Lottery Paradoxes if we identify *belief* with *absolute certainty*. Such an identification they take to amount to skepticism. But the reduction can take place, without skepticism, if we treat belief as full belief, whose aim is knowledge.

4. See Williamson (1996): 506. He claims that the account works for believing, but this is so only if we can find a property of belief that mirrors the factiveness of knowledge.

5. For rich reflections on this feature, see Moran (1997).

6. The proof does not require addition of any new assumption or principle. Contrast with Hintikka's (1962: 64–78) analysis.

7. We can thus circumvent treacherous questions as to what inferences one is committed to by virtue of one's explicit assertions (beliefs).

8. I put aside sorites-type borderline statements, and proposals for deviant (three- or many-valued) logics to handle them.

9. See Dummett (1973): 330, 356.

10. Thus I agree with the conclusion Collins (1996) reaches, but I deny that he is treating the genuine Moore's Paradox. He focuses on "I believe that p, and $\sim p$," which is an instance not of (1), but of (3).

11. See Urmson (1966) and Williams (1973), "Deciding to Believe".

12. The disanalogy is observed by Stalnaker (1987): 92.

13. Another difference is that the individual statements in the book are not in competition, as they are in the Lottery Paradox.

14. Stalnaker (1987: 90–96), while broadly endorsing rejection of the conjunction rule, offers a more complex picture. Acceptance includes belief, but, as well, other truth-aiming attitudes.

15. This view of the Preface Paradox is close to that of Kaplan (1996) and Ryan (1991). However, Ryan's argument is insufficient for handling the Preface Paradox as applied to what is already accepted, rather than the act of accepting the individual statements in the book.

16. See especially Harman (1973): 118–120, 155–161 and for an extended defense Nelkin (2000).

17. See Harman (1973), DeRose (1996), Nelkin (2000), and Fogelin (1994): part I, appendix A. Fogelin connects this claim to the Preface Paradox. On some contextualist accounts, discussed in chap. 9, we can know in lottery situations (when, roughly, the existence of a lottery is not salient). See Cohen (1998).

18. In fact, to grant that the tape is conceivable or epistemically possible is already to concede the point.

19. It might be responded that although "I am almost sure that" may not express modesty, the expressing of it would. However, to preserve the contrast, this would be so only if others did not so express their modesty. As noted further on in this chapter, even then the assertion misleadingly suggests that the author has specific undermining evidence.

20. A weaker relation like "implicates" will not do because Moore's Paradox itself (1) is precisely a failed attempt to "cancel" the implicature. See Grice (1989): 41–42.

21. Compare with Hume's (1975: 181–182) skepticism in regard to reason, briefly discussed in chap. 10.

22. This is obviously fundamental for Kyburg (1997).

Chapter 8

1. I allow that a closer reading would reveal special reasons for Elizabeth to be more cautious. If so, my use of the example presumes that a variant case could still be presented as realistic, where Elizabeth lacks clues to treat Wickham's testimony more skeptically, such as her own disposition against Darcy.

2. For an argument against the possibility of the suspension of all belieflike attitudes, see Burnyeat (1983).

3. Of course, awareness of constraints is difficult to maintain simultaneously with judgments subject to them. But it cannot be a condition of participation in these practices that we regularly attend to their conceptual foundations.

4. On some views, all emotions are judgments, e.g., Solomon (1980).

5. On a related point, see Williams (1973): 210–212, and Nozick (1993): 11. It is by treating the italicized phrase below as an embedded conditional that I would handle the following troublesome example suggested by L. J. Cohen (pers. comm.):

If I *even suspected that* Jones molested my neighbor's son, I would be furious at him.

6. The problem is the flip slide to advantages of committee judgments. Social friction is eased by virtue of making negative decisions more impersonal and creating uncertainty or doubt as to which individuals did judge one negatively.

7. Such a hybrid attitude should be distinguished from those implied by "Probably, John resents . . ." and "John probably resents . . . ," which mean either

John resents something. Probably, it is the fact that p.

or

John knows that p. Probably, he resents it.

The Kiparskys (1971: 354–355) observe that when a nonfactive verb qualifies a factive one, the factive remains dominant.

8. Imagination helps, but it is subject to bias when our emotions are passionately engaged.

9. One of the reasons for the success of the tit-for-tat strategy in iterated Prisoner's Dilemmas is that it is quickly provoked to retaliation (Axelrod 1984: 184–85).

10. For related worries, see Harman (1986): 23.

11. The value being ascribed to simple formulations is restricted to the elimination of epistemic qualifications. Even the advances in argumentation that are marked by modification (the admission of exceptions, the more nuanced presentation of conclusions) are not the withdrawing of a thesis, as would be the case with epistemic qualification.

12. On the importance of variety and competition in science, see Kitcher (1990) and Railton (1994).

13. Even when the issue is explicitly debated, there is "polarization" (84), which is evidence of pressure toward full belief. See "What Caused the Mass Extinction?" *Scientific American,* October 1990: 76–92. The authors of the article defending the comet-impact hypothesis write in regard to the extinction of the dinosaurs: "We now believe that we have solved the mystery. . . . Other suspects, such as sea level changes, climatic shifts and volcanic eruptions, have alibis that appear to rule them out" (78). The very next article defends the volcanic eruption hypothesis. However, for a challenge to the place of full belief in theoretical science, see van Fraassen (1980).

14. On a related point, see Morton (1988).

15. A fundamental result from iterated Prisoner's Dilemmas when a modicum of trust and certain other conditions are met. (See Axelrod 1984.)

16. Kant recommends strongly against teaching morality by looking for "motives to be morally good" (Kant 1981: AK 411, n. 2). The Golden Rule appeals to children's sense of equality or fairness, not strict reciprocity. It rings true even when a child knows that the envisaged role reversal will not actually take place.

Chapter 9

1. The cases are restricted to first-person parenthetical uses of epistemic qualifiers. See Urmson (1966).

2. On the two notions of probability, see Hacking (1975) and Carnap (1962): chap. 2.

3. Because full belief reflects a demand on us to economize, betting behavior poorly captures the logic of full belief. The objective of a bet is presumed to be winning alone, which is determined just by correctness. Initially, it is attractive to measure belief by willingness to bet. If I believe that Seattle is north of New York City, I should be willing to wager on its truth (setting aside my finances and my attitude toward gambling). I should be willing to put my money where my mouth is. (For an excellent defense, see Mellor 1971.) But betting taps only the aim of belief as correct judgment, not the existence of full belief as a mechanism of economy. One might as well measure the value of automobiles only by speed. It is along these lines, as well through application of the belief/confidence distinction of chapter 10, that I would hope to exempt full belief from van Fraassen's (1984) "reflection principle."

4. Also, partial belief is burdensome by having to represent the negation of a belief. See Gilbert (1991).

5. Additionally, Harman (1986: 25–27) observes that memory would be greatly burdened in operating on partial beliefs. For related criticisms, see Goldman (1986): chaps 15 and 16.

6. They also rule out acceptance as in "accept *p* for the sake of argument" or weakenings (adding disjuncts) to accommodate limited evidence or treating it as governed by an epistemic qualifier "It's approximately true that *p.*"

7. On these uses of acceptance, see Cohen (1992) and Stalnaker (1987): chap. 5. Railton (1994) raises difficulties for van Frassen's (1980) view that scientists accept a theory (to work on) without full belief in its theoretical posits.

8. The psychology alluded to is the basis for Pascal's (1966: 418) famous recommendation for becoming a religious believer on prudential grounds.

9. On markedness and related issues, see Horn (1989): chap. 3. As is standard, these claims about markedness are meant comparatively—e.g., significantly less frequent than without the qualifier.

10. However, as discussion indicates, I disagree with Toulmin's assimilation of assertion and guarded assertion as either both or neither referring to the speaker's mental state.

11. For this, and related reasons, I disagree with Searle's (1979: 33–35) claim that inferences toward grasping speaker's meaning in indirect speech acts is probabilistic. The inference is defeasible, as shown by cancellability tests, but it does not follow that the conclusion (not merely the inference) is probabilistic as Searle claims. Specifically, in his own example of responding "I have to study" to the proposal "Let's go to the movies tonight," the conclusion that the speaker probably intends to reject the proposal would not yet settle the proposal ("OK, you probably will not go. But now, will you or won't you?").

12. "Transparent" does not imply that the content of the belief is fully understood. See Burge (1987).

13. On the difference in direction of fit between belief and desire, see Searle (1983): chaps. 1 and 6.

14. See, among others, DeRose (1992, 1995), Lewis (1983, 1996), and Unger (1984).

15. On the special-reasons requirement, see Austin (1970), Cherniak (1986), and Harman (1986).

16. Austin (1970): 84.

17. For discussion of burdens of proof in argument, see Walton (1996).

18. Some hold that it is enough that conditions are normal—you need no reason to believe that they are. For reasons offered in chapter 5, this is too weak and a stronger condition need not entail a regress. For related discussion, see Williams (1991): chap. 8.

Chapter 10

1. The belief/confidence distinction would handle, I think, Roorda's (1997) cases of "epistemic ambivalence" without the apparatus he introduces.

2. The centrality given to "weight" in the theory of inductive support of Cohen (1977) has greatly influenced my discussion. See also his (1986b). But it can be inferred from his (1991), which is a response to Logue (1991), that he would not accept the role I give to the notion.

3. For a further example and related discussion, see Gardenfors and Sahlin (1988).

4. Popper (1959): 406–419. However, he claims only that the paradox applies to a particular way of understanding probability.

5. Specifically, divergence arises in conditional probability judgments, which represent dispositions to change belief. The greater number of trials increases the resistance to change (or "resilience") of the judgment. See Skyrms's (1977) development of Jeffrey's view. Other developments invoke levels or second-order probabilities, which is an approach closer to what I have to say about full belief and confidence. See, for example, Hacking (1978) and van Fraassen (1984).

6. Keynes also concentrated on positive evidence and weight as the proportion of evidence gathered ("based upon a greater amount of relevant evidence"). He did not consider significant variations in the importance of different kinds of negative evidence.

7. Another serviceable example: You receive a letter of recommendation for a job candidate, and it is very positive. However, you become aware that the letter writer is not terribly trustworthy for recommendations (Griffin and Tversky 1992).

8. A slight variation on the same point can be put in more abstract, but theoretically familiar, terms: Were the conditions met for betting behavior to yield a measure of partial belief, the amount one is willing to stake on a proposition varies with the weight one ascribes to one's evidence. The variation has similar practical consequences as an alteration in the probability one assigns to that proposition. (However, I do not imply that partial belief should be measured by appropriate stakes rather than betting quotients. See Mellor 1971: 34.)

9. There is a correlative distinction between having reasons to doubt and actually doubting. For a similar distinction, although in the context of skepticism, see Moore (1962).

10. For a contemporary version of this pragmatist reasoning, see Cohen (1988).

11. As previously noted, there is also the skepticism inherent in not treating way-out possibilities of error as dismissable ones. I can know that the normal coin I flip will land heads or tails, even though there is a tiny probability that it will land on its side.

12. Hume's argument is held to violate the weight/force distinction in Hacking (1978); and, following Hacking, in Fogelin (1985): 17–19. (Some of their criticisms are anticipated by Reid 1969: essay VII, section IV.) Influenced by Hacking and Fogelin's critique there has been a vigorous debate in *Hume Studies*. See Morris (1989) and Dauer (1996). Of obvious pertinence is Karlsson's (1990) response that "when I [err], it is as often in placing too little confidence in my judgment as in placing too much."

13. A conversational source of the reasoning's plausibility is set out in chapter 4. When, in regard to a specific assertion, it is said that the speaker might be mistaken, the possibility of error is taken as applicable to what is asserted or the reasons for it. If the possibility is taken as genuine, in deference to the speaker, then it is misconstrued as implying a specific failing for which the challenger has grounds.

14. The debate was initiated by Cohen (1981). A major portion of Kahneman, Slovic, and Tversky (1982) is devoted to the base rate studies.

15. To borrow Rey's (1997) term, discussions influenced by the focal assumption suffer from "superficialism" (328). All epistemic questions are reduced to only the most salient ones.

16. Examples due to Radford (1970) could also be adopted to serve our purposes, though he offers them to refute the view that knowledge implies belief or even the right to be sure.

17. A nonevidential ground for withdrawing an assertion not discussed here, but treated in section 8 below, based on the discussion in chapter 9, is when standards in the context are altered. However, since the standards are altered, the withdrawal of the assertion is not under the same conditions as when the assertion is originally entered.

18. The intuitive and unavoidable notion of "defeaters" is discussed in many works in epistemology. For extended treatment, see Klein (1981): chap. 2.

19. This point is overlooked by Nisbett and Ross (1980): 271.

Chapter 11

1. See the initial characterization by Mele (1987): chap. 4.

2. Roughly, "epistemic self-control" may be thought of as Goldman's (1991) "epistemic paternalism" in the first person.

3. Bracketing is roughly complementary to Stalnaker's (1987: 79–81) notion of acceptance.

4. On this theme, see Kitcher (1990, 1993).

5. Judgments that are also subject to the "fundamental attribution error." See Nisbett and Ross (1980).

6. The dogmatism paradox introduced in Harman (1973: 148) can be viewed as an instance of the "each, but some not" structure. His solution—undermining the paradox—has been supported by a careful analysis of Ginet (1980). Although I am unsure the solution works for the question of whether I can have reason to admit putative counterevidence, I shall skirt around it.

7. A striking example from the history of medicine that can be understood in these terms is offered by Cherniak (1986).

8. A similar criticism applies to another recommended role in chapter 3 for explicitness to block a "cold" motivational account of the proposed extension of the dissonance study to the dynamic setting. We selected what to be explicit about to serve subjects' ends. But the subjects could not have done the same from their point of view. Otherwise the experiment would not have worked, since it depended on nonconscious or surreptitious influence on subjects' judgments. Discussion here is meant to correct for this criticism by filling in the claim of chapter 3 that "explicitness is advantageous only if highly selective."

9. On the general theme of inherent and necessary conflicts between internal (or subjective) and external (or objective) views, see Nagel (1986).

10. This kind of conundrum is suggested repeatedly in the studies of reasoning and judgment in psychology as reviewed in Nisbett and Ross (1980: chap. 5). But it is an old theme. Here's a famed worry from Meditation One: "since I judge that others sometimes make mistakes in matters that they believe they know most perfectly, may I not, in like fashion, be deceived every time I add two and three or count the sides of a square, or perform an even simpler operation?" (Descartes 1996).

11. Commenting on Helen's beauty, the elders declare in the *Iliad:* "Her face is uncannily like the faces of the immortal goddesses. But, beautiful though she is, let her depart in the ships; may she not be left behind to cause grief to us and our children" (iii, 156–160; cited in Irwin's commentary on Aristotle 1985: 315).

12. Sidgwick (1981: 203) observes that we may misconstrue an act when we evaluate it in itself, rather than for its contribution to an overall goal.

13. On strategic (self-control) problems with dieting, see Ainslie (1985).

14. There are also situations where one is moved to belief, and yet one's will is weak in sticking to or acting on the belief. One's confidence is low or one vacillates.

15. This role for reason, in allowing independent voice to emotions, is overlooked by Adams (1985): 10.

16. Surprisingly, Blanshard (1984) thinks that the main enemy of reasonableness is prejudice. But prejudice alone does not have sufficient explanatory reach given Blanshard's shrewd observation that though the standards for reasonableness are not high, they are still often not met.

References

(Dates are to the works cited, which may not be the original editions.)

Adams, Robert Merrihew. 1985. "Involuntary Sins." *The Philosophical Review* 94: 3–31.

———. 1995. "Moral Faith." *The Journal of Philosophy* 92: 75–95.

Adler, Jonathan E. 1981. "Skepticism and Universalizability." *The Journal of Philosophy* 77: 143–156.

———. 1983. "The Rationality of the (Lay) Scientist: Toward Reconciliation." *The Behavioral and Brain Sciences* 6.

———. 1984. "Abstraction Is Uncooperative." *Journal for the Theory of Social Behavior* 14: 165–181.

———. 1990. "Conservatism and Tacit Confirmation." *Mind* 99: 559–570.

———. 1991. "An Optimist's Pessimism: Conversation and Conjunction." In *Probability and Rationality*, E. Eells and T. Maruszewski, eds. (Amsterdam: Poznan): 251–282.

———. 1994a. "Fallacies and Alternative Interpretations." *Australasian Journal of Philosophy* 74: 271–282.

———. 1994b. "Testimony, Trust, Knowing." *The Journal of Philosophy* 91: 264–275.

———. 1996. "An Overlooked Argument for Epistemic Conservatism." *Analysis* 56: 80–84.

———. 1997. "Fallacies Not Fallacious: Not!" (and "Reply by Repetition and Reminder"). *Philosophy and Rhetoric* 30: 333–350; 367–375.

———. 1998. "Open Minds and the Argument from Ignorance." *Skeptical Inquirer* 22: 41–44.

———. 1999. "The Ethics of Belief: Off the Wrong Track." *Midwest Studies in Philosophy: New Directions in Philosophy* 23 (Oxford: Blackwell's): 267–285.

Ainslie, George. 1985. "Beyond Microeconomics: Conflict among Interests in a Multiple Self as a Determinant of Value." In *The Multiple Self*, Jon Elster, ed. (Cambridge: Cambridge University Press): 133–175.

Albert, Hans. 1985. *Treatise on Critical Reason.* M.V. Rorty, trans. (Princeton: Princeton University Press.)

Alston, William P. 1983. "Christian Experience and Christian Belief." In Plantinga and Wolterstorff, eds., 1983: 103–134.

———. 1989. *Epistemic Justification* (Ithaca: Cornell University Press).

———. 1993. *The Reliability of Sense Perception* (Ithaca: Cornell University Press).

Aristotle. 1984. *Sophistical Refutations.* In *The Complete Works of Aristotle,* volume one (The revised Oxford translation), Jonathan Barnes, ed. (Princeton: Princeton University Press).

———. 1985. *Nichomachean Ethics* Terence Irwin, ed. (Indianapolis: Hackett).

Armstrong, D. M. 1973. *Belief, Truth, and Knowledge* (Cambridge: Cambridge University Press).

Audi, Robert. 1982. "Believing and Affirming." *Mind* 91: 115–120.

———. 1997. "The Place of Testimony in the Fabric of Knowledge and Justification." *American Philosophical Quarterly* 34: 405–422.

Audi, Robert and William J. Wainwright, eds. 1986. *Rationality, Religious Belief, and Moral Commitment* (Ithaca: Cornell University Press).

Austin, J. L. 1970. "Other Minds." In his *Philosophical Papers,* second edition (Oxford: Oxford University Press): 76–116.

Axelrod, Robert. 1984. *The Evolution of Cooperation* (New York: Basic Books).

Bach, Kent. 1981. "An Analysis of Self-Deception." *Philosophy and Phenomenological Research* 41: 351–370.

———. 1984. "Default Reasoning: Jumping to Conclusions and Knowing When to Think Twice." *Pacific Philosophical Quarterly* 65: 37–58.

Baier, Annette. 1986. "Trust and Anti-Trust." *Ethics* 96: 231–260.

———. 1994. "Sustaining Trust." In her *Moral Prejudices* (Cambridge: Harvard University Press): 152–182.

Bem, D. J. 1967. "Self-Perception: An Alternative Interpretation of Cognitive Dissonance Phenomena." *Psychological Review* 74: 183–200.

Bennett, Jonathan. 1974. "The Conscience of Huckleberry Finn." *Philosophy* 69: 123–134.

———. 1990. "Why is Belief Involuntary?" *Analysis* 50: 87–107.

Blais, Michael. 1987. "Epistemic Tit for Tat." *The Journal of Philosophy* 84: 363–375.

Blanshard, Brand. 1973. "Can Men Be Reasonable?" In his *The Uses of Liberal Education,* E. Freeman, ed. (La Salle, Ill.: Open Court): 127–151.

———. 1974. *Reason and Belief* (London: George Allen and Unwin).

———. 1984. *Four Reasonable Men* (Middletown, Connecticut: Wesleyan University Press).

Bonjour, Laurence. 1985. *The Structure of Empirical Knowledge* (Cambridge: Harvard University Press).

Braithwaite, Richard B. 1932–33. "The Nature of Believing." *Proceedings of the Aristotelian Society* 33: 129–146.

Brandom, Robert B. 1994. *Making It Explicit* (Cambridge: Harvard University Press).

Bratman, Michael E. 1987. *Intentions, Plans, and Practical Reason* (Cambridge: Harvard University Press).

Bryan, C. D. B. 1995. *Close Encounters of the Fourth Kind: Alien Abduction, UFOs, and the Conference at M.I.T.* (New York: Knopf).

Burge, Tyler, 1987. "Intellectual Norms and the Philosophy of Mind." *The Journal of Philosophy* 83: 697–720.

———. 1993. "Content Preservation." *The Philosophical Review* 102: 457–488.

———. 1997. "Interlocution, Perception, and Memory." *Philosophical Studies* 86: 21–47.

Burnyeat, Myles F. 1983. "Can the Skeptic Live His Skepticism?" In *The Skeptical Tradition*, Myles Burnyeat, ed. (Berkeley: University of California Press): 117–148.

Carey, Susan. 1990. "Cognitive Development." In *Thinking: An Invitation to Cognitive Science*, volume 3, D. N. Osherson and E. E. Smith, eds. (Cambridge: The MIT Press).

Carnap, Rudolf. 1962. *Logical Foundations of Probability,* second edition (Chicago: University of Chicago Press).

Carroll, Lewis. 1895. "What the Tortoise Said to Achilles." *Mind* 4: 278–280.

Cherniak, Christopher. 1986. *Minimal Rationality* (Cambridge: The MIT Press).

Clifford, W. K. 1999. "The Ethics of Belief." In *Ethics of Belief and Other Essays* (Amherst, New York: Prometheus Books): 70–96.

Coady, C. A. J. 1992. *Testimony: A Philosophical Study* (Oxford: Oxford University Press).

Code, Lorraine. 1987. *Epistemic Responsibility* (Hanover: University of New England Press): 77–83.

Cohen, L. Jonathan. 1977. *The Probable and the Provable* (Oxford: Oxford University Press).

———. 1981. "Can Human Irrationality Be Experimentally Demonstrated?" *Behavioral and Brain Sciences* 4: 317–370.

———. 1986. "Twelve Questions about Keynes's Concept of Weight." *British Journal for the Philosophy of Science* 37: 263–278.

———. 1991. "Some Comments by L. J. C." (on Logue). In *Probability and Rationality*, E. Eells and T. Maruszewski, eds. (Amsterdam: Rodopi): 329–332.

———. 1992. *An Essay on Belief and Acceptance* (Oxford: Oxford University Press).

Cohen, Stewart. 1988. "How to Be a Fallibilist." *Philosophical Perspectives* 2: 581–605.

———. 1998. "Contextualist Solutions to Epistemological Problems: Scepticism, Gettier, and the Lottery." *Australasian Journal of Philosophy* 76: 289–306.

Collins, Arthur W. 1996. "Moore's Paradox and Epistemic Risk." *The Philosophical Quarterly* 49: 308–319.

Cook, J. Thomas. 1987. "Deciding to Believe without Self-Deception." *The Journal of Philosophy* 84: 441–446.

Crimmins, Mark. 1992. *Talk about Beliefs* (Cambridge: The MIT Press).

Curley, E. M. 1975. "Descartes, Spinoza, and the Ethics of Belief." In *Spinoza: Essays in Interpretation,* Eugene Freeman and Maurice Mandelbaum, eds. (LaSalle, Ill.: Open Court): 159–189.

Damasio, Antonio R. 1994. *Descartes' Error* (New York: G. P. Putnam's Sons).

Danto, Arthur. 1968. "Basic Actions." In *Readings in the Theory of Action,* N. S. Care and C. Landesman, eds. (Indiana: Indiana University Press): 93–112.

Darmstadter, Howard. 1971. "Consistency of Belief." *The Journal of Philosophy* 68: 301–310.

Dauer, Francis W. 1996. "Hume's Scepticism with Regard to Reason: A Reconsideration." *Hume Studies* 22: 211–229.

Davidson, Donald. 1982. *Essays on Actions and Events* (Oxford: Oxford University Press).

———. 1984. *Inquiries into Truth and Interpretation* (Oxford: Oxford University Press).

———. 1986. "A Coherence Theory of Truth and Knowledge." In *Truth and Interpretation,* E. LePore, ed. (Oxford: Blackwell's): 307–319.

Dennett, Daniel C. 1978. *Brainstorms* (Cambridge: The MIT Press).

———. 1984. *Elbow Room* (Cambridge: The MIT Press).

———. 1987. *The Intentional Stance* (Cambridge: The MIT Press).

———. 1987. "Cognitive Wheels: The Frame Problem in AI." In *The Robot's Dilemma,* Z. Pylysyn, ed. (Norwood, NJ: Ablex).

De Rose, Keith. 1991. "Epistemic Possibilities." *The Philosophical Review* 100: 581–605.

———. 1992. "Contextualism and Knowledge Attributions." *Philosophy and Phenomenological Research* 52: 913–929.

———. 1995. "Solving the Sceptical Problem." *The Philosophical Review* 104: 1–52.

———. 1996. "Knowledge, Assertion, and Lotteries." *Australasian Journal of Philosophy* 74: 568–579.

Descartes, Rene. 1996. *Meditations on First Philosophy,* J. Cottingham, ed. (Cambridge: Cambridge University Press).

De Sousa, Ronald B. 1971. "How to Give a Piece of Your Mind: Or, the Logic of Belief and Assent." *Review of Metaphysics* 25: 52–79.

———. 1987. *Rationality of the Emotions* (Cambridge: The MIT Press).

di Sessa, A. 1982. "Students' Understanding of Ordinary Physics." *Cognitive Science* 6: 37–75.

Donaldson, Margaret. 1978. *Children's Minds* (New York: W.W. Norton).

Dretske, Fred. 1970. "Epistemic Operators." *The Journal of Philosophy* 69: 1015–1016.

———. 1971. "Conclusive Reasons." *Australasian Journal of Philosophy* 49: 1–22.

———. 1981. *Knowledge and the Flow of Information* (Cambridge: The MIT Press).

———. 1990. "Seeing, Believing, and Knowing." In *An Invitation to Cognitive Science, Visual Cognition and Action,* volume 2, D. N. Osherson, S. M. Kosslyn, and J. M. Hollerbach, eds. (Cambridge: The MIT Press): 129–148.

———. 1991. *Explaining Behavior* (Cambridge: The MIT Press).

Drosnin, Michael. 1997. *The Bible Code* (New York: Simon and Schuster).

Duhem, Pierre. 1954. *The Aim and Structure of Physical Theory* (Princeton: Princeton University Press).

Dummett, Michael. 1973. *Frege: The Philosophy of Language* (London: Duckworth).

Elgin, Catherine Z. 1996. *Considered Judgment* (Princeton: Princeton University Press).

———. 1997. *Between the Absolute and the Arbitrary* (Ithaca: Cornell University Press).

Elster, Jon. 1984. *Ulysses and the Sirens,* second edition (Cambridge: Cambridge University Press).

Evans, Gareth. 1982. *The Varieties of Reference.* John McDowell, ed. (Oxford: Oxford University Press).

Evnine, Simon. 1999. "Believing Conjunctions." *Synthese* 118: 201–227.

Faulkner, Paul. 2000. "The Social Character of Testimonial Knowledge." *The Journal of Philosophy* 197: 581–601.

Feldman, Richard and Earl Conee. 1985. "Evidentialism." *Philosophical Studies* 48: 15–34.

Festinger, L. and Carlsmith, J. M. 1959. "Cognitive Consequences of Forced Compliance." *Journal of Abnormal and Social Psychology* 58: 203–210.

Festinger, Leon, Riecken, Henry W., and Schachter, Stanley. 1956. *When Prophecy Fails* (New York: Harper and Row).

Field, Hartry. 1998. "Epistemological Nonfactualism and the A Prioricity of Logic." *Philosophical Studies* 92: 1–24.

———. (unpublished.) "A Prioricity as an Evaluative Notion."

Fingarette, Herbert. 1969. *Self-Deception* (London: Routledge and Kegan Paul).

Fischer, John Martin. 1994. *The Metaphysics of Free Will* (Oxford: Blackwell).

Flanagan, Owen. 1991. *Varieties of Moral Personality* (Cambridge: Harvard University Press).

Flew, Antony. 1955. "Theology and Falsification." In *New Essays in Philosophical Theology*, A. Flew and A. MacIntyre, eds. (New York: Macmillan): 96–99.

Fogelin, Robert J. 1985. *Hume's Skepticism* (London: Routledge and Kegan Paul).

———. 1994. *Pyrrhonian Reflections on Knowledge and Justification* (New York: Oxford University Press).

Foley, Richard. 1987. *The Theory of Epistemic Rationality* (Cambridge: Harvard University Press).

———. 1993. *Working without A Net* (New York: Oxford University Press).

———. 1994. "Egoism in Epistemology." In *Socializing Epistemology,* Frederick F. Schmitt, ed. (Maryland: Rowman and Littlefield): 53–73.

Frege, Gottlob. 1967. "*Begriffsschrift,* a Formula Language, Modeled Upon That of Arithmetic, for Pure Thought." In *From Frege to Godel,* Jean van Heijenoort, ed. (Cambridge: Harvard University Press): 1–82.

French, P. A., Uehling, T. E., Jr., and Wettstein, H. K. 1980. *Midwest Studies in Philosophy V* (Minneapolis: University of Minnesota Press).

Fricker, Elizabeth. 1987. "The Epistemology of Testimony." *Proceedings of the Aristotelian Society,* supplementary volume 61: 57–83.

———. 1994. "Against Gullibility." *Knowing from Words,* B. K. Matilal and A. Chakrabarti, eds. (Boston: Kluwer): 125–161.

Gardenfors, Peter and Sahlin, Nils-Eric. 1988. "Unreliable probabilities, risk taking, and decision making." In *Decision, Probability, and Utility,* Peter Gardenfors and Nils-Eric Sahlin, eds. (Cambridge: Cambridge University Press): 313–334.

Garver, Eugene. 1994. *Aristotle's* Rhetoric: *An Art of Character* (Chicago: University of Chicago Press).

Gettier, Edmund L. 1970. "Is Justified True Belief Knowledge?" In *Knowing,* M. D. Roth and L. Galis, eds. (New York: Random House): 35–38.

Gigerenzer, Gerd, Ulrich Hoffrage, and Heinz Kleinbolting. 1991. "Probabilistic Mental Models: A Brunswikian Theory of Confidence." *Psychological Review* 98: 506–528.

Gilbert, Daniel T. 1991. "How Mental Systems Believe." *American Psychologist* 46: 107–119.

———. 1993. "The Assent of Man: Mental Representation and the Control of Belief." In *Handbook of Mental Control,* Wegner and Pennebaker, eds. (Englewood Cliffs, NJ: Prentice-Hall): 57–87.

Gilovich, T. 1991. *How We Know What Isn't So: The Fallibility of Human Reason in Everyday Life* (New York: The Free Press).

Ginet, Carl. 1980. "Knowing Less by Knowing More." *Midwest Studies in Philosophy V* (Minneapolis: University of Minnesota Press): 151–161.

————. 2001. "Deciding to Believe." In *Knowledge, Truth, and Duty*, M. Steup, ed. (Oxford: Oxford University Press): 63–76.

Goldman, Alvin I. 1986. *Epistemology and Cognition* (Cambridge: Harvard University Press, 1986).

————. 1991. "Epistemic Paternalism." *The Journal of Philosophy* 88: 113–131.

————. 1993. "Reliabilism: What Is Justified Belief." In *The Theory of Knowledge,* Louis P. Pojman, ed. (Belmont, California: Wadsworth): 292–306.

————. 1999. "Internalism Exposed." *The Journal of Philosophy* 96: 271–293.

Goodman, Nelson. 1983. *Fact, Fiction, and Forecast* (Cambridge: Harvard University Press).

Govier, Trudy. 1976. "Belief, Values, and the Will." *Dialogue* 15: 642–663.

————. 1993. "Trust and Testimony: Nine Arguments on Testimonial Knowledge." *International Journal of Moral and Social Studies* 8: 21–39.

Greenspan, Patricia S. 1988. *Emotions and Reasons* (London: Routledge).

Grice, Paul. 1989. *Studies in the Way of Words* (Cambridge: Harvard University Press).

Griffin, Dale and Tversky, Amos. 1992. "The Weighing of Evidence and the Determinants of Confidence." *Cognitive Psychology* 24: 411–435.

Gutting, Gary. 1982. *Religious Belief and Religious Skepticism* (Notre Dame: University of Notre Dame Press).

Haack, Susan. 1993. *Evidence and Inquiry* (Oxford: Blackwell).

Hacking, Jan. 1967. "Possibility." *The Philosophical Review* 76: 143–168.

————. 1975. *The Emergence of Probability* (Cambridge: Cambridge University Press).

————. 1978. "Hume's Species of Probability." *Philosophical Studies* 33: 21–37.

Hamblin, C. L. 1970 *Fallacies* (London: Methuen).

Hardwig, John. 1991. "The Role of Trust in Knowledge." *The Journal of Philosophy* 88: 693–708.

Hare, Richard M. 1981. *Moral Thinking: Its Levels, Method, and Point* (Oxford: Oxford University Press).

Harman, Gilbert. 1973. *Thought* (Princeton: Princeton University Press).

————. 1986. *Change in View: Principles of Reasoning* (Cambridge: The MIT Press).

————. 1997 "Pragmatism and Reasons for Belief." In *Realism/Antirealism and Epistemology*, C. B. Kulp, ed. (Lanham, Maryland: Rowman and Littlefield): 123–147.

Hawthorne, James and Bovens, Luc. 1999. "The Preface, the Lottery, and the Logic of Belief." *Mind* 108: 241–264.

Heil, John. 1984. "Doxastic Incontinence." *Mind* 93: 56–70.

Helm, Paul. 1984. *Belief Policies* (Cambridge: Cambridge University Press).

Hempel, Carl G. 1965. *Aspects of Scientific Explanation* (New York: The Free Press): 3–46.

Hintikka, Jaakko. 1962. *Knowledge and Belief* (Ithaca: Cornell University Press).

Hogarth, R. M. 1986. "Beyond Discrete Biases: Functional and Dysfunctional Aspects of Judgmental Heuristics." In Arkes and Hammond (1986): 680–704.

Holton, Richard. 1994. "Deciding to Trust, Coming to Believe." *Australasian Journal of Philosophy* 72: 63–76.

———. 1999. "Intention and Weakness of Will." *The Journal of Philosophy* 96: 241–262.

Hook, Sidney. 1980. "The Ethics of Controversy." In his *Philosophy and Public Policy* (Carbondale: Southern Illinois University Press): 117–123.

Horn, Laurence R. 1989. *A Natural History of Negation* (Chicago: University of Chicago Press).

Horwich, Paul. 1990. *Truth* (Oxford: Blackwell).

Hume, David. 1975. *A Treatise of Human Nature.* L. A. Selby-Bigge, ed. (Oxford: Oxford University Press).

———. 1977. "Of Miracles." In *An Enquiry Concerning Human Understanding,* E. Steinberg, ed. (Indianapolis: Hackett).

James, William. 1951. "The Will to Believe." In *Essays on Pragmatism,* A. Castelli, ed. (New York: Harner): 88–109.

Janis, I. 1972. *Victims of Groupthink* (Boston: Houghton Mifflin).

Jeffrey, Richard C. 1970. "Dracula meets Wolfman: Acceptance vs. Partial Belief." in *Induction, Acceptance, and Rational Belief,* M. Swain, ed. (Dordrecht: D. Reidel): 157–185.

———. 1983. *The Logic of Decision,* second edition. (Chicago: The University of Chicago Press).

Jones, Karen. 1999. "Second-Hand Moral Knowledge." *The Journal of Philosophy* 96: 55–78.

Jordan, Jeff. 1996. "Pragmatic Arguments and Belief." *American Philosophical Quarterly* 33: 409–420.

Kagan, Jerome and Lamb, Sharon, eds. 1987. *The Emergence of Morality in Young Children* (Chicago: University of Chicago).

Kahneman, D. and Tversky, A. 1982. "On the Psychology of Prediction." In Kahneman, Slovic, and Tversky (1982): 48–68.

———. 1990. "Prospect Theory: An Analysis of Decision under Risk." In Moser (1990): 140–170.

Kahneman, D., Slovic, P., and Tversky, A., eds. 1982. *Judgment under Uncertainty: Heuristics and Biases* (Cambridge: Cambridge University Press).

Kamin, Leon. 1974. *The Science and Politics of IQ* (Potomac, Md.: Erlbaum).

Kant, Immanuel. 1981. *Groundwork for the Metaphysics of Morals.* J. W. Ellington, trans. (Indianapolis: Hackett).

————. 1991. *The Metaphysics of Morals.* Mary Gregor, trans. (Cambridge: Cambridge University Press).

Kaplan, Mark. 1996. *Decision Theory as Philosophy* (Cambridge: Cambridge University Press).

Karlsson, Mikael. 1990. "Epistemic Leaks and Epistemic Meltdowns: A Response to William Morris on Scepticism with Regard to Reason." *Hume Studies* 16: 121–130.

Katz, Jerrold J. 1998. *Realistic Rationalism* (Cambridge: The MIT Press).

Katzoff, Charlotte. 2000. "Counter-Evidence and the Duty to Critically Reflect." *Analysis* 60: 89–96.

Kelley, H. H. 1967. "Attribution theory in social psychology." In *Nebraska Symposium on Motivation,* vol. 15 (University of Nebraska Press): 192–238.

Kevles, Daniel J. 1996. "The Assault on David Baltimore." *The New Yorker,* May 27, 1996: 94–109.

Keynes, John Maynard. 1962. *A Treatise on Probability* (New York: Harper and Row).

Kim, Jaegwon. 1993. "What Is 'Naturalized Epistemology'?" In Pojman (1993): 329–340.

Kiparsky, Paul and Kiparsky, Carol. 1971. "Fact." In *Semantics,* Danny D. Steinberg and Leon A. Jakovits, eds. (New York: Cambridge University Press): 345–369.

Kirkham, Richard L. 1992. *Theories of Truth* (Cambridge: The MIT Press).

Kitcher, Philip. 1990. "The Division of Cognitive Labor." *The Journal of Philosophy* 87: 5–22.

————. 1993. *The Advancement of Science* (Oxford: Oxford University Press).

Klein, Peter D. 1981. *Certainty: A Refutation of Skepticism* (Minneapolis: University of Minnesota Press).

Kornblith, Hilary. 1983. "Justified Belief and Epistemically Responsible Action." *The Philosophical Review* 92: 33–48.

————. 1986. "Naturalizing Rationality." In *Naturalism and Rationality,* Newton Garver and Peter H. Hare, eds. (Buffalo, New York: Prometheus Books): 115–133.

Kretzmann, Norman. 1992. "Evidence against Anti-Evidentialism." In *Our Knowledge of God,* K. J. Clark, ed. (Dordrecht: Kluwer Academic Publishers): 17–38.

Kripke, Saul. 1972. *Naming and Necessity* (Cambridge: Harvard University Press).

Kyburg, Henry E., Jr. 1961. *Probability and the Logic of Rational Belief* (Middletown: Wesleyan University Press).

————. 1970. "Conjunctivitis." In *Induction, Acceptance, and Rational Belief,* M. Swain, ed. (Dordrecht-Holland: D. Reidel): 55–82.

————. 1997. "The Rule of Adjunction and Reasonable Inference." *The Journal of Philosophy* 94: 109–125.

Laudan, Larry. 1983. "The Demise of the Demarcation Problem." In *Physics, Philosophy and Psychoanalysis*, R. S. Cohen and L. Laudan, eds. (Boston: D. Reidel): 111–127.

Levi, Isaac. 1980. *The Enterprise of Knowledge* (Cambridge: The MIT Press).

Levin, Michael E. 1998. *Why Race Matters* (New York: Plenum Press).

Lewis, David. 1969. *Convention* (Cambridge: Harvard University Press).

————. 1983. *Philosophical Papers,* volume I (Oxford: Oxford University Press).

————. 1996. "Elusive Knowledge." *Australasian Journal of Philosophy* 74: 549–567.

Locke, John. 1975. *An Essay Concerning Human Understanding.* P. H. Nidditch, ed. (Oxford: Oxford University Press).

Loewer, Barry 1993. "The Value of Truth" in *Nature and Normativity* E. Villanueva, ed. (Atascadero, California: Ridgeview): 265–280.

Logue, James. 1991. "Weight of Evidence, Resiliency, and Second-Order Probabilities." In *Probability and Rationality,* E. Eells and T. Maruszewski, eds. (Amsterdam: Rodopi): 147–172.

Lycan, William. 1994. *Meaning and Modality* (Boston: D. Reidel).

MacIntyre, Alasdair. 1988. *After Virtue* (Notre Dame: University of Notre Dame Press).

Makinson, D. C. 1964. "The Paradox of the Preface." *Analysis* 25: 205–207.

Malcolm, Norman. 1992. "The Groundlessness of Belief." In *Contemporary Perspectives on Religious Epistemology,* R. Douglas Geivett and Brendan Sweetman, eds. (New York: Oxford University Press): 92–103.

Marcus, Ruth Barcan. 1990. "Some Revisionary Proposals about Belief and believing." *Philosophy and Phenomenological Research* 50: 133–153.

Margolis, Howard. 1987. *Patterns, Thinking, and Cognition* (Chicago: The University of Chicago Press).

McCloskey, Michael. 1983. "Intuitive Physics." *Scientific American* 247: 122–130.

McLaughlin, Brian P. 1988. "Exploring the Possibility of Self-Deception in Belief." In McLaughlin and Rorty (1988): 29–62.

McLaughlin, B. P. and Rorty, A. O., eds. 1988. *Perspectives on Self-Deception* (Berkeley: University of California Press).

Meiland, Jack. 1993. "What Ought We to Believe?" In Pojman (1993): 514–525.

Mele, Alfred R. 1987. *Irrationality* (Oxford: Oxford University Press).

Mellor, Hugh. 1971. *The Matter of Chance* (Cambridge: Cambridge University Press).

————. 1980. "Consciousness and Degrees of Belief" In *Prospects for Pragmatism: Essays in Memory of Frank Ramsey,* D. H. Mellor, ed. (Cambridge: Cambridge University Press): 139–173.

Milgram, Stanley. 1974. *Obedience to Authority* (New York: Harper and Row).

Mill, John Stuart. 1978. *On Liberty.* E. Rapaport, ed. (Indianapolis: Hackett).

Millar, Alan. 1991. *Reasons and Experience* (Oxford: Oxford University Press).

Millgram, Elijah. 1997. *Practical Induction* (Cambridge: Harvard University Press).

Mitchell, Basil. 1955 "Theology and Falsification." In Flew and MacIntyre (1955): 103–105.

Moore, G. E. 1962. "Four Forms of Scepticism." In his *Philosophical Papers* (New York: Collier Books): 193–222.

Moran, Richard. 1997. "Self-Knowledge: Discovery, Resolution, and Undoing." *European Journal of Philosophy* 5: 141–161.

Morris, William E. 1989. "Hume's Scepticism about Reason." *Hume Studies* 15: 39–60.

Morton, Adam. 1988. "Partisanship." In McClaughlin and Rorty (1988): 170–182.

Nagel, Thomas. 1986. *The View from Nowhere* (Oxford: Oxford University Press).

Nelkin, Dana K. 2000. "The Lottery Paradox, Knowledge, and Rationality." *The Philosophical Review* 109: 373–409.

Nisbett, R. and Ross, L. 1980. *Human Inference: Strategies and Shortcomings of Social Judgment* (Englewood Cliffs, N.J.: Prentice Hall).

Nisbett, Richard E. and Wilson, Timothy DeCamp. 1977. "Telling More Than We Can Know: Verbal Reports on Mental Processes." *Psychological Review* 84: 231–259.

Nozick, Robert. 1974. *Anarchy, State, and Utopia* (New York: Basic Books).

————. 1981. *Philosophical Explanations* (Cambridge: Harvard University Press).

————. 1993. *The Nature of Rationality* (Princeton: Princeton University Press).

E. Ochs and B. Schiefflein, eds. 1979. *Developmental Pragmatics* (New York: Academic Press).

Pascal, Blaise. 1966. *Pensees.* A. J. Krailsheimer, trans. (Harmondsworth: Penguin).

Peacocke, Christopher. 1992. *A Study of Concepts* (Cambridge: The MIT Press).

————. 2001. "Does Perception Have a Nonconceptual Content?" *The Journal of Philosophy* 98: 239–264.

Peirce, Charles S. 1957. "The Fixation of Belief." In his *Essays in the Philosophy of Science,* V. Thomas, ed. (New York: Bobbs-Merrill): 3–30.

Petit, Philip and Smith, Michael. 1996. "Freedom in Belief and Desire." *The Journal of Philosophy* 93: 429–449.

Pinker, Stephen. 1997. *How the Mind Works* (New York: W.W. Norton).

Plantinga, Alvin. 1983. "Reason and Belief in God." In Plantinga and Wolterstorff (1983): 16–93.

———. 1986. "Coherentism and the Evidentialist Objection to Belief in God." In Audi and Wainwright (1986): 109–138.

———. 1993. *Warrant and Proper Function*. (Oxford: Oxford University Press, 1993).

Plantinga, Alvin and Wolterstorff, Nicholas. eds. 1983. *Faith and Rationality* (Notre Dame: University of Notre Dame Press).

Plato. 1981. *Euthyphro, Apology, Crito, Meno* in *Five Dialogues*. G. M. A. Grube, trans. (Indianapolis: Hackett).

———. 1990. *The Theaetetus of Plato*. M. J. Levett, trans., revised by Myles Burnyeat (Indianapolis: Hackett).

Pojman, Louis P., ed. 1993a. *The Theory of Knowledge* (Belmont, California: Wadsworth).

———. 1993b. "Believing, Willing, and the Ethics of Belief." In L. P. Pojman (1993a): 525–544.

Pollock, John and Cruz Joseph. 1999. *Contemporary Theories of Knowledge*, second edition (Lanham, Maryland: Rowman and Littlefield).

Popper, Karl R. 1959. *The Logic of Scientific Discovery* (New York: Harper).

Post, John F. 1980. "Infinite Regresses of Justification and of Explanation." *Philosophical Studies* 38: 31–52.

Post, John F. and Turner, Derek. 2000. "Sic Transitivity: Reply to McGrew and McGrew." *Journal of Philosophical Research* 25: 67–82.

Priest, Graham. 1998. "What Is So Bad about Contradictions?" *The Journal of Philosophy* 95: 410–426.

Putnam, Hilary. 1975. "The Meaning of 'Meaning.' " In his *Mind, Language and Reality: Philosophical Papers,* volume 2 (Cambridge: Cambridge University Press): 215–271.

———. 1978. *Meaning and the Moral Sciences* (London: Routledge and Kegan Paul).

Quine, W. v. O. 1960. *Word and Object* (Cambridge: The MIT Press).

———. 1980. "Two Dogmas of Empiricism." In his *From a Logical Point of View,* second edition (Cambridge: Harvard University Press): 20–46.

Quine, W. v. O. and Ullian, J. S. 1978. *The Web of Belief,* second edition (New York: Random House).

Radcliffe, Dana. 1997. "Scott-Kakures on Believing at Will." *Philosophy and Phenomenological Research* 57: 145–151.

Radford, Colin. 1970. "Knowledge—By Examples." In *Knowing: Essays in the Analysis of Knowledge,* M. D. Roth and L. Galis, eds. (New York: Random House): 171–185.

Railton, Peter. 1994. "Truth, Reason, and the Regulation of Belief." *Philosophical Issues* 5: 72–93.

Ramsey, F. P. 1978a. "Facts and Propositions." In his *Foundations,* D. H. Mellor, ed. (London: Routledge and Kegan Paul): 40–57.

———. 1978b. *Foundations.* D. H. Mellor, ed. (London: Routledge and Kegan Paul): 133–141.

Rawls, John. 1968. "Two Concepts of Rules." In *Readings in the Theory of Action,* N. S. Care and C. Landesman, eds. (Bloomington: Indiana University Press): 306–340.

———. 1971. *A Theory of Justice* (Cambridge: Harvard University Press).

Raz, Joseph. 1990. *Practical Reason and Norms,* second edition (Princeton: Princeton University Press).

———. 2000. "When We Are Ourselves." In his *Engaging Reason* (Oxford: Oxford University Press): 5–21.

Reeve, C. D. C. 1989. *Socrates in the* Apology (Indianapolis: Hackett).

Reid, Thomas. 1969. *Essays on the Intellectual Powers of Man* (Cambridge: The MIT Press).

Rey, Georges. 1988. "Toward a Computational Account of *Akrasia* and Self-Deception." in *Perspectives on Self-Deception,* B. P. McLaughlin and A. O. Rorty, eds. (Berkeley: University of California Press): 264–296.

———. 1997. *Contemporary Philosophy of Mind* (Oxford: Blackwell).

Robinson, Richard. 1971. "Arguing from Ignorance." *The Philosophical Quarterly* 21: 97–108.

Rogoff, Barbara. 1990. *Apprenticeship in Thinking: Cognitive Development in Social Context* (Oxford: Oxford University Press).

Roorda, Jonathan. 1997. "Fallibilism, Ambivalence, and Belief." *The Journal of Philosophy* 94: 126–155.

Rorty, Richard. 1979. *Philosophy and the Mirror of Nature* (Princeton: Princeton University Press).

Ross, Angus. 1986. "Why Do We Believe What We Are Told?" *Ratio* 27: 69–88.

Ross, Lee. 1988. "Situationist Perspectives on the Obedience Experiments." *Contemporary Psychology* 33: 101–104.

Ross, Lee and Anderson, Craig A. 1982. "Shortcomings in the Attribution Process: On the Origins and Maintenance of Erroneous Social Assessments." In Kahneman, Slovic, and Tversky (1982): 129–152.

Ross, Lee, Lepper, M. R., and Hubbard, M. 1975. "Perseverance in Self-Perception and Social Perception: Biased Attributional Processes in the Debriefing Paradigm." *Journal of Personality and Social Psychology* 32: 880–892.

Russell, Bertrand. 1948. *Human Knowledge: Its Scope and Limits* (New York: Simon and Schuster).

Ryan, Sharon. 1991. "The Preface Paradox." *Philosophical Studies* 64: 293–307.

Ryle, Gilbert. 1949. *The Concept of Mind* (New York: Barnes and Noble).

Sahlin, Nihls-Eric. 1986. "How to Be 100% Certain 99.5% of the Time." *The Journal of Philosophy* 83: 91–111.

Schick, Frederic. 1992. "Allowing for Understandings." *The Journal of Philosophy* 89: 30–41.

Schiffer, Stephen R. 1972. *Meaning* (Oxford: Oxford University Press).

———. 1998. "Two Issues of Vagueness." *The Monist* 81:193–214.

Schmitt, Frederick F. 1987. "Justification, Sociality, and Autonomy." *Synthese* 73: 43–85.

———. 1994. "Introduction" to his collection *Socializing Epistemology* (Rowman and Littlefield): 1–27.

———. 1999. "Social Epistemology." In *The Blackwell Guide to Epistemology*, J. Greco and E. Sosa, eds. (Oxford: Blackwell): 354–382.

Shklar, J. N. 1984. *Ordinary Vices* (Cambridge, MA: Harvard University Press).

Scott-Kakures, Dion. 1994. "On Belief and the Captivity of the Will." *Philosophy and Phenomenological Research* 54: 77–103.

Searle, John. 1979. "Indirect Speech Acts." In his *Expression and Meaning* (Cambridge: Cambridge University Press): 30–57.

———. 1983. *Intentionality* (Cambridge: Cambridge University Press).

Sellars, Wilfrid. 1963. "Empiricism and the Philosophy of Mind." In his *Science, Perception, and Reality* (London: Routledge and Kegan Paul): 127–196.

Shoemaker, Sydney. 1996. "Moore's Paradox and Self-Knowledge." In his *The First-Person Perspective and Other Essays* (Cambridge: Cambridge University Press): 74–93.

Shubik, Martin. 1971. "The Dollar Auction Game: A Paradox in Noncooperative Behavior and Escalation." *Journal of Conflict Resolution* 15: 109–111.

Sidgwick, Henry. 1981. *The Methods of Ethics*, seventh edition (Indianapolis: Hackett).

Skyrms, Brian. 1977. "Resiliency, Propensities, and Causal Necessity." *The Journal of Philosophy* 74: 704–713.

Smith, Edward E. 1995. "Categorization." In *Thinking: An Invitation to Cognitive Science*, vol. 3, Edward E. Smith and Daniel N. Osherson, eds. (Cambridge: The MIT Press): 3–33.

Solomon, Robert C. 1980. "Emotions and Choice." In *Explaining Emotions*, Amelie Oksenberg Rorty, ed. (Berkeley: University of California Press): 251–281.

Sorensen, Roy. 1988. *Blindspots* (Oxford: Oxford University Press).

Sosa, Ernest. 1999. "The Raft and the Pyramid." In Pojman (1999): 251–266.

Sperber, Dan. 1985. "Apparently Irrational Beliefs." In His *On Anthropological Knowledge* (Cambridge: Cambridge University Press, 1985): 35–63.

Spinoza, Baruch. 1982. *The Ethics and Selected Letters.* S. Shirley, trans.; S. Feldman, ed. and intro. (Indianapolis: Hackett).

Stalnaker, Robert C. 1987. *Inquiry* (Cambridge: The MIT Press).

Stevenson, Leslie. 1993. "Why Believe What People Say?" *Synthese* 94: 429–451.

Stich, Stephen P. 1990. *The Fragmenation of Reason* (Cambridge, Mass.: The MIT Press).

Stocker, Michael. 1982. "Responsibility Especially for Beliefs." *Mind* 91: 398–417.

———. 1990. *Plural and Conflicting Values* (Oxford: Oxford University Press).

Stone, Tony and Young, Andrew G. 1997. "Delusions and Brain Injury: The Philosophy and Psychology of Belief." *Mind and Language* 12: 327–364.

Strawson, Peter F. 1952. *Introduction to Logical Theory* (London: Methuen).

———. 1982. "Freedom and Resentment." In *Free Will,* Gary Watson, ed. (Oxford: Oxford University Press): 59–80.

Stroll, Avrum. 1994. *Moore and Wittgenstein on Certainty* (New York: Oxford University Press).

Stroud, Barry. 1971. "Wittgenstein and Logical Necessity." In *Essays on Wittgenstein,* E. D. Klemke, ed. (Urbana: University of Illinois Press): 447–463.

———. 1984. *The Significance of Philosophical Scepticism* (Oxford: Oxford University Press).

Swinburne, Richard. 1981. *Faith and Reason* (Oxford: Oxford University Press).

———. 1985. "Review of Plantinga and Wolterstorff, eds. (and other works)." *The Journal of Philosophy* 82: 46–53.

Tarksi, Alfred. 1983. "The Concept of Truth in Formalized Languages." In his *Logic, Semantics, and Meta-Mathematics,* second edition, J. H. Woodger, trans.; J. Corcoran, ed. (Indianapolis: Hackett): 152–278.

Taylor, Charles. 1982. "Responsibility for Self." In *Free Will,* Gary Watson, ed. (Oxford: Oxford University Press): 111–126.

Thomas, David E. 1997. "Hidden Messages and the Bible Code." *Skeptical Inquirer* Nov./Dec.: 30–36.

Thomson, Judith Jarvis. 1986. "Remarks on Causation and Liability." In her *Rights, Restitution, and Risk: Essays in Moral Theory,* William Parent, ed. (Cambridge: Harvard University Press): 192–224.

Toulmin, Stephen. 1958. *The Uses of Argument* (Cambridge: Cambridge University Press).

Tversky. A. and Kahneman, D. 1983. "Extensional versus Intuitive Reasoning: The Conjunction Fallacy in Probability Judgment." *Psychological Review* 90: 293–315.

Ullmann-Margalit, Edna. 1983. "On Presumption." *The Journal of Philosophy* 80: 143–163.

Ullmann-Margalit, Edna and Morgenbesser, Sidney. 1977. "Picking and Choosing." *Social Research* 44: 757–785.

Unger, Peter. 1975. *Ignorance* (Oxford: Oxford University Press).

———. 1984. *Philosophical Relativity* (Minneapolis: University of Minnesota Press).

Urmson, J. O. 1966. "Parenthetical Verbs." In *Essays in Conceptual Analysis,* Antony Flew, ed. (New York: St. Martin's Press): 192–212.

van Fraassen, Bas C. 1980. *The Scientific Image* (Oxford: Oxford University Press).

———. 1984. "Belief and the Will." *The Journal of Philosophy* 81: 235–256.

Velleman, J. David. 1989. *Practical Reflection* (Princeton: Princeton University Press, 1989).

———. 2000. *The Possibility of Practical Reason* (Oxford: Oxford University Press).

Vogel, Jonathan. 1990. "Are There Counterexamples to the Closure Principle?" In *Doubting,* Michael D. Roth and Glenn Ross, eds. (Dordrecht: Kluwer Academic Publishers): 13–27.

Walton, Douglas. 1996. *Arguments from Ignorance* (University Park, Pa.: The Pennsylvania State University Press).

Walton, Kendall. 1978. "Fearing Fictions." *The Journal of Philosophy* 75: 5–27.

Wason, P. C. 1977. "Self-Contradictions." In *Thinking: Readings in Cognitive Science,* P.N. Johnson-Laird and P. C. Wason, eds. (Cambridge: Cambridge University Press): 114–128.

Webb, Mark Owen. 1993. "Why I Know about as Much as You: A Reply to Hardwig." *The Journal of Philosophy* 90: 260–270.

Welbourne, Michael. 1986. *The Community of Knowledge* (Aberdeen University Press).

Whyte, J. T. 1990. "Success Semantics." *Analysis* 50: 149–157.

Wiggins, David. 1970. "Freedom, Knowledge, Belief, and Causality." In *Knowledge and Necessity,* Royal Institute of Philosophy Lectures vol. 3, G. N. A. Vesey, ed. (London: Macmillan): 132–154.

Williams, B. A. O. 1973. *Problems of the Self* (Cambridge: Cambridge University Press).

———. 1978. *Descartes: The Project of Pure Enquiry* (New York: Penguin).

———. 1981. "Moral Luck." In his *Moral Luck* (Cambridge: Cambridge University Press): 20–39.

Williams, Michael. 1977. *Groundless Beliefs* (New Haven: Yale University Press).

———. 1991. *Unnatural Doubts* (Oxford: Blackwell).

Williamson, Timothy. 1996. "Knowing and Asserting." *The Philosophical Review* 105: 489–523.

Winch, Peter. 1970. "Understanding a Primitive Society." In *Rationality*, B. R. Wilson, ed. (New York: Harper and Row): 78–111.

Winters, Barbara 1979. "Willing to Believe." *The Journal of Philosophy* 76: 243–256.

Wittgenstein, Ludwig. 1953. *Philosophical Investigations*. G. E. M. Anscombe, trans. (New York: Macmillan).

———. 1956. *Remarks on the Foundation of Mathematics*. G. H. von Wright, R. Rhees, and G. E. M. Anscombe, eds.; G. E. M. Anscombe, trans. (Cambridge: The MIT Press).

———. 1969. *On Certainty*. G. E. M. Anscombe and G. H. von Wright, eds.; Denis Paul and G. E. M. Anscombe, trans. (New York: Harper and Row).

Wolterstorff, Nicholas 1983. "Can Belief in God Be Rational if It Has No Foundations?" In Plantinga and Wolterstorff (1983): 135–186.

———. 1986. "The Migration of the Theistic Arguments: From Natural Theology to Evidentialist Apologetics." In Audi and Wainwright (1986): 38–81.

———. 1996. *John Locke and the Ethics of Belief* (Cambridge: Cambridge University Press).

Wood, Allen W. 1988. "Self-Deception and Bad Faith." In *Perspectives on Self-Deception*, B. P. McLaughlin and A. O. Rorty, eds. (Berkeley: University of California Press): 207–227.

Woods, John and Walton, Douglas. 1978. "The Fallacy of 'Ad Ignorantiam.'" *Dialectica* 32: 87–99.

Yablo, Stephen. 1993. "Is Conceivability a Guide to Possibility?" *Philosophy and Pheomenological Research* 53: 1–42.

Zemach, Eddy. 1997. "Practical Reasons for Belief?" *Nous* 31: 525–527.

Index